Extraintestinal Manifestations of Coeliac Disease

Extraintestinal Manifestations of Coeliac Disease

Special Issue Editors

Marios Hadjivassiliou
David Sanders

MDPI • Basel • Beijing • Wuhan • Barcelona • Belgrade

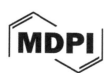

Special Issue Editors
Marios Hadjivassiliou
University of Sheffield
UK

David Sanders
University of Sheffield
UK

Editorial Office
MDPI
St. Alban-Anlage 66
4052 Basel, Switzerland

This is a reprint of articles from the Special Issue published online in the open access journal *Nutrients* (ISSN 2072-6643) from 2018 to 2019 (available at: https://www.mdpi.com/journal/nutrients/special_issues/Coeliac_Disease)

For citation purposes, cite each article independently as indicated on the article page online and as indicated below:

LastName, A.A.; LastName, B.B.; LastName, C.C. Article Title. *Journal Name* **Year**, *Article Number*, Page Range.

ISBN 978-3-03897-798-8 (Pbk)
ISBN 978-3-03897-799-5 (PDF)

Contents

About the Special Issue Editors vii

Preface to "Extraintestinal Manifestations of Coeliac Disease" ix

Camilla Pasternack, Eriika Mansikka, Katri Kaukinen, Kaisa Hervonen, Timo Reunala, Pekka Collin, Heini Huhtala, Ville M. Mattila and Teea Salmi
Self-Reported Fractures in Dermatitis Herpetiformis Compared to Coeliac Disease
Reprinted from: *Nutrients* 2018, 10, 351, doi:10.3390/nu10030351 1

Luis Rodrigo, Nuria Álvarez, Enrique Fernández-Bustillo, Javier Salas-Puig, Marcos Huerta and Carlos Hernández-Lahoz
Efficacy of a Gluten-Free Diet in the Gilles de la Tourette Syndrome: A Pilot Study
Reprinted from: *Nutrients* 2018, 10, 573, doi:10.3390/nu10050573 11

Timo Reunala, Teea T. Salmi, Kaisa Hervonen, Katri Kaukinen and Pekka Collin
Dermatitis Herpetiformis: A Common Extraintestinal Manifestation of Coeliac Disease
Reprinted from: *Nutrients* 2018, 10, 602, doi:10.3390/nu10050602 26

Eriika Mansikka, Kaisa Hervonen, Katri Kaukinen, Pekka Collin, Heini Huhtala, Timo Reunala and Teea Salmi
Prognosis of Dermatitis Herpetiformis Patients with and without Villous Atrophy at Diagnosis
Reprinted from: *Nutrients* 2018, 10, 641, doi:10.3390/nu10050641 35

Panagiotis Zis, Ptolemaios Georgios Sarrigiannis, Dasappaiah Ganesh Rao and Marios Hadjivassiliou
Quality of Life in Patients with Gluten Neuropathy: A Case-Controlled Study
Reprinted from: *Nutrients* 2018, 10, 662, doi:10.3390/nu10060662 45

Hilary Jericho and Stefano Guandalini
Extra-Intestinal Manifestation of Celiac Disease in Children
Reprinted from: *Nutrients* 2018, 10, 755, doi:10.3390/nu10060755 53

Luis Rodrigo, Valia Beteta-Gorriti, Nuria Alvarez, Celia Gómez de Castro, Alvaro de Dios, Laura Palacios and Jorge Santos-Juanes
Cutaneous and Mucosal Manifestations Associated with Celiac Disease
Reprinted from: *Nutrients* 2018, 10, 800, doi:10.3390/nu10070800 64

George J. Kahaly, Lara Frommer and Detlef Schuppan
Celiac Disease and Glandular Autoimmunity
Reprinted from: *Nutrients* 2018, 10, 814, doi:10.3390/nu10070814 84

Michael D. E. Potter, Marjorie M. Walker, Stephen Hancock, Elizabeth Holliday, Gregory Brogan, Michael Jones, Mark McEvoy, Michael Boyle, Nicholas J. Talley and John Attia
A Serological Diagnosis of Coeliac Disease Is Associated with Osteoporosis in Older Australian Adults
Reprinted from: *Nutrients* 2018, 10, 849, doi:10.3390/nu10070849 93

Mahmoud Slim, Fernando Rico-Villademoros and Elena P. Calandre
Psychiatric Comorbidity in Children and Adults with Gluten-Related Disorders: A Narrative Review
Reprinted from: *Nutrients* 2018, 10, 875, doi:10.3390/nu10070875 105

Iva Hoffmanová, Daniel Sánchez, Ludmila Tučková and Helena Tlaskalová-Hogenová
Celiac Disease and Liver Disorders: From Putative Pathogenesis to Clinical Implications
Reprinted from: *Nutrients* **2018**, *10*, 892, doi:10.3390/nu10070892 134

Pilvi Laurikka, Samuli Nurminen, Laura Kivelä and Kalle Kurppa
Extraintestinal Manifestations of Celiac Disease: Early Detection for Better
Long-Term Outcomes
Reprinted from: *Nutrients* **2018**, *10*, 1015, doi:10.3390/nu10081015 151

Ana Vinagre-Aragón, Panagiotis Zis, Richard Adam Grunewald and Marios Hadjivassiliou
Movement Disorders Related to Gluten Sensitivity: A Systematic Review
Reprinted from: *Nutrients* **2018**, *10*, 1034, doi:10.3390/nu10081034 165

Xuechen B. Yu, Melanie Uhde, Peter H. Green and Armin Alaedini
Autoantibodies in the Extraintestinal Manifestations of Celiac Disease
Reprinted from: *Nutrients* **2018**, *10*, 1123, doi:10.3390/nu10081123 179

**Giulia De Marchi, Giovanna Zanoni, Maria Cristina Conti Bellocchi, Elena Betti,
Monica Brentegani, Paola Capelli, Valeria Zuliani, Luca Frulloni, Catherine Klersy and
Rachele Ciccocioppo**
There Is No Association between Coeliac Disease and Autoimmune Pancreatitis
Reprinted from: *Nutrients* **2018**, *10*, 1157, doi:10.3390/nu10091157 195

**Marios Hadjivassiliou, Richard A Grünewald, David S Sanders, Panagiotis Zis, Iain Croal,
Priya D Shanmugarajah, Ptolemaios G Sarrigiannis, Nick Trott, Graeme Wild and
Nigel Hoggard**
The Significance of Low Titre Antigliadin Antibodies in the Diagnosis of Gluten Ataxia
Reprinted from: *Nutrients* **2018**, *10*, 1444, doi:10.3390/nu10101444 206

Panagiotis Zis, Thomas Julian and Marios Hadjivassiliou
Headache Associated with Coeliac Disease: A Systematic Review and Meta-Analysis
Reprinted from: *Nutrients* **2018**, *10*, 1445, doi:10.3390/nu10101445 213

Lars-Petter Jelsness-Jørgensen, Tomm Bernklev and Knut E. A. Lundin
Fatigue as an Extra-Intestinal Manifestation of Celiac Disease: A Systematic Review
Reprinted from: *Nutrients* **2018**, *10*, 1652, doi:10.3390/nu10111652 225

Alina Popp and Markku Mäki
Gluten-Induced Extra-Intestinal Manifestations in Potential Celiac Disease—Celiac Trait
Reprinted from: *Nutrients* **2019**, *11*, 320, doi:10.3390/nu11020320 233

**Elizabeth S. Mearns, Aliki Taylor, Kelly J. Thomas Craig, Stefanie Puglielli,
Allie B. Cichewicz, Daniel A. Leffler, David S. Sanders, Benjamin Lebwohl and
Marios Hadjivassiliou**
Neurological Manifestations of Neuropathy and Ataxia in Celiac Disease: A Systematic Review
Reprinted from: *Nutrients* **2019**, *11*, 380, doi:10.3390/nu11020380 245

About the Special Issue Editors

Marios Hadjivassiliou is a Consultant Neurologist and the Academic Director of the Department of Neurosciences, Sheffield Teaching Hospitals NHS Trust, Sheffield, UK. His primary research interest is in the neurological manifestations of gluten-related diseases and ataxias, areas that he initially studied for his MD thesis and which subsequently became the focus of his research career over the last 24 years. He has a particular interest in autoimmune neurological diseases and runs joint clinics with rheumatologists, managing patients with neurological manifestations of connective tissue diseases. He has published extensively in high-impact journals, including 3 first author papers in the Lancet. He runs a weekly gluten sensitivity/neurology, vasculitis/autoimmunity, and ataxia clinics, and receives referrals from all over the United Kingdom and internationally. He is the director of the Sheffield Ataxia Centre, caring for over 2000 patients with ataxias, and is a founding member of the Sheffield Institute of Gluten-Related Diseases (SIGReD).

David Sanders is a Professor of Gastroenterology and a Consultant Gastroenterologist at the Royal Hallamshire Hospital and the University of Sheffield. He has published ¿400 peer-reviewed papers (H-score > 60). He is internationally recognised for his work in coeliac disease, percutaneous gastrostomy feeding (PEG), and small bowel endoscopy. His other research interests include pancreatic exocrine insufficiency, irritable bowel syndrome and gastrointestinal bleeding. He has received a number of research awards, including the European Rising Star Award (2010), Cuthbertson Medal in 2011 and Silver Medal in 2017 (both awards from the UK Nutrition Society), Swedish Gastroenterology Society Bengt Ihre Medal (2017) and, most recently, the BSG Hopkins prize for Endoscopy (2019). His clinical work with patients who have coeliac disease has resulted in him being awarded the Coeliac UK Healthcare Professional of the Year Award (2010) and the inaugural Complete Nutrition Coeliac Health Care Professional Award (2013). He is fortunate to work as part of the Sheffield Gastroenterology Team, which has been recognised for their standards of clinical care. The Small Bowel Endoscopy Service won one of the inaugural British Society of Gastroenterology National GI Care awards (2011) and the Medipex award (2013). In 2012, the PEG team won both the Health Service Journal's Primary Care and Integrated Clinical Care awards. In 2014, the Sheffield Gastroenterology team won one of the SAGE (Shire Awards for Gastrointestinal Excellence) awards for their primary care and GI bleed unit services. In 2017, because of his diverse clinical nutrition interests, he was voted (by patients and healthcare professionals) as the Clinical Nutrition Healthcare Professional of the Year. Professor Sanders has chaired both the British Society of Gastroenterology (BSG) Small Bowel and Nutrition Section (2006–2012) and the BSG Audit Committee (2010–2013). He is the current Chair of the Coeliac UK Health Advisory Council, BSG Council Member, and President of the International Society for the Study of Coeliac Disease (ISSCD). The Sheffield Unit has recently been recognised as the Rare Disease Collaborative Network on refractory coeliac disease (NHS England). http://www.profdavidsanders.co.uk/

Preface to "Extraintestinal Manifestations of Coeliac Disease"

Gluten-related disorders (GRDs) is the term used to describe a spectrum of diverse immune-mediated manifestations triggered by the ingestion of gluten. Coeliac disease (CD), also known as gluten sensitive enteropathy, is perhaps the most well-recognized and characterized entity within this spectrum. Extraintestinal manifestations have, up until recent years, been largely neglected and often wrongly presumed to be secondary to nutrient deficiencies. This is despite the fact that the recognition of one of such manifestation affecting the skin, known as dermatitis herpetiformis, goes back to the early 1960s. Apart from isolated case reports, neurological manifestations have been the subject of intense study during the last 20 years. This has resulted in well-characterized conditions, such as gluten ataxia, gluten neuropathy and gluten encephalopathy. Furthermore, the realisation that gluten sensitivity may exist in the absence of enteropathy has gained credence amongst gastroenterologists. The diagnosis of the whole spectrum of GRDs no longer relies on tests that are specific to the presence of enteropathy (endomysium and tissue transglutaminase 2 antibodies) but on additional serological testing with anti-gliadin antibodies. This means that GRDs account for much more than 1% of cases, which is the prevalence rate of CD in the population. Finally, although identification of tissue transglutaminase 2 (TG2) as the autoantigen in CD has led the way in clarifying the pathophysiology of this disease, TG3, an epidermal transglutaminase, and TG6, a neural transglutaminase, have been shown to be respectively implicated in dermatitis herpetiformis and neurological manifestations.This Special Issue of Nutrients has, as its focus, the extraintestinal manifestations of GRDs, covering the whole spectrum from skin to neurological manifestations to endocrine, bone, and also liver and pancreatic involvement. Included are original research and systematic reviews from a range of experts in the field.

Marios Hadjivassiliou, David Sanders

Special Issue Editors

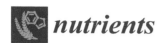

Article

Self-Reported Fractures in Dermatitis Herpetiformis Compared to Coeliac Disease

Camilla Pasternack [1], Eriika Mansikka [1,2], Katri Kaukinen [1,3], Kaisa Hervonen [1,2], Timo Reunala [1,2], Pekka Collin [4], Heini Huhtala [5], Ville M. Mattila [6] and Teea Salmi [1,2,*]

1   Coeliac Disease Research Center, Faculty of Medicine and Life Sciences, University of Tampere, 33014 Tampere, Finland; pasternack.m.camilla@student.uta.fi (C.P.); mansikka.eriika.k@student.uta.fi (E.M.); katri.kaukinen@staff.uta.fi (K.K.); kaisa.hervonen@staff.uta.fi (K.H.); timo.reunala@uta.fi (T.R.)
2   Department of Dermatology, Tampere University Hospital, 33521 Tampere, Finland
3   Department of Internal Medicine, Tampere University Hospital, 33521 Tampere, Finland
4   Department of Gastroenterology and Alimentary Tract Surgery, Tampere University Hospital, 33521 Tampere, Finland; pekka.collin@uta.fi
5   Faculty of Social Sciences, University of Tampere, 33014 Tampere, Finland; heini.huhtala@staff.uta.fi
6   Division of Orthopedics and Traumatology, Department of Trauma, Musculoskeletal Surgery and Rehabilitation, Tampere University Hospital, 33521 Tampere, Finland; ville.mattila@staff.uta.fi
*   Correspondence: teea.salmi@uta.fi; Tel.: +358-40-586-3818

Received: 15 February 2018; Accepted: 12 March 2018; Published: 14 March 2018

Abstract: Dermatitis herpetiformis (DH) is a cutaneous manifestation of coeliac disease. Increased bone fracture risk is known to associate with coeliac disease, but this has been only scantly studied in DH. In this study, self-reported fractures and fracture-associated factors in DH were investigated and compared to coeliac disease. Altogether, 222 DH patients and 129 coeliac disease-suffering controls were enrolled in this study. The Disease Related Questionnaire and the Gastrointestinal Symptom Rating Scale and Psychological General Well-Being questionnaires were mailed to participants; 45 out of 222 (20%) DH patients and 35 out of 129 (27%) of the coeliac disease controls had experienced at least one fracture ($p = 0.140$). The cumulative lifetime fracture incidence did not differ between DH and coeliac disease patients, but the cumulative incidence of fractures after diagnosis was statistically significantly higher in females with coeliac disease compared to females with DH. The DH patients and the coeliac disease controls with fractures reported more severe reflux symptoms compared to those without, and they also more frequently used proton-pump inhibitor medication. To conclude, the self-reported lifetime bone fracture risk is equal for DH and coeliac disease. After diagnosis, females with coeliac disease have a higher fracture risk than females with DH.

Keywords: dermatitis herpetiformis; coeliac disease; fracture; bone health; quality of life

1. Introduction

Coeliac disease is a systemic autoimmune disorder triggered by gluten and characterized by small-bowel mucosal villous atrophy. It has a highly heterogeneous clinical picture including intestinal, extraintestinal, and asymptomatic manifestations [1]. A number of comorbidities are associated with coeliac disease, one of which is metabolic bone disease predisposing to bone fractures [2]. At the time of diagnosis, coeliac disease patients frequently suffer from decreased bone mineral density (BMD) [2,3], which in turn may be a risk factor for fractures. Decreased BMD is not limited to only patients with severe gastrointestinal symptoms; it also occurs in subclinical and asymptomatic coeliac disease patients [4–6]. Once diagnosed, coeliac disease is treated with a life-long gluten-free diet (GFD). Strict adherence to a GFD typically improves bone health in coeliac disease, but full bone recovery is often not reached in adult coeliac disease patients [7]. Fracture risk in coeliac disease has been studied extensively, and based on a recent meta-analysis, it can be concluded that the risk of fractures in coeliac disease is increased by 30% for any fractures and by 69% for hip fractures [8].

Dermatitis herpetiformis (DH) is one of the well-established extraintestinal manifestations of coeliac disease [9]. In DH, dietary gluten induces an itchy, blistering rash, which responds to a GFD [10]. Since a GFD often alleviates the intensively itching rash fairly slowly, patients with severe symptoms are additionally treated with dapsone medication at the beginning of the dietary treatment to alleviate the skin symptoms more quickly [11]. At diagnosis, DH patients also suffer from coeliac disease-type small-bowel mucosal villous atrophy or inflammation. Occasionally gastrointestinal symptoms also occur, but they are often minor [9,12]. It seems presumable that the increased risk of bone fractures would also be associated with DH, but bone complications in DH have been studied scantily and the results are thus far conflicting [13–17]. The only study focusing on the fracture risk in DH found no increase in risk [13]. The aim of the current study was to discover whether DH patients have an increased bone fracture risk similar to the one known to exist in coeliac disease. A further objective was to study the factors associated with increased bone fracture risk in DH, and to assess the burden related to fractures.

2. Materials and Methods

2.1. Patients, Controls, and Study Design

All patients with DH within the catchment area of the city of Tampere are diagnosed and treated at a special outpatient clinic at Tampere University Hospital's Department of Dermatology. The diagnosis of DH is based on clinical symptoms and the demonstration of granular immunoglobulin A deposits in perilesional skin biopsies studied with direct immunofluorescence [18]. From 1970 onwards, data have been prospectively collected from all patients diagnosed with DH. All adult DH patients alive in December 2015 and diagnosed before December 2014 ($n = 413$) were recruited to the study. The control group comprised 222 biopsy-proven coeliac disease patients diagnosed at Tampere University Hospital over the same time period who were suffering from abdominal symptoms at the time of diagnosis.

Self-administered study questionnaires (see below for more detail) were mailed to the patients and controls. A second round of questionnaires were sent to all non-respondent patients and controls under 80 years old. For the DH patients, the total response rate was 56% (237 out of 413). Of these responders, 15 patients were excluded for having a coeliac disease diagnosis made more than one year prior to the DH diagnosis. The remaining 222 DH patients constituted the study cohort. For the coeliac disease controls, the final response rate was 59% (130 out of 222), and one patient was excluded because of a DH diagnosis. The patients' medical records were reviewed and the clinical, serological, and histological severity of the disease and the use of dapsone were recorded.

The DH patients and coeliac disease controls received a full written explanation of the aims of the study and they gave their written informed consent. The Regional Ethics Committee of Tampere University Hospital approved the study protocol.

2.2. Questionnaires

Three self-administrated questionnaires were used in this study: the Disease Related Questionnaire (DRQ), which was specifically designed for this study, and the general Psychological General Well-Being (PGWB) and Gastrointestinal Symptom Rating Scale (GSRS) questionnaires, which have been widely used in coeliac disease studies. The DRQ includes both open questions and multiple-choice questions. Patients were asked to report all experienced bone fractures during their lifetime, the year of each fracture, and the type of trauma causing the fracture. The DRQ also includes questions about the respondent's sociodemographic and lifestyle characteristics, presence of comorbidities, use of long-term medication, and current weight and height. In addition, the questionnaire also enquires about previous and current clinical symptoms related to coeliac disease and DH and the strictness of the respondent's GFD.

The PGWB is a 22-item questionnaire used to evaluate quality of life and well-being [19,20]. It covers six emotional states: anxiety, depressed mood, self-control, positive well-being, general health, and vitality. All of the items use a six-grade Likert scale, where value one represents the poorest and value six the best possible well-being. The total PGWB score thus ranges from 22 to 132 points, with a higher score indicating a better quality of life.

The GSRS is a 15-item questionnaire used to assess the severity of five groups of gastrointestinal symptoms: diarrhoea, indigestion, constipation, abdominal pain, and reflux [21]. The questionnaire uses a seven-grade Likert scale for each item, one symbolizing no symptoms and seven indicating the most severe symptoms. The final scores are calculated as a mean for each sub-dimension and the total GSRS score as the mean of all 15 items. A higher score indicates more severe symptoms.

2.3. Fractures

The self-reported fractures were categorized based on whether they had occurred before or after the DH or coeliac disease diagnosis. The traumas causing the fractures were evaluated, and if the trauma was considered sufficient to cause a bone fracture in any person (traffic accidents, high-energy sports fractures), the fracture was excluded from further analysis. Fractures diagnosed as stress fractures were also excluded from all further analysis.

2.4. Statistical Analysis

Median values, minimum and maximum values, and interquartile ranges (IQR) were used to describe the continuous variables. All testing was two-sided and $p < 0.05$ was considered statistically significant. The chi-squared test was used in cross-tabulations and the Mann–Whitney U test was used for assessing changes between groups. Kaplan–Meier survival analysis was used to compare the cumulative incidence of fractures between the groups. The odds ratios (OR) and 95% confidence intervals (CI) were calculated by using binary logistic regression analysis. For fracture incidence rates, 95% CI were calculated assuming the number of fractures to have a Poisson distribution. All of the statistical analyses were performed with SPSS version 20 (IBM SPSS Statistics for Windows, Version 20.0. IBM Corp., Armonk, NY, USA) in cooperation with a statistician.

3. Results

In total, 101 of the 222 DH patients (45%) and 104 of the 129 coeliac disease controls (81%) were female. The DH patients were younger at the time of diagnosis than the coeliac disease controls (Table 1). At the time of the study, there were no differences in age or body mass index between the groups. The median follow-up time after diagnosis was 23 years (range 2–53) for the DH patients and 20 years (range 1–43) for the coeliac disease controls. The DH patients and the coeliac disease controls reported a total of 128 fractures, of which 9 excess-trauma fractures and 5 stress fractures were excluded from further analysis. There were no statistical differences between the groups in terms of the number of study participants who reported a fracture (Table 1).

The fracture incidence rate per 10^5 person-years for the first fracture was 317 (95% CI 228–431) for the DH patients and 388 (95% CI 259–558) for the coeliac disease controls. For the first fracture after DH or coeliac disease diagnosis, the fracture incidence rates per 10^5 person-years were 629 (95% CI 427–894) for the DH patients and 1083 (95% CI 707–1589) for the coeliac disease controls. In the binary logistic regression analysis, the risk of fracture for the coeliac disease group did not statistically significantly differ from the DH group before (OR 1.47, 95% CI 0.88–2.43, $p = 0.141$) or after adjustment for gender and age at the time of the study (adjusted OR 1.04, 95% CI 0.60–1.79, $p = 0.891$). In the Kaplan–Meier analysis, neither the cumulative lifetime fracture incidence (Figure 1A) nor the incidence before diagnosis ($p = 0.127$) significantly differed between the groups. The cumulative incidence of fractures after the diagnosis was statistically significantly higher in the coeliac disease group than in the DH group (Figure 1B). When the genders were analysed separately the difference was observed for female ($p = 0.021$) but not for male patients ($p = 0.291$).

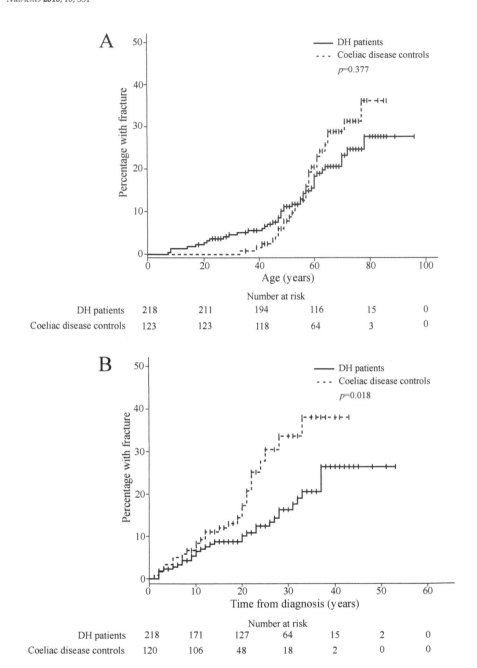

Figure 1. Kaplan–Meier cumulative incidence of the first fracture (**A**) and for first fracture after diagnosis (**B**) for the dermatitis herpetiformis (DH) patients and the coeliac disease controls.

In both study groups, patients with fractures were more often female, had more often been diagnosed with osteoporosis, and more often had multiple long-term illnesses (Table 2). At the time of the study, those with fractures were more often using proton-pump inhibitors (PPI) and vitamin D and calcium supplementation than those with no reported fractures (Table 2). The current usage of hormone replacement therapy and diuretics was more common among the DH patients with reported fractures than those without, but this was not seen in the coeliac disease controls. There were no differences in the smoking habits or current adherence to a GFD, the amount of weekly exercise, or the use of glucocorticoids or bisphosphonates between those with and without fractures in either groups (Table 2). Compared to coeliac disease controls with fractures, DH patients with fractures were statistically significantly more often male, and they were younger at the time of the diagnosis (Table 2) and at the time of the first fracture (median 48 years vs. 57 years, $p = 0.048$).

The DH patients with fractures more frequently had severe villous atrophy in the small bowel at the time of the diagnosis than those without fractures, but the difference in the histological severity of the disease did not reach statistical difference (Table 3). There were no differences in the duration of skin symptoms before DH diagnosis, the severity of skin symptoms, or the presence of gastrointestinal symptoms at diagnosis between DH patients with fractures and those without, but DH patients with fractures had used dapsone medication statistically significantly longer after diagnosis than those without fractures (Table 3).

The severity of the gastrointestinal symptoms as measured with the GSRS total score did not differ between DH patients or coeliac disease controls with and without fractures (Table A1). However, DH patients with fractures reported higher GSRS reflux subscores than those without fractures (median 1.5 vs. 1.0, $p = 0.012$). This was also seen in the coeliac disease controls, although without reaching statistical significance (median 1.5 vs. 1.0, $p = 0.083$). The quality of life measured with the PGWB questionnaire was decreased in DH patients with fractures compared to those without in total score (median 106 vs. 112, $p = 0.006$) and in all other subscores except depression (Table A1). This same phenomenon was not observed in the coeliac disease controls (Table A1).

Table 1. Demographic data and reported fractures among 222 dermatitis herpetiformis (DH) patients and the 129 coeliac disease controls.

	DH Patients (*n* = 222)		Coeliac Disease Controls (*n* = 129)		*p*-Value
	n	%	*n*	%	
Female	101	45	104	81	<0.001
Age at diagnosis, median (range), years	37 (5–78)		42 (7–72)		0.027
Age at the time of the study, median (range), years	65 (18–96)		66 (35–86)		0.654
BMI [1] at the time of the study, median (range), kg/m^2	26 (17–40)		26 (15–46)		0.714
Reported fractures	45	20	35	27	0.140
Before diagnosis	13	6	3	3	0.143
After diagnosis	31	14	26	22	0.080
Reported multiple fractures	15	7	12	9	0.388

[1] BMI, Body mass index.

Table 2. Demographic data, strictness of gluten-free diet (GFD), and clinical data for the dermatitis herpetiformis (DH) patients and the coeliac disease controls with and without fractures.

	DH Patients (n = 222)			Coeliac Disease Controls (n = 129)		
	With Fracture (n = 45)	Without Fracture (n = 177)	p-Value	With Fracture (n = 35)	Without Fracture (n = 94)	p-Value
Female, %	58 *	42	0.064	97	74	0.002
Age at diagnosis, median (range), years	34 (7–78) *	37 (5–78)	0.652	45 (23–59)	40 (7–72)	0.428
Age at the time of the study, median (range), years	68 (22–85)	65 (18–96)	0.343	68 (51–82)	63 (35–86)	0.020
Smoking at the time of the study, %			0.581			0.218
Non-smoker	69	68		66	70	
Ex-smoker	17	22		31	20	
Current smoker	14	10		3	10	
Exercise at the time of the study, %			0.341			0.396
Not at all	11	11		6	10	
1 to 3 times per week	55	43		57	44	
4 to 7 times per week	34	46		37	46	
Dietary adherence to GFD at the time of the study, %			0.858			0.646
Strict [1]	70	73		80	86	
Dietary lapses less than once a month	21	18		17	10	
Dietary lapses more than once a month	7	8		3	3	
Normal diet	2	1		0	1	
Diagnosed with osteoporosis, %	11 *	2	0.024	40	11	0.001
Multiple long-term illnesses [2], %	33	19	0.033	43	26	0.057
Use of long-term medication at the time of the study, %						
Proton-pump inhibitor	21	9	0.029	26	11	0.034
Hormone replacement therapy	14	4	0.008	3	11	0.155
Any glucocorticoid medication	18	12	0.349	26	16	0.205
Vitamin D and calcium supplementation	39	10	<0.001	43	25	0.045
Bisphosphonates	5	3	0.545	9	6	0.506
Diuretics	21	9	0.028	11	8	0.491

[1] No dietary lapses, [2] Two or more of the following diseases: thyroid disease, diabetes, hypercholesterolaemia, hypertension, rheumatoid disease, coronary artery disease. * $p < 0.05$ when the DH patients with fractures were compared to the coeliac disease patients with fractures.

Table 3. Disease-related characteristics presented as percentages, median values, and interquartile ranges (IQR) for the dermatitis herpetiformis (DH) patients with fractures and those without fractures.

	DH Patients		*p*-Value
	With Fracture (*n* = 45)	Without Fracture (*n* = 177)	
Year of DH diagnosis, median (IQR)	1990 (1976–2000)	1991 (1982–2002)	0.076
Duration of skin symptoms prior to DH diagnosis, median (IQR), months	12 (6–60)	10 (5–24)	0.183
Severity of skin symptom at diagnosis, %			0.818
Mild	19	15	
Moderate	46	50	
Severe	35	35	
Presence of gastrointestinal symptoms at the time of diagnosis, %	47	49	0.886
Small-bowel histology at diagnosis, %			0.405
Normal	16	24	
PVA [1]	35	39	
SVA/TVA [2]	49	37	
Use of dapsone after diagnosis, %	79	77	0.854
Duration of dapsone, median (IQR), months	60 (12–171)	24 (12–60)	0.031

[1] PVA, Partial villous atrophy; [2] SVA/TVA, Subtotal or total villous atrophy.

4. Discussion

In the current study, the lifetime fracture risk in DH was found not to differ from that in coeliac disease, which is well known to be linked to increased bone fracture risk [8]. However, it was found that females with coeliac disease had more fractures after coeliac disease was diagnosed than females with DH after DH diagnosis. The sole previous study addressing bone fracture risk in DH, with a respectable 846 DH patients from the United Kingdom, found no increased fracture risk in DH compared to the general population (hazard ratio 1.1) [13]. However, the study had limitations, as their observation period was rather short (median 3.7 years, 3496 person-years) and the data collected regarding adherence to GFD treatment was scanty. In the current study, the fracture incidence was smaller than in the work by Lewis et al. but the results are not comparable, as different study methods and follow-up times were used. In addition, our study groups had good adherence to a GFD, which is likely to decrease the fracture incidence. Other than the study by Lewis et al., bone health in DH has been investigated in four small studies focusing on the DH patients' BMD. Two studies found that DH patients have a decreased BMD compared to non-DH controls but better BMD than coeliac disease controls [14,15], and two studies found that the BMD in DH patients did not differ from that expected [16,17].

It is acknowledged that strict adherence to a GFD increases BMD in coeliac disease patients [2,7], and thus probably decreases the risk of bone fractures in the long term. In the current study, there were no differences in the strictness of GFD at the time of the study in the DH patients and the coeliac disease controls with and without fractures (Table 2). Overall, the GFD in this study cohort was strict, showing that bone fractures also tend to occur when the patients adhere to the diet well. However, we do not have short-term data about the strictness of the diet after the diagnosis. The duration of dapsone use after diagnosis was longer for DH patients reporting fractures compared to those who did not (Table 3). Longer requirement of dapsone usage suggests more active and prolonged rash, which might be a consequence of ongoing gluten consumption from dietary lapses on GFD. Less strict GFD after diagnosis in turn would be a logical cause for increased risk of fractures.

Bone deterioration in coeliac disease is considered a consequence of autoimmune reaction. The autoimmune reaction causes local and systemic chronic inflammation, which in turn causes micronutrient deficiency and activates a network of cytokines that have deleterious consequences for bone remodeling [22]. As DH and coeliac disease principally share the same pathogenetic mechanisms, it is accurate to assume that the same mechanisms explain the increased fracture risk also observed in DH. However, our study showed that after diagnosis, the female coeliac disease controls experienced more fractures than the female DH patients. This difference could be caused by the on-going small-bowel inflammation that remains in coeliac disease even after the recovery of the mucosal architecture [23]. In addition, the age at diagnosis was higher for the coeliac disease controls compared to the DH patients. The higher age at diagnosis has been linked to less complete bone recovery following GFD, and it seems that the ability to bone recovery is the least satisfactory for peri- and post-menopausal women [3,24]. The higher age at diagnosis might also indicate that coeliac disease patients have suffered from the untreated disease longer than DH patients, and untreated disease particularly before puberty would have unfavorable effects on bone health.

The prevalence of gastrointestinal symptoms at the time of diagnosis was not linked to reported fractures, nor was any symptom other than reflux in the GSRS questionnaire at the time of the study. Consistently with more severe reflux symptoms detected, both the DH patients and the coeliac disease controls with fractures reported using PPI as a long-term medication more often than those without fractures. The usage of PPI medication has been reported to increase the risk of fractures at any site in a recent meta-analysis [25]. Thus, caution with PPI medications should be advised, although based on the experienced reflux symptoms, there is a clear need for PPI medication in certain individuals with DH and coeliac disease.

This study showed that the DH patients who reported fractures had a decreased quality of life compared to those with no fractures. Although we do not know if this decrease in life quality is caused by the burden of fractures or simply explained by a higher rate of multiple long-term illnesses detected in patients with fractures, we think that more attention should be directed to fractures in DH. In this study cohort, very few of the DH patients with fractures had been diagnosed with osteoporosis, which suggests that BMD measurements may not have been carried out systematically in the presence of fractures. This limits the awareness and motivation to adequately treat patients suffering from low BMD, and thus it also limits the prevention of additional fractures.

The strengths of this study are the large cohorts of patients with biopsy-proven DH and coeliac disease with strict inclusion and exclusion criteria, and thus a minimal possibility for misclassification bias. The cohorts were diagnosed and treated by specialists during the same time period, and they included patients with different severities of the disease from the same geographic area. The limitations of this study should be recognized, however. The fractures in this study were self-reported, which is not ideal. Nevertheless, questionnaire studies have in fact proven to be rather reliable [26], and although we know that the results are underestimations of the true occurrence due to recall bias [27], the groups in this study are comparable because they were both studied in a similar manner. Another limitation is that we have not taken the site of the fracture into account in our analysis, so we do not know how this would have differed between the groups. The study also compared only the fractures between DH and coeliac disease, and we did not enrol healthy controls. The gender distributions between our cohorts were unequal, but they correspond to the true distributions in both diseases and therefore the cohorts cannot be considered unrepresentative.

5. Conclusions

In conclusion, the fracture risk in DH is analogous to that in coeliac disease, which is a disease widely documented to be associated with increased bone fracture risk. However, after the diagnosis, the fracture risk was higher in coeliac disease than in DH for female patients. The severity of the skin disease did not correlate with the fracture risk in DH, but the reflux symptom and usage of PPI medication were linked to an increased fracture risk. The quality of life was shown to be decreased in DH patients with a history of fractures, which indicates that more attention should be directed to the fracture risk in DH, and BMD measurements should not be overlooked.

Acknowledgments: This work was supported by the Academy of Finland; the Sigrid Juselius Foundation; the Finnish Medical Foundation; and the Competitive State Research Financing of the Expert Responsibility area of Tampere University Hospital under Grants 9U019, 9T018, and 9U053.

Author Contributions: C.P., E.M., K.H., T.R., K.K., P.C., V.M.M. and T.S. conceived and designed the experiments; C.P., E.M., K.H. and T.S. performed the experiments; C.P. and H.H. analyzed the data; K.H., T.R, K.K., P.C. and T.S. contributed reagents/materials/analysis tools; all authors wrote, reviewed and commented on the paper.

Conflicts of Interest: The authors declare no conflict of interest.

Appendix A

Table A1. Median values and interquartile ranges for the Psychological General Well-Being (PGWB) and Gastrointestinal Symptoms Rating Scale (GSRS) totals and subscores for the dermatitis herpetiformis (DH) patients and the coeliac disease controls with and without fractures. In the PGWB, a higher score indicates a better quality of life, and in the GSRS, a higher score indicates more severe symptoms.

	DH Patients ($n = 222$)			Coeliac Disease Controls ($n = 129$)		
	With Fracture ($n = 45$)	Without Fracture ($n = 177$)	*p*-Value	With Fracture ($n = 35$)	Without Fracture ($n = 94$)	*p*-Value
GSRS						
Total	1.9 (1.3–2.3)	1.6 (1.3–2.1)	0.191	1.9 (1.5–2.5)	1.7 (1.4–2.5)	0.472
Diarrhoea	1.7 (1.0–2.3)	1.3 (1.0–2.0)	0.116	2.0 (1.0–2.7)	1.7 (1.0–2.5)	0.635
Indigestion	2.0 (1.3–2.5) *	1.8 (1.5–2.5)	0.630	2.4 (1.8–2.8)	2.0 (1.5–3.0)	0.343
Constipation	1.3 (1.0–2.3)	1.3 (1.0–2.3)	0.568	1.7 (1.3–2.5)	1.7 (1.0–2.7)	0.572
Pain	1.7 (1.2–2.3)	1.3 (1.0–2.0)	0.130	1.7 (1.3–2.3)	1.7 (1.3–2.3)	0.517
Reflux	1.5 (1.0–2.0)	1.0 (1.0–1.5)	0.012	1.5 (1.0–2.5)	1.0 (1.0–2.0)	0.083
PGWB						
Total	106 (94–113)	112 (101–119)	0.006	110 (93–120)	106 (97–116)	0.629
Anxiety	25 (22–27)	26 (23–28)	0.020	27 (21–29)	25 (23–28)	0.757
Depression	17 (16–18)	18 (16–18)	0.311	17 (15–18)	17 (15–18)	0.948
Well-being	17 (15–19)	18 (16–20)	0.007	18 (15–19)	17 (16–20)	0.941
Self control	16 (15–17)	16 (15–17)	0.052	16 (13–17)	16 (14–17)	0.888
General health	13 (11–15)	15 (13–16	0.012	13 (11–16)	13 (11–15)	0.712
Vitality	18 (17–21)	20 (17–21)	0.029	19 (17–20)	18 (16–20)	0.665

* $p < 0.05$ when the DH patients with fractures were compared to the coeliac disease patients with fractures.

References

1. Ludvigsson, J.F.; Bai, J.C.; Biagi, F.; Card, T.R.; Ciacci, C.; Ciclitıra, P.J.; Green, P.H.R.; Hadjivassiliou, M.; Holdoway, A.; Van Heel, D.A.; et al. Diagnosis and management of adult coeliac disease: Guidelines from the British Society of Gastroenterology. *Gut* **2014**, *63*, 1210–1228. [CrossRef] [PubMed]
2. Zanchetta, M.B.; Longobardi, V.; Bai, J.C. Bone and Celiac Disease. *Curr. Osteoporos Rep.* **2016**, *14*, 43–48. [CrossRef] [PubMed]
3. Di Stefano, M.; Mengoli, C.; Bergonzi, M.; Corazza, G.R. Bone mass and mineral metabolism alterations in adult celiac disease: Pathophysiology and clinical approach. *Nutrients* **2013**, *5*, 4786–4799. [CrossRef] [PubMed]
4. Mazure, R.; Vazquez, H.; Gonzalez, D.; Mautalen, C.; Pedreira, S.; Boerr, L.; Bai, J.C. Bone mineral affection in asymptomatic adult patients with celiac disease. *Am. J. Gastroenterol.* **1994**, *89*, 2130–2134. [CrossRef] [PubMed]
5. Mustalahti, K.; Collin, P.; Sievänen, H.; Salmi, J.; Mäki, M. Osteopenia in patients with clinically silent coeliac disease warrants screening. *Lancet* **1999**, *354*, 744–745. [CrossRef]
6. Corazza, G.R.; Di Sario, A.; Cecchetti, L.; Tarozzi, C.; Corrao, G.; Bernardi, M.; Gasbarrini, G. Bone mass and metabolism in patients with celiac disease. *Gastroenterology* **1995**, *109*, 122–128. [CrossRef]
7. Szymczak, J.; Bohdanowicz-Pawlak, A.; Waszczuk, E.; Jakubowska, J. Low bone mineral density in adult patients with coeliac disease. *Endokrynol. Pol.* **2012**, *63*, 270–276. [PubMed]
8. Heikkilä, K.; Pearce, J.; Mäki, M.; Kaukinen, K. Celiac disease and bone fractures: A systematic review and meta-analysis. *J. Clin. Endocrinol. Metab.* **2015**, *100*, 25–34. [CrossRef] [PubMed]

9. Collin, P.; Salmi, T.T.; Hervonen, K.; Kaukinen, K.; Reunala, T. Dermatitis herpetiformis: A cutaneous manifestation of coeliac disease. *Ann. Med.* **2016**, 1–25. [CrossRef] [PubMed]
10. Fry, L.; Riches, D.J.; Seah, P.P.; Hoffbrand, A.V. Clearance of skin lesions in dermatitis herpetiformis after gluten withdrawal. *Lancet* **1973**, *301*, 288–291. [CrossRef]
11. Hervonen, K.; Alakoski, A.; Salmi, T.T.; Helakorpi, S.; Kautiainen, H.; Kaukinen, K.; Pukkala, E.; Collin, P.; Reunala, T. Reduced mortality in dermatitis herpetiformis: A population-based study of 476 patients. *Br. J. Dermatol.* **2012**, *167*, 1331–1337. [CrossRef] [PubMed]
12. Alakoski, A.; Salmi, T.T.; Hervonen, K.; Kautiainen, H.; Salo, M.; Kaukinen, K.; Reunala, T.; Collin, P. Chronic gastritis in dermatitis herpetiformis: A controlled study. *Clin. Dev. Immunol.* **2012**, *2012*, 640630. [CrossRef] [PubMed]
13. Lewis, N.R.; Logan, R.F.A.; Hubbard, R.B.; West, J. No increase in risk of fracture, malignancy or mortality in dermatitis herpetiformis: A cohort study. *Aliment. Pharmacol. Ther.* **2008**, *27*, 1140–1147. [CrossRef] [PubMed]
14. Di Stefano, M.; Jorizzo, R.A.; Veneto, G.; Cecchetti, L.; Gasbarrini, G.; Corazza, G.R. Bone mass and metabolism in dermatitis herpetiformis. *Dig. Dis. Sci.* **1999**, *44*, 2139–2143. [CrossRef] [PubMed]
15. Lorinczy, K.; Juhász, M.; Csontos, Á.; Fekete, B.; Terjék, O.; Lakatos, P.L.; Miheller, P.; Kocsis, D.; Kárpáti, S.; Tulassay, Z.; et al. Does dermatitis herpetiformis result in bone loss as coeliac disease does? A cross sectional study. *Rev. Esp. Enferm. Dig.* **2013**, *105*, 187–193. [CrossRef] [PubMed]
16. Abuzakouk, M.; Barnes, L.; O'Gorman, N.; O'Grady, A.; Mohamed, B.; McKenna, M.J.; Freaney, R.; Feighery, C. Dermatitis herpetiformis: No evidence of bone disease despite evidence of enteropathy. *Dig. Dis. Sci.* **2007**, *52*, 659–664. [CrossRef] [PubMed]
17. Lheure, C.; Ingen-Housz-Oro, S.; Guignard, S.; Inaoui, R.; Jolivet, B.; Chevalier, X.; Wolkenstein, P.; Fautrel, B.; Chosidow, O. Dermatitis herpetiformis and bone mineral density: Analysis of a French cohort of 53 patients. *Eur. J. Dermatol.* **2017**, *27*, 353–358. [CrossRef] [PubMed]
18. Zone, J.J.; Meyer, L.J.; Petersen, M.J. Deposition of granular IgA relative to clinical lesions in dermatitis herpetiformis. *Arch. Dermatol.* **1996**, *132*, 912–918. [CrossRef] [PubMed]
19. Dimenäs, E.; Carlsson, G.; Glise, H.; Israelsson, B.; Wiklund, I. Relevance of norm values as part of the documentation of quality of life instruments for use in upper gastrointestinal disease. *Scand. J. Gastroenterol. Suppl.* **1996**, *221*, 8–13. [CrossRef] [PubMed]
20. Roos, S.; Kärner, A.; Hallert, C. Psychological well-being of adult coeliac patients treated for 10 years. *Dig. Liver Dis.* **2006**, *38*, 177–180. [CrossRef] [PubMed]
21. Svedlund, J.; Sjodin, I.; Dotevall, G. GSRS-A clinical rating scale for gastrointestinal symptoms in patients with irritable bowel syndrome and peptic ulcer disease. *Dig. Dis. Sci.* **1988**, *33*, 129–134. [CrossRef] [PubMed]
22. Larussa, T.; Suraci, E.; Nazionale, I.; Abenavoli, L.; Imeneo, M.; Luzza, F. Bone mineralization in celiac disease. *Gastroenterol. Res. Pract.* **2012**, *2012*. [CrossRef] [PubMed]
23. Ilus, T.; Lähdeaho, M.-L.; Salmi, T.; Haimila, K.; Partanen, J.; Saavalainen, P.; Huhtala, H.; Mäki, M.; Collin, P.; Kaukinen, K. Persistent duodenal intraepithelial lymphocytosis despite a long-term strict gluten-free diet in celiac disease. *Am. J. Gastroenterol.* **2012**, *107*, 1563–1569. [CrossRef]
24. Kemppainen, T.; Kroger, H.; Janatuinen, E.; Arnala, I.; Kosma, V.M.; Pikkarainen, P.; Julkunen, R.; Jurvelin, J.; Alhava, E.; Uusitupa, M. Osteoporosis in adult patients with celiac disease. *Bone* **1999**, *24*, 249–255. [CrossRef]
25. Zhou, B.; Huang, Y.; Li, H.; Sun, W.; Liu, J. Proton-pump inhibitors and risk of fractures: An update meta-analysis. *Osteoporos. Int.* **2016**, *27*, 339–347. [CrossRef] [PubMed]
26. Honkanen, K.; Honkanen, R.; Heikkinen, L.; Kröger, H.; Saarikoski, S. Validity of self-reports of fractures in perimenopausal women. *Am. J. Epidemiol.* **1999**, *150*, 511–516. [CrossRef] [PubMed]
27. Mock, C.; Acheampong, F.; Adjei, S.; Koepsell, T. The effect of recall on estimation of incidence rates for injury in Ghana. *Int. J. Epidemiol.* **1999**, *28*, 750–755. [CrossRef] [PubMed]

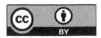

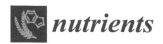

Article

Efficacy of a Gluten-Free Diet in the Gilles de la Tourette Syndrome: A Pilot Study

Luis Rodrigo [1,*], Nuria Álvarez [1], Enrique Fernández-Bustillo [2], Javier Salas-Puig [3], Marcos Huerta [4] and Carlos Hernández-Lahoz [5]

1   Gastroenterology Unit, Hospital Universitario Central de Asturias (HUCA), Avda. de Roma s/n, 33011 Oviedo, Spain; nuriaalvarezh@gmail.com
2   Technical Department, Hospital Universitario Central de Asturias (HUCA), Avda. de Roma s/n, 33011 Oviedo, Spain; bustillo.e@telefonica.net
3   Neurology Service, Hospital del Valle de Hebrón, Paseo del Valle de Hebrón 119, 08035 Barcelona, Spain; jsalasp@meditex.es
4   Psychiatry Service, Mental Health Center, Pedro Pablo 42, 33209 Gijón, Spain; marcoshuerta47@gmail.com
5   Neurology Service, Hospital Universitario Central de Asturias (HUCA), Avda. de Roma s/n, 33011 Oviedo, Spain; carloshlahoz@gmail.com
*   Correspondence: lrodrigosaez@gmail.com; +34-985-23-44-16

Received: 27 March 2018; Accepted: 4 May 2018; Published: 7 May 2018

Abstract: The Gilles de la Tourette syndrome (GTS) and Non-Coeliac Gluten Sensitivity (NCGS) may be associated. We analyse the efficacy of a gluten-free diet (GFD) in 29 patients with GTS (23 children; six adults) in a prospective pilot study. All of them followed a GFD for one year. The Yale Global Tics Severity Scale (YGTSS), the Yale-Brown Obsessive-Compulsive Scale—Self Report (Y-BOCS) or the Children's Yale-Brown Obsessive-Compulsive Scale—Self Report (CY-BOCS), and the Cavanna's Quality of Life Questionnaire applied to GTS (GTS-QOL) were compared before and after the GFD; 74% of children and 50% of adults were males, not significant (NS). At the beginning of the study, 69% of children and 100% of adults had associated obsessive-compulsive disorder (OCD) (NS). At baseline, the YGTSS scores were 55.0 ± 17.5 (children) and 55.8 ± 19.8 (adults) (NS), the Y-BOCS/CY-BOCS scores were 15.3, (standard deviation (SD) = 12.3) (children) and 26.8 (9.2) (adults) ($p = 0.043$), and the GTS-QOL scores were 42.8 ± 18.5 (children) and 64 ± 7.9 (adults) ($p = 0.000$). NCGS was frequent in both groups, with headaches reported by 47.0% of children and 83.6% of adults ($p = 0.001$). After one year on a GFD there was a marked reduction in measures of tics (YGTSS) ($p = 0.001$), and the intensity and frequency of OCD (Y-BOCS/CY-BOCS) ($p = 0.001$), along with improved generic quality of life ($p = 0.001$) in children and adults. In conclusion, a GFD maintained for one year in GTS patients led to a marked reduction in tics and OCD both in children and adults.

Keywords: Gilles de la Tourette syndrome (GTS); children and adults; motor and vocal/phonic tics; obsessive-compulsive disorder (OCD); non-coeliac gluten sensitivity (NCGS); gluten-free diet; one-year adherence

1. Introduction

The Gilles de la Tourette syndrome (GTS) is a chronic neuropsychiatric process of unknown cause. It is characterised by the presence of multiple motor tics and at least one vocal or phonic tic. Both types of tic are usually intermittent, although not necessarily concurrently. They are of variable frequency, with periods of intensification and remission, persisting for more than a year, from the appearance of the first tic [1].

This disorder begins in childhood or adolescence before the age of 18 years [1]. Tic severity worsens throughout childhood and for most patients, the worst ever period of tics occurs between 8 and 12 years of age [2,3]. Although up to 80% of patients with GTS have a significant tic decrease during adolescence, and by age 18 years tic intensity and frequency have decreased to such an extent that the person no longer experiences any impairment from their tics, objective ratings indicate that up to 90% of adults continue to exhibit mild tics, although they may occasionally pass unnoticed [3,4]. Its prevalence in school-age children worldwide is around 1%, with a clear predominance in males compared with females on average (3:1). The GTS may be associated with other comorbidities in up to 90% of cases, including obsessive-compulsive disorder (OCD) and those related with attention-deficit/hyperactivity disorder (ADHD) [5]. When comorbid OCD debuts during childhood, it tends to remit in adulthood in only about 40% of cases. It also can develop during adolescence or early adulthood [3,6].

Non-coeliac gluten sensitivity (NCGS) was first described in 1980 [7], but it was classified as part of the spectrum of gluten-related disorders, which also includes coeliac disease (CD) and wheat allergy (WA), until being recognised as a separate clinical entity in 2010. The NCGS is the most frequent of these and is estimated to occur at a prevalence as high as 13% in the general population [8,9].

The clinical presentations of NCGS are varied and overlap with those of CD. It is diagnosed through the prior exclusion of CD, because the serological and histological markers of gluten are usually negative and show a positive response to the withdrawal of gluten from the diet [10,11]. The extra-intestinal symptoms may be the only manifestations of the NCGS, affecting the skin and the musculoskeletal and nervous systems in general [12]. All the associated symptoms improve notably, even disappearing with prolonged adherence to a gluten-free diet (GFD), in a similar manner to what occurs in coeliac patients [13].

The spectrum of neurological processes associated with gluten has progressively broadened in recent years [14–16]. We might expect that the neurological symptoms in certain patients with GTS would maintain a certain relation with the presence of a previously unknown associated NCGS. For this reason, the GFD could have a beneficial effect on their general symptomatology, including neurological symptoms. At present, there is little evidence of its utility in these patients and only isolated cases have provided evidence of the efficacy of a GFD, showing that it could be beneficial [17–19], as has been reported in patients with autism; in these cases, milk casein was also eliminated from the diet of many of them [20]. Its long-term efficacy has been described in one isolated case of GTS treated with GFD for 3 years, whose neurological and general symptomatology completely recovered. Currently, no controlled studies are available of series of patients. A recent systematic review of the literature on the influence of different dietary interventions in patients with GTS found nine articles and one book chapter, none of which included isolated comparative or inter-group studies [21].

The aim of the current study was to analyse and evaluate the efficacy of the GFD, followed for a year by a series of child and adult patients with GTS. The evolution of the neurological and other symptoms associated with NCGS, and the changes observed in their quality of life were evaluated, enabling the comparison of existing clinical aspects before starting the GFD and after 1 year of adherence to it.

2. Materials and Methods

We carried out a prospective pilot study at the national level in Spain of patients diagnosed with GTS to evaluate the efficacy of following a GFD in children and adults. Participants were recruited as voluntary in the study through the online invitation from the National Forum for Tourette's Syndrome. Adults or children's parents gave their written informed consent before they participated in the study. Children are considered to be those younger than 14 years before inclusion in the study. A fundamental inclusion criterion for all patients was that they exhibited motor tics and at least one vocal/phonic tic that had lasted for more than one year.

Thirty-four consecutive patients with GTS began the study, comprising 26 children and eight adults diagnosed, evaluated and followed up various specialists (paediatricians, neurologists, general practitioners, psychiatrists and psychologists). Five patients (three children and two adults) were withdrawn, three due to prolonged interruptions of the diet (one child and two adults) and two children due to voluntary abandonment of the diet. The final sample therefore comprised 29 patients (23 children and six adults).

The children's parents and the adults voluntarily agreed to take part in the study, having been provided with detailed information about the characteristics of the GFD and control criteria. The study was carried out in accordance with Good Clinical Practice, in accordance with the Personal Data Protection and Confidentiality Law, thereby maintaining the anonymity of patients at all times. This study received the ethical approval for the Committee of the Hospital Universitario Central de Asturias (HUCA) with the ethical code number 6265481/16.

Patients were recommended to follow a strict and permanent GFD, as was explained in detail to the parents and adults, and to avoid all types of contamination, for a minimum period of adherence of one year. The observed differences in clinical evolution were compared, and the findings and data collected during the period before starting the GFD and at the end of the year adhering to the diet.

Upon joining the study, patients were asked to undergo a wide range of blood tests, including a complete blood count, general biochemistry, levels of serum anti-tissue transglutaminase antibodies (TGt), the CD genetic markers Human Leukocyte Antigen-DQ2 and Human Leukocyte Antigen-DQ8 (HLA-DQ2 and HLA-DQ8), and serum levels of thyroid hormone and of 25(OH)-Vit. D.

Four questionnaires were administered upon commencement and after 1 year on the GFD. Two of these covered different aspects of GTS, with respect to tics and to OCD. The other two addressed quality of life: a generic one and another one specific to GTS. All the questionnaires were supervised by the parents of the children or filled in by the adults themselves. Information was collected about the principal symptoms related to the patients' neurological characteristics and the signs and symptoms associated with the presence of NCGS.

Our team reviewed all the questionnaires received to ensure that they were complete and contained no contradictory responses. Contact by regular e-mails, telephone calls and/or face-to-face meetings was maintained throughout the study with the parents of the children and with the adults themselves to resolve queries and check the data.

2.1. Questionnaires Used in the Study

2.1.1. Questionnaire to Assess the Severity of Tics Using the Yale Global Tics Severity Scale (YGTSS)

The YGTSS is a widely used instrument for evaluating the intensity and clinical severity of tics in patients with GTS. A variety of tics are enumerated and scored to derive three subscales: motor tics, vocal/phonic tics, and the impairment caused by the tics. For each tics scale, the mean number, total frequency, intensity, complexity and interference are scored between 0 (no affectation) and 5 (maximum affectation). The highest possible overall score for motor tics is 25 and for phonic tics is 25. The score for the impairment arising varies between 0 (none) and 50 (maximum). The total score for the YGTSS is obtained by summing the results obtained from the three subscales and has a maximum value of 100. We used the validated Spanish version of the YGTSS [22,23].

2.1.2. Questionnaires for Evaluating OCD Using the Yale-Brown Obsessive-Compulsive Scale—Self Report (Y-BOCS) and the Children's Yale-Brown Obsessive-Compulsive Scale—Self Report (CY-BOCS)

The Y-BOCS and the CY-BOCS are used to evaluate obsessions and compulsions in children and adults, respectively. They comprise ten items, scored from 0 (no symptoms) to 4 (severe symptoms), to evaluate three components: (a) Obsessions: obtained as the sum of the first five items: Time occupied by the main obsession, its interference in daily life, the distress caused, the resistance against them, and the control over them; (b) Compulsions: comprising the latter five items, which likewise evaluate the time, interference, distress, resistance and control of the principal compulsion presented by the individual; (c) Overall evaluation of obsessions and compulsions: obtained as the sum of the two previous measures. The overall score varies between 0 (minimum) and 40 (maximum). We used the validated Spanish version [24,25].

2.1.3. EuroQol-5D (EQ-5D) Generic Quality of Life Questionnaire

The EQ-5D is a generic instrument for evaluating a person's state of general health. It analyses five dimensions (mobility, self-care, usual activities, pain/discomfort, anxiety/depression), each scored on a scale of 1–3, representing best and worst health. The final evaluation includes a summary index, whose maximum value is 1 (indicating a state of full health). It also includes a visual analogue scale (VAS) from 0 to 100, where a value of 100 represents the best imaginable health state. We used the validated Spanish version [26].

2.1.4. Cavanna's Quality of Life Questionnaire Applied to GTS (GTS-QOL)

This is a specific instrument for evaluating the quality of life of patients with GTS. It comprises 27 items covering six dimensions, each scored from 0 (minimum possible value) to four (maximum possible value): cognitive (eight items); psychological (six items); obsessive-compulsive (four items); physical (three items); coprophenomena (three items); activities of daily living (three items). The results from the six dimensions are evaluated by summing the scores of all the items and, for ease of interpretation, transforming the total to give a value between 0 and 108. It also includes a VAS, scored from 0 to 100, for which the maximum value represents the best possible health. The validated scale in English was administered in Spanish [27].

2.2. Evaluation of Other Neurological Characteristics

Other data of GTS were collected at the time of inclusion, including age of onset and duration of the different symptoms of the disease, number of family members affected, and types of medication consumed. The changes that had occurred with respect to the various aspects under investigation by the end of the year on the GFD were analysed.

2.3. Evaluation of NCGS Symptoms

The signs and symptoms related to the NCGS were evaluated with a questionnaire comprising several items with a variable number of possible responses. Clinical characteristics of NCGS were collected at the time of inclusion, along with information about family background, analytical results and complementary tests and their evolution after the GFD. A group of questions designed to evaluate the different symptoms distributed by organs and apparatus, each with a variable number of possible responses, and a general score between 0 (absence of symptoms) and 3 (maximum possible intensity) was included.

2.4. Evaluation of GFD Compliance

The evaluation and follow up of the diet compliance were carried out through questionnaires filled in by the patients (in the case of adults) or their parents (in the case of children) and regular contact by telephone, e-mail or, in some cases, face-to-face consultation.

2.5. Audio-Visual Monitoring Evaluation

For the assessment of tics and following the recommendations of the European clinical guidelines for Tourette Syndrome and other tic disorders, we ask our patients for some audiovisual recordings, reflecting spontaneous situations of everyday life [3]. The parents of one of our patients gave their written informed consent to attach a demonstration video of their child's evolution for scientific purposes in this study, whose details are specified in the Supplementary Material Section.

2.6. Statistical Methods

Data were analysed with SPSS (v15.0 for Windows; SPSS Inc., Chicago, IL, USA). Descriptive analyses were used to characterize the study population. Categorical variables were expressed as absolute frequencies and percentages. Quantitative variables were expressed as the mean or median, if normally or non-normally distributed, respectively, and were compared within and between groups using Student's two-tailed independent samples t-test. To compare the proportions (frequencies) of qualitative variables between the groups, contingency test methods (chi-squared (χ^2) or Fisher's exact tests) were used, as appropriate. Student's t-test and Mann-Whitney were used for independent (unpaired) samples (children vs. adults). When the number of observations of any of the groups compared was small, always the parametric tests (Student) were used; otherwise, the tests used were Mann-Whitney and Wilcoxon. When the data were quantitative of low rank (for example, scores from 1 to 5) nonparametric tests were always used. For samples of repeated measurements, the McNemar test has been used. The paired Wilcoxon signed-rank test was used to compare differences in the medians of continuous non-parametric variables. The tests used and the variables of the groups in which they have been applied are specified at the beginning of the foot of each table. In all cases, a value of $p < 0.05$ was considered to indicate a statistically significant difference.

3. Results

3.1. Baseline Demographic Characteristics of Children and Adults

Comparing the baseline characteristics of child and adult patients included in the study, showed that 74% of the children and 50% of the adults were male (NS). 69% of children and 100% of adults presented an associated OCD (NS). ADHD was present in 52.2% of children and 66.2% of adults (NS).

The total tic score, as measured by the YGTSS questionnaire, was similar in the two groups (NS). Conversely, the total OCD score assessed with the Y-BOCS/CY-BOCS questionnaires, was lower in the children 15.3 (12.3) than in the adults 26.8 (9.2) ($p = 0.043$). The generic quality of life score at the beginning of the study was similar in the two groups. However, GTS-specific quality of life was lower in the children 42.8 (18.5) than in the adults 64.0 (7.9) ($p = 0.000$). There was no difference in the consumption of medication between the groups, either overall or with respect to Non-Steroidal Anti-Inflammatory Drugs (NSAIDs). However, many fewer children than adults took psychotropics (34.8% vs. 100%) ($p = 0.006$) (Table 1).

Table 1. Baseline demographic characteristics of children and adults.

Parameters	Children ($n = 23$)	Adults ($n = 6$)	p
Males, n (%)	17 (74)	3 (50)	NS
Mean age, years, ($X \pm$ SD)	8.3 ± 2.7	32.2 ± 11.9	NA
Age at commencement, years, ($X \pm$ SD)	3.8 ± 2.0	7.7 ± 3.4	NA
Duration of symptoms of GTS, years, ($X \pm$ SD)	4.5 ± 2.4	24.5 ± 10.9	NA
Associated OCD, n (%)	16 (69)	6 (100)	NS
Associated ADHD, n (%)	11 (52.2)	4 (66.2)	NS
Total YGTSS score, ($X \pm$ SD)	55.0 ± 17.5	55.8 ± 19.8	NS
Total Y-BOCS score, ($X \pm$ SD)	15.3 ± 12.3	26.8 ± 9.2	=0.043
Total EQ-5D score, ($X \pm$ SD)	0.6 ± 0.2	0.5 ± 0.2	NS
Total GTS-QOL score, ($X \pm$ SD)	42.8 ± 18.5	64.0 ± 7.9	=0.000
Drug consumption, n (%)	21 (91.3)	6 (100)	NS
-NSAIDs, n (%)	21 (91.3)	6 (100)	NS
-Psychotropics, n (%)	8 (34.8)	6 (100)	=0.006

The Mann Whitney or Fisher tests were used when the variances were different and when they were similar, the Student test was employed. X = Mean; SD = Standard Deviation; OCD = Obsessive Compulsive Disorder; ADHD = Attention-Deficit/Hyperactivity Disorder; YGTSS = Yale Global Tics Severity Scale; Y-BOCS = Yale-Brown Obsessive-Compulsive Scale; EQ-5D = EuroQol-5D; GTS-QOL = Gilles de la Tourette Syndrome-Quality of Life Scale; NSAIDs = Non-Steroidal Anti-Inflammatory Drugs; NS = Non-Significant; NA = Not Applicable.

3.2. Baseline Characteristics of the Symptoms and Signs of Gluten Sensitivity in Children and Adults

Upon entering the study, a series of symptoms and signs related to the presence of NCGS, which were present in the individual participants, were compared between the two groups. No significant differences were found for any characteristics, except for the presence of headaches and/or migraines, which were more common in the adults than the children (83.3% vs. 47.8%) ($p = 0.1$), and of behavioural disorders, which were also more common in adults (100% vs. 95.6%) ($p = 0.001$) (Table 2).

Table 2. Baseline characteristics of the symptoms and signs of NCGS in children and adults.

Parameters	Children ($n = 23$)	Adults ($n = 6$)	p
Upper respiratory tract infections, n (%)	20 (86.9)	4 (66.7)	NS
Lower respiratory tract infections, n (%)	15 (65.2)	2 (33.3)	NS
Associated allergies, n (%)	12 (52.2)	2 (33.3)	NS
Headaches and/or migraines, n (%)	11 (47.8)	5 (83.3)	NS *
Infectious oral processes, n (%)	20 (86.9)	4 (66.7)	NS
Other dental changes, n (%)	18 (78.3)	6 (100.0)	NS
Musculoskeletal affectation, n (%)	21 (91.3)	5 (83.3)	NS
Dermatitis, n (%)	20 (86.9)	5 (83.3)	NS
Anaemia and/or ferropaenia, n (%)	17 (73.9)	5 (83.3)	NS
Sleep disorders, n (%)	21 (91.3)	6 (100.0)	NS
Behavioural disorders, n (%)	22 (95.6)	6 (100.0)	NS **
Urinary disorders, n (%)	13 (56.5)	4 (66.7)	NS
Dietary disorders, n (%)	20 (86.9)	6 (100.0)	NS
Change in intestinal habit, n (%)	22 (95.6)	6 (100.0)	NS
Change in stool consistency, n (%)	11 (47.8)	1 (16.7)	NS

The Mann Whitney or Fisher tests were used when the variances were different and when they were similar, the Student test was employed. * Comparing intensity, Mann-Whitney U, $p = 0.1$; ** Comparing intensity, Mann-Whitney, $p = 0.001$ NCGS = Non-Coeliac Gluten Sensitivity; n = number; NS = Non-Significant.

3.3. Evolution of Neurological Symptoms and Quality of Life after 1 Year of a GFD

After one year of following a GFD, the improvement in neurological symptoms was very striking, with a significant reduction in tics and OCD in both children and adults ($p = 0.001$). The same occurred with the improvement found in the generic and specific quality of life ($p = 0.001$), whereby there was no difference between the children and adults. This translated into a reduction in the consumption of medication in both groups, the effect being very pronounced in children ($p = 0.001$) but more moderate in adults ($p = 0.072$); the reduction among the adults was mainly a consequence of a decrease in the consumption of psychotropics ($p = 0.071$) (Table 3).

Table 3. Evolution of neurological symptoms and quality of life after 1 year of a GFD.

Parameters	Pre-GFD	Post-GFD	p
Total YGTSS score, ($X \pm$ SD), (Maximum 100)			
-Children	55.0 ± 17.5	27.3 ± 22.3	$=0.000$
-Adults	55.8 ± 19.8	20.7 ± 13.5	$=0.001$
Total Y-BOCS/CY-BOCS score, ($X \pm$ SD), (Maximum 40)			
-Children	15.3 ± 12.3	5.4 ± 8.6	$=0.000$
-Adults	26.8 ± 9.2	8.0 ± 8.9	$=0.001$
Total EQ-5D score, ($X \pm$ SD), (Maximum 1)			
-Children	0.62 ± 0.23	0.88 ± 0.17	$=0.000$
-Adults	0.50 ± 0.22	0.87 ± 015	$=0.004$
Total GTS-QOL score, ($X \pm$ SD), (Maximum 108)			
-Children	42.8 ± 18.5	22.4 ± 19.9	$=0.000$
-Adults	64.0 ± 7.9	20.5 ± 12.2	$=0.001$
Drug consumption *			
-Children: -Total consumption, n (%)	21 (91.3)	16 (69.6)	$=0.001$
-NSAIDs, n (%)	21 (91.3)	12 (52.2)	$=0.002$
-Psychotropics, n (%)	8 (34.8)	7 (30.4)	$=0.190$

Table 3. *Cont.*

Parameters	Pre-GFD	Post-GFD	*p*
-Adults: -Total consumption, *n* (%)	6 (100)	6 (100)	=0.072
-NSAIDs, *n* (%)	6 (100)	5 (83.3)	=0.100
-Psychotropics, *n* (%)	6 (100)	4 (66.7)	=0.071

The tests used were the Wilcoxon signed-rank test for adults, the Student paired test for children and the McNemar test for drugs consumption. * Comparing intensity, Wilcoxon test, GFD = Gluten-free diet; X = Mean; SD = Standard Deviation; YGTSS = Yale Global Tics Severity Scale; Y-BOCS = Yale-Brown Obsessive-Compulsive Scale; EQ-5D = EuroQol-5D; GTS-QOL = Gilles de la Tourette Syndrome-Quality of Life Scale; NSAIDs = Non-Steroidal Anti-Inflammatory Drugs.

3.4. Evolution after 1 Year of a GFD of the Various Components of Motor and Phonic Tics, Obsessions and Compulsions

The evolution of the different components of the motor and vocal/phonic tics, and of OCD, was assessed, comparing the results obtained before beginning and a year after following the GFD. With respect to the evolution of the characteristics of the motor tics, we found a notable decrease in their various components (number, intensity, frequency, complexity and interference), that was more significant in children (p = 0.000) than in adults (p = 0.027). The evaluation of the vocal/phonic tics revealed a reduction in their principal characteristics in both groups, again being more pronounced in children (p = 0.001) than in adults (p = 0.028). This was maintained with an identical significance when jointly evaluating the motor and vocal/phonic tics, this improvement being somewhat smaller in the adults than in the children. The evolution of the disability associated to the motor tics was significantly reduced in the children (p = 0.000), but less so in the adults (p = 0.059). Likewise, a clear improvement in the evolution of the disability related to the vocal/phonic tics was confirmed, the effect being more significant in the children (p = 0.001) than in the adults (p = 0.041). The decrease in the overall degree of disability along with the motor and vocal/phonic tics was significant in both groups, though slightly higher in the children (p = 0.000) than in the adults (p = 0.027). Equally, after one year on the GFD the various components of the obsessions (time, interference, distress, resistance and control) were significantly reduced, which was somewhat more marked in children (p = 0.001) than in adults (p = 0.028). The same components of the compulsions after a year on a GFD confirmed a significant improvement in both groups, again being slightly greater in children (p = 0.008) than in adults (p = 0.027) (Table 4).

Table 4. Evolution after 1 year of a GFD of the various components of motor and phonic tics, obsessions and compulsions.

Parameters	Pre-GFD	Post-GFD	*p*
Evaluation of motor tics (number, frequency, intensity, complexity and interference), ($X \pm$ SD), (Maximum 25)			
-Children	18.7 ± 4.3	10.1 ± 6.3	=0.000
-Adults	17.3 ± 7.1	9.0 ± 4.7	=0.027
Evaluation of phonic tics (number, frequency, intensity, complexity and interference), ($X \pm$ SD), (Maximum 25)			
-Children	14.4 ± 5.6	7.4 ± 7.1	=0.001
-Adults	15.2 ± 5.8	5.8 ± 3.9	=0.028
Overall evaluation of motor and phonic tics (number, frequency, intensity, complexity and interference), ($X \pm$ SD), (Maximum 50)			
-Children	33.1 ± 8.3	17.5 ± 12.1	=0.000
-Adults	32.5 ± 9.5	14.8 ± 7.7	=0.028
Overall disability of motor tics, ($X \pm$ SD), (Maximum 5)			
-Children	2.3 ± 1.1	1.0 ± 1.1	=0.000
-Adults	2.5 ± 1.6	0.7 ± 0.8	=0.059

Table 4. *Cont.*

Parameters	Pre-GFD	Post-GFD	*p*
Overall disability of phonic tics, ($X \pm$ SD), (Maximum 5)			
-Children	2.0 ± 1.2	1.0 ± 1.2	=0.001
-Adults	2.2 ± 1.3	0.5 ± 0.8	=0.041
Overall disability of motor and phonic tics, ($X \pm$ SD), (Maximum 10)			
-Children	4.4 ± 2.0	1.9 ± 2.1	=0.000
-Adults	4.7 ± 2.2	1.2 ± 1.6	=0.027
Evaluation of obsessions (time, interference, discomfort, resistance and control), ($X \pm$ SD), (Maximum 20)			
-Children	8.7 ± 6.6	3.0 ± 4.7	=0.001
-Adults	13.5 ± 4.4	4.0 ± 4.5	=0.028
Evaluation of compulsions (time, interference, discomfort, resistance and control), ($X \pm$ SD), (Maximum 20)			
-Children	6.6 ± 6.3	2.4 ± 4.5	=0.008
-Adults	13.3 ± 4.9	4.0 ± 4.3	=0.027

The tests used were the Wilcoxon signed-rank test for adults and the Student paired test for children. GFD = Gluten-free diet; X = Mean; SD = Standard Deviation.

3.5. Evolution of Symptoms of Non-Coeliac Gluten Sensitivity after 1 Year of a GFD

The evolution of the symptoms associated with NCGS after one year on a GFD was also very favourable. The number and intensity of upper airway infections were significantly reduced in both groups, though more notably in the children ($p = 0.000$) than in the adults ($p = 0.068$). The same pattern was found for the lower airway, with children showing a more significant reduction ($p = 0.001$) than the adults ($p = 0.180$). Conversely, no significant differences were found in the number of associated allergies. Fewer episodes of headaches/migraines were observed, the effect being slightly more significant in children ($p = 0.013$) than in adults ($p = 0.068$). Infectious or inflammatory oral processes were notably reduced in children ($p = 0.000$) but were unchanged in adults ($p = 0.104$). Musculoskeletal affectation decreased significantly in children ($p = 0.002$) and slightly less significantly in adults ($p = 0.042$). Associated dermatitis also decreased strikingly in children ($p = 0.002$), more significantly than in the adults ($p = 0.058$). Anaemia and iron deficiency improved notably in children ($p = 0.004$) but was unchanged in adults ($p = 0.131$). Likewise, sleep disorders reduced significantly in the children ($p = 0.000$) and in a smaller proportion of adults ($p = 0.046$). No significant changes in urinary disorders were noted in children ($p = 0.082$) or adults ($p = 0.109$). Behavioural disorders decreased significantly in children ($p = 0.000$) and to a lesser degree in adults ($p = 0.028$). The improvement achieved in the dietary disorders was more evident in children ($p = 0.000$) than in adults ($p = 0.027$), as was the case for the improvement in intestinal habit, which was greater in children ($p = 0.001$) than in adults ($p = 0.075$) (Table 5).

Table 5. Evolution of symptoms of non-coeliac gluten sensitivity after 1 year of a GFD.

Parameters	Pre-GFD	Post-GFD	*p*
Upper respiratory tract infections, ($X \pm$ SD), (Maximum 18)			
-Children	3.2 ± 2.1	0.6 ± 0.9	=0.000
-Adults	4.5 ± 4.9	0.2 ± 0.4	=0.680
Lower respiratory tract infections, ($X \pm$ SD), (Maximum 9)			
-Children	2.1 ± 2.2	0.1 ± 0.4	=0.001
-Adults	1.3 ± 2.1	0.3 ± 0.8	=0.180
Associated allergies, ($X \pm$ SD), (Maximum 27)			
-Children	1.8 ± 3.4	1.7 ± 2.4	=0.782
-Adults	1.3 ± 2.8	2.2 ± 3.7	=0.285

Table 5. *Cont.*

Parameters	Pre-GFD	Post-GFD	*p*
Headaches and/or migraines, (X ± SD), (Maximum 18)			
-Children	1.7 ± 2.7	0.4 ± 0.6	=0.013
-Adults	4.8 ± 4.9	0.8 ± 1.2	=0.068
Infectious oral processes, (X ± SD), (Maximum 15)			
-Children	3.0 ± 2.3	1.0 ± 1.3	=0.000
-Adults	3.8 ± 4.2	0.5 ± 0.8	=0.104
Other dental changes, (X ± SD), (Maximum 15)			
-Children	2.1 ± 1.6	1.6 ± 1.3	=0.105
-Adults	2.8 ± 2.1	1.8 ± 1.0	=0.276
Musculoskeletal affectation, (X ± SD), (Maximum 36)			
-Children	5.0 ± 5.7	1.4 ± 2.5	=0.002
-Adults	9.0 ± 12.7	1.3 ± 2.0	=0.042
Dermatitis, (X ± SD), (Maximum 45)			
-Children	4.8 ± 6.3	1.4 ± 1.9	=0.002
-Adults	6.3 ± 4.9	2.0 ± 2.1	=0.058
Anaemia and/or ferropaenia, (X ± SD), (Maximum 24)			
-Children	2.8 ± 3.1	0.8 ± 1.4	=0.004
-Adults	4.0 ± 3.6	1.2 ± 1.5	=0.131
Sleep disorders, (X ± SD), (Maximum 27)			
-Children	6.2 ± 6.4	1.6 ± 2.0	=0.000
-Adults	8.7 ± 5.3	2.0 ± 1.3	=0.046
Behavioural disorders, (X ± SD), (Maximum 24)			
-Children	7.2 ± 5.6	2.6 ± 4.1	=0.002
-Adults	16.0 ± 3.0	3.0 ± 4.5	=0.028
Urinary disorders, (X ± SD), (Maximum 21)			
-Children	1.8 ± 2.7	0.7 ± 1.3	=0.082
-Adults	3.3 ± 5.3	0.5 ± 0.8	=0.109
Dietary disorders, (X ± SD), (Maximum 45)			
-Children	9.5 ± 9.5	1.3 ± 1.9	=0.000
-Adults	10.5 ± 9.4	1.8 ± 1.2	=0.027
Change in intestinal habit, (X ± SD), (Maximum 33)			
-Children	9.1 ± 6.8	3.7 ± 4.8	=0.001
-Adults	7.7 ± 5.2	2.3 ± 2.1	=0.075

The tests used were the Wilcoxon signed-rank test for adults, the Student paired test for children and the McNemar test for drugs consumption. GFD = Gluten-free diet; X = Mean; SD = Standard Deviation.

4. Discussion

At the beginning of the study, the presence of motor and vocal/phonic tics was similar in children and adults. The generic quality of life was similar in the two groups; however, specifically GTS-related quality of life was worse in children than in adults. Nevertheless, the adults were taking a higher proportion of psychotropics than the children, with significant differences. Our results coincide with those of other authors, in the sense that during childhood the intensity and frequency of tics are usually higher in children than in adults, while OCD usually predominates in adults compared with children, which accounts for the more widespread consumption of psychotropics among adults than children [2,28,29].

People with NCGS usually exhibit a variety of associated symptoms such as headaches or migraines, "brain fog", fatigue, fibromyalgia, joint and muscle pain, leg or arm numbness, tingling of the extremities, dermatitis (eczema or skin rash), allergies, atopic disorders, depression, anxiety, anaemia, iron-deficiency anaemia, folate deficiency, asthma, rhinitis, eating disorders, or autoimmune diseases. Among the extra-intestinal manifestations, NCGS has been implicated in some neuropsychiatric disorders, such as schizophrenia, autism, peripheral neuropathy, ataxia, ADHD, mood swings, sensory symptoms, disturbed sleep patterns, and hallucinations ("gluten psychosis") [9,16,30–35].

Many coeliac patients or those with undiagnosed NCGS underestimate their multiple and frequent discomfort from digestive and more general causes because they have grown accustomed to living with a state of chronic poor health as though it were normal. They are only able to recognise that they really did have symptoms related to the consumption of gluten when they start the GFD and the improvement becomes obvious [36,37].

The disproportionately common occurrence in patients with GTS of immunologically determined illnesses, such as allergic processes, rhinitis, asthma, dermatitis and conjunctivitis, frequently with raised IgE and a positive family history of autoimmune diseases has been reported. Likewise, the presence of migraines, autistic spectrum disorders, anxiety, depression, sleep disorders, behavioural problems and hallucinations have frequently been noted [38–40].

At the beginning of our study, various symptoms and signs associated with NCGS were present in similar proportions in both groups, with a slight predominance of headaches and/or migraines and behavioural disorders in adults. After a year on the GFD a significant improvement was observed in most of these symptoms and signs, both in children and adults, similar to what generally occurs in patients with NCGS without associated GTS [8,34,41].

We found a significant improvement in the neurological signs of GTS after one year on the GFD, with a notable reduction in motor and vocal/phonic tics and OCD symptoms, both in children and adults. A probable explanation lies in the presence of an increase in intestinal permeability of patients with NCGS, as happens in coeliac patients. This enables the passage of gluten peptides and other related peptides to the bloodstream, crossing the blood-brain barrier and reaching different areas of the brain, provoking the appearance of inflammatory processes localised in various structures within the brain, which might explain the presence of the symptoms and signs related to the GTS [34]. This would explain why the withdrawal of gluten from the diet produces a reduction in such deposits and thereby gives rise to significant clinical improvement in the evolution of motor and vocal/phonic tics and OCD symptoms. As Hadjivassiliou stated more than 15 years ago, "Gluten sensitivity can be primarily and at times exclusively a neurological disease. The absence of an enteropathy should not preclude patients from treatment with a gluten-free diet. Early diagnosis and removal of the trigger factor by the introduction of gluten-free diet is a promising therapeutic intervention" and consequently the fact "that gluten sensitivity is regarded as principally a disease of the small bowel is a historical misconception" [42–44].

The GFD produced a clear improvement in generic and specific quality of life in both groups, accompanied by a reduction in the overall consumption of drugs, this being more pronounced in adults than children, largely due to the notable reduction in the consumption of psychotropics in the former group, but not significant.

The improvement found with respect to the presence of tics was maintained upon evaluating the degree of disability generated for the motor and vocal/phonic tics, although it was somewhat higher in the children than the adults.

As confirmed by a systematic review, the risk of developing neurological complications in coeliac patients is lower in children than in adults and their response to a GFD is generally quicker and stronger, probably because they have spent less of their life eating gluten [45,46].

Likewise, an improvement was observed in the disability related to the presence of OCD, which is also more striking in children than in adults. We have only found two previous reports in the literature, one of a patient with OCD associated with GTS, and another of an isolated case, both of which showed an improvement in symptoms along with a reduction in their previous disability [17,18].

The patients with GTS, as well as presenting motor and phonic tics, may develop multiple behavioural problems in response to the impact of the symptoms that affect their relationships with family members, friends, class-mates and teachers. Furthermore, it has been estimated that around

90% present other comorbidities, including, amongst others, OCD and those related to ADHD, which exacerbate the disorders of character and behaviour they already had that arose from the presence of tics [47,48].

We can conclude that the improvement of the patients cannot be justified solely by the passage of time because the children were in the stage of worse evolution of the GTS and the adults belong to the subgroup of people whose disorder does not ameliorate or even get worse. In addition, the follow-up period was only a year and the majority of patients had associated comorbidities. In the evaluation and follow-up of diet compliance, 22 of the 29 patients indicated that they had suffered clearly identified occasional contaminations due to errors in their diet. The tics reappeared or worsened in all cases (16 cases with phonic and motor tics, 4 cases with only motor tics, 2 cases with only phonic tics); all of the cases who previously had comorbid OCD experienced its reappearance or intensification. The exacerbation was resolved after days or even weeks of resetting the gluten-free diet. It is interesting to note that since these are inadvertent and involuntary contaminations verified *a posteriori*, mainly associated with misinterpretations of labelling, eating out at restaurants or in family homes, the nocebo effect can also be ruled out, especially in the case of children because they do not know the detailed information about the diet. These data indicate a clear relationship between the improvement of GTS symptoms and the withdrawal of gluten from the diet that is not conditioned by the passage of time or hypothetical spontaneous remission.

We evaluated the symptoms related to the tics and the OCD using questionnaires that are widely validated and accepted internationally. However, we did not evaluate the symptoms related to ADHD, although we also found that they improved while on the GFD, as has been confirmed in a recent systematic review of this subject [49].

This paper presents the results of a prospective uncontrolled cohort study, designed as a pilot, and is the first of its kind, as far as we know. It has certain limitations, since the sample size of the study was small, especially in the group of adults, and we have not been able to include a control group. Our initial intention was to include it, but this was not possible. The patients who contacted us presented significant affectation of their quality of life and all of them wanted to try the diet. This prevents us from drawing definitive conclusions, added the fact that we cannot be sure that either the children or the adults followed the GFD fully. Gluten is ubiquitous and removing it strictly from the diet is difficult, especially when eating outside the home [50]. Ensuring fulfilment of the GFD is complicated, as other authors have found [20,50–53] and we cannot be certain that it was achieved in this study. Current studies show that compliance with the diet in patients with gluten sensitivity is much worse than was formerly considered, demonstrating that approximately 79% of them continue to present intestinal lesions, despite maintaining treatment with the GFD [52]. None of the methods used to evaluate the strict compliance of the GFD has proved to be sufficiently accurate: questionnaires filled in by patients; evaluation of symptoms; determination of gluten-specific antibodies; and findings in duodenal biopsies [51,54]. Frequently, people with a poor educational level and a poor understanding of how to follow a GFD believe that they are strictly following the diet, when in fact they are frequently making mistakes [50,52]. This leads patients to overestimate their compliance when they fill in the questionnaire, making their results unreliable. Neither the absence of digestive symptoms nor the negativity of the antibodies guarantees that the intestinal mucosa recovers, which is complicated to determine with biopsies because the intestinal lesions usually consist of minimal changes without villous atrophy, and that are frequently patched and difficult to identify [51,54,55]. Recently, new methods have been developed to monitor strict adherence to the diet, based on the determination of the presence of gluten peptides in faeces or urine, which seem to offer a realistic alternative, but have not yet been validated or become available for use in daily clinical practice [55]. We gave detailed information to the patients about how to comply fully with the GFD. Although in the case of the children we always recommend to parents that the whole family adopt a GFD, avoiding the consumption of foodstuffs containing gluten at home, in school canteens and elsewhere cannot always be fully achieved. We used questionnaires filled in by the patients (in the case of adults) or their parents (in the case of children) and had regular contact by telephone, e-mail or, in some cases, face-to-face consultation, to monitor compliance and clarify doubts. However, for all the reasons stated above, we conclude that we cannot guarantee that compliance with the gluten-free diet was entirely strict.

5. Conclusions

In conclusion, we have shown that following a GFD opens up a new line of therapy for patients with GTS. It is entirely innocuous but requires a strict and prolonged adherence. It seems to be useful for reducing the frequency and intensity of motor and vocal/phonic tics, and OCD symptoms. It is also accompanied by an improved quality of life, both generally and specifically, and a reduction in the consumption of NSAID drugs by children and of antipsychotics by adults.

Subsequent controlled and/or multi-centre studies including more patients and with a prolonged period on the GFD will enable the efficacy of the diet to be determined more exactly.

Supplementary Materials: The following are available online at http://www.mdpi.com/2072-6643/10/5/573/s1, Video S1: A 7 years old child with GTS and OCD-evolution after 1 year of GFD. We include one video of the evolution of an seven-year-old child, recorded before and after 1 year on the GFD, and the scores he obtained. A clear improvement in his symptomatology can be seen. The child was not taking any medication.

Author Contributions: L.R. and N.Á. designed the study and wrote the Introduction and Discussion. E.F.-B. analysed and interpreted the results and performed the statistical analysis. J.S.-P., M.H. and C.H.-L. made substantial technical contributions to the design and interpretation of the results.

Conflicts of Interest: The authors declare no conflict of interest.

References

1. American Psychiatric Association. *Diagnostic and Statistical Manual of Mental Disorders*, 5th ed.; American Psychiatric Association: Washington, DC, USA, 2013.
2. Robertson, M.M. A personal 35 year perspective on Gilles de la Tourette syndrome: Prevalence, phenomenology, comorbidities, and coexistent psychopathologies. *Lancet Psychiatry* **2015**, *2*, 68–87. [CrossRef]
3. Cath, D.C.; Hedderly, T.; Ludolph, A.G.; Stern, J.S.; Murphy, T.; Hartmann, A.; Czernecki, V.; Robertson, M.M.; Martino, D.; Munchau, A.; et al. ESSTS Guidelines Group. European clinical guidelines for Tourette syndrome and other tic disorders. Part I: Assessment. *Eur. Child Adolesc. Psychiatry* **2011**, *20*, 155–171. [CrossRef] [PubMed]
4. Hassan, N.; Cavanna, A.E. The prognosis of Tourette syndrome: Implications for clinical practice. *Funct. Neurol.* **2012**, *27*, 23–27. [PubMed]
5. Robertson, M.M.; Eapen, V.; Cavanna, A.E. The international prevalence, epidemiology, and clinical phenomenology of Tourette syndrome: A cross-cultural perspective. *J. Psychosom. Res.* **2009**, *67*, 475–483. [CrossRef] [PubMed]
6. Bloch, M.H.; Leckman, J.F. Clinical course of Tourette syndrome. *J. Psychosom. Res.* **2009**, *67*, 497–501. [CrossRef] [PubMed]
7. Cooper, B.T.; Holmes, G.K.; Ferguson, R.; Thompson, R.A.; Allan, R.N.; Cooke, W.T. Gluten-sensitive diarrhea without evidence of celiac disease. *Gastroenterology* **1980**, *79*, 801–806. [PubMed]
8. Molina-Infante, J.; Santolaria, S.; Sanders, D.S.; Fernández-Bañares, F. Systematic review: Noncoeliac gluten sensitivity. *Aliment. Pharmacol. Ther.* **2015**, *41*, 807–820. [CrossRef] [PubMed]
9. Catassi, C.; Bai, J.C.; Bonaz, B.; Bouma, G.; Calabrò, A.; Carroccio, A.; Castillejo, G.; Ciacci, C.; Cristofori, F.; Dolinsek, J.; et al. Nonceliac gluten sensitivity: The new frontier of gluten related disorders. *Nutrients* **2013**, *5*, 3839–3853. [CrossRef] [PubMed]
10. Mansueto, P.; Seidita, A.; D'Alcamo, A.; Carroccio, A. Non-celiac gluten sensitivity: Literature review. *J. Am. Coll. Nutr.* **2014**, *33*, 39–54. [CrossRef] [PubMed]
11. Fasano, A.; Catassi, C. Clinical practice. Celiac disease. *N. Engl. J. Med.* **2012**, *367*, 2419–2426. [CrossRef] [PubMed]

12. Volta, U.; Caio, G.; Karunaratne, T.B.; Alaedini, A.; De Giorgio, R. Non-coeliac gluten/wheat sensitivity: Advances in knowledge and relevant questions. *Expert Rev. Gastroenterol. Hepatol.* **2017**, *11*, 9–18. [CrossRef] [PubMed]

13. Sapone, A.; Bai, J.C.; Ciacci, C.; Dolinsek, J.; Green, P.H.; Hadjivassiliou, M.; Kaukinen, K.; Rostami, K.; Sanders, D.S.; Schumann, M.; et al. Spectrum of gluten-related disorders: Consensus on new nomenclature and classification. *BMC Med.* **2012**, *10*, 13. [CrossRef] [PubMed]

14. Jackson, J.R.; Eaton, W.W.; Cascella, N.G.; Fasano, A.; Kelly, D.L. Neurologic and psychiatric manifestations of celiac disease and gluten sensitivity. *Psychiatr. Q.* **2012**, *83*, 91–102. [CrossRef] [PubMed]

15. Bushara, K.O. Neurologic presentation of celiac disease. *Gastroenterology* **2005**, *128*, S92–S97. [CrossRef] [PubMed]

16. Lebwohl, B.; Ludvigsson, J.F.; Green, P.H. Celiac disease and non-celiac gluten sensitivity. *BMJ* **2015**, *351*, h4347. [CrossRef] [PubMed]

17. Rodrigo, L.; Huerta, M.; Salas-Puig, J. Tourette syndrome and non-celiac gluten sensitivity. Clinical remission with a gluten-free diet: A description case. *J. Sleep Disord. Ther.* **2015**, *4*, 183. [CrossRef]

18. Couture, D.C.; Chung, M.K.; Shinnick, P.; Curzon, J.; McClure, M.J.; LaRiccia, P.J. Integrative Medicine Approach to Pediatric Obsessive-Compulsive Disorder and anxiety: A Case-report. *Glob. Adv. Health Med.* **2016**, *5*, 117–121. [CrossRef] [PubMed]

19. Warsi, Q.; Kirby, C.; Beg, M. Pediatric Tourette Syndrome: A Tic Disorder with a Tricky Presentation. *Case Rep. Gastroenterol.* **2017**, *11*, 89–94. [CrossRef] [PubMed]

20. Millward, C.; Ferriter, M.; Calver, S.; Connell-Jones, G. Gluten-and casein-free diets for autistic spectrum disorder. *Cochrane Database Syst. Rev.* **2008**, CD003498. [CrossRef] [PubMed]

21. Ludlow, A.K.; Rogers, S.L. Understanding the impact of diet and nutrition on symptoms of Tourette syndrome: A scoping review. *J. Child Health Care* **2017**, *22*, 68–83. [CrossRef] [PubMed]

22. Leckman, J.F.; Riddle, M.A.; Hardin, M.T.; Ort, S.I.; Swartz, K.L.; Stevenson, J.; Cohen, D.J. The Yale Global Tics Severity Scale: Initial testing of a clinician-rated scale of tic severity. *J. Am. Acad. Child Adolesc. Psychiatry* **1989**, *28*, 566–573. [CrossRef] [PubMed]

23. García-López, R.; Perea-Milla, E.; Romero-González, J.; Rivas-Ruiz, F.; Ruiz-García, C.; Oviedo-Joekes, E.; de las Mulas-Bejar, M. Spanish adaptation and diagnostic validity of the Yale Global Tics Severity Scale. *Rev. Neurol.* **2008**, *46*, 261–266. [PubMed]

24. Goodman, W.K.; Price, L.H.; Rasmussen, S.A.; Mazure, C.; Delgado, P.; Heninger, G.R.; Charney, D.S. The Yale-Brown Obsessive Compulsive Scale. II. Validity. *Arch. Gen. Psychiatry* **1989**, *46*, 1012–1016. [CrossRef] [PubMed]

25. Godoy, A.; Gavino, A.; Valderrama, L.; Quintero, C.; Cobos, M.P.; Casado, Y.; Sosa, M.D.; Capafons, J.I. Factor structure and reliability of the Spanish adaptation of the Children's Yale-Brown Obsessive-Compulsive Scale–Self Report (CY-BOCS-SR). *Psicothema* **2011**, *23*, 330–335. [PubMed]

26. Badia, X.; Roset, M.; Montserrat, S.; Herdman, M.; Segura, A. The Spanish version of EuroQol: A description and its applications. European Quality of Life scale. *Med. Clin.* **1999**, *112*, 79–85.

27. Cavanna, A.E.; Schrag, A.; Morley, D.; Orth, M.; Robertson, M.M.; Joyce, E.; Critchley, H.D.; Selai, C. The Gilles de la Tourette Syndrome-Quality of Life Scale (GTS-QOL): Development and validation. *Neurology* **2008**, *71*, 1410–1416. [CrossRef] [PubMed]

28. Kompoliti, K. Sources of Disability in Tourette Syndrome: Children vs. Adults. *Tremor Other Hyperkinet Mov.* **2016**, *5*, 318. [CrossRef]

29. Leckman, J.F. Tic disorders. *BMJ* **2012**, *344*, d7659. [CrossRef] [PubMed]

30. Volta, U.; De Giorgio, R. New understanding of gluten sensitivity. *Nat. Rev. Gastroenterol. Hepatol.* **2012**, *9*, 295–299. [CrossRef] [PubMed]

31. Aziz, I.; Hadjivassiliou, M.; Sanders, D.S. The spectrum of noncoeliac gluten sensitivity. *Nat. Rev. Gastroenterol. Hepatol.* **2015**, *12*, 516–526. [CrossRef] [PubMed]

32. Fasano, A.; Sapone, A.; Zevallos, V.; Schuppan, D. Nonceliac gluten sensitivity. *Gastroenterology* **2015**, *148*, 1195–1204. [CrossRef] [PubMed]

33. Volta, U.; Caio, G.; De Giorgio, R.; Henriksen, C.; Skodje, G.; Lundin, K.E. Non-celiac gluten sensitivity: A work-in-progress entity in the spectrum of wheat-related disorders. *Best Pract. Res. Clin. Gastroenterol.* **2015**, *29*, 477–491. [CrossRef] [PubMed]

34. Catassi, C.; Elli, L.; Bonaz, B.; Bouma, G.; Carroccio, A.; Castillejo, G.; Cellier, C.; Cristofori, F.; de Magistris, L.; Dolinsek, J.; et al. Diagnosis of Non-Celiac Gluten Sensitivity (NCGS): The Salerno Experts' Criteria. *Nutrients* **2015**, *7*, 4966–4977. [CrossRef] [PubMed]

35. Catassi, C. Gluten Sensitivity. *Ann. Nutr. Metab.* **2015**, *67* (Suppl. 2), 16–26. [CrossRef] [PubMed]

36. Lionetti, E.; Gatti, S.; Pulvirenti, A.; Catassi, C. Celiac disease from a global perspective. *Best Pract. Res. Clin. Gastroenterol.* **2015**, *29*, 365–379. [CrossRef] [PubMed]

37. Ludvigsson, J.F.; Card, T.R.; Kaukinen, K.; Bai, J.; Zingone, F.; Sanders, D.S.; Murray, J.A. Screening for celiac disease in the general population and in high-risk groups. *United Eur. Gastroenterol. J.* **2015**, *3*, 106–120. [CrossRef] [PubMed]

38. Hornig, M.; Lipkin, W.I. Immune-mediated animal models of Tourette syndrome. *Neurosci. Biobehav. Rev.* **2013**, *37*, 1120–1138. [CrossRef] [PubMed]

39. Chang, Y.T.; Li, Y.F.; Muo, C.H.; Chen, S.C.; Chin, Z.N.; Kuo, H.T.; Lin, H.C.; Sung, F.C.; Tsai, C.H.; Chou, I.C. Correlation of Tourette syndrome and allergic disease: Nationwide population-based case-control study. *J. Dev. Behav. Pediatr.* **2011**, *32*, 98–102. [CrossRef] [PubMed]

40. Palumbo, D.; Kurlan, R. Complex obsessive compulsive and impulsive symptoms in Tourette's syndrome. *Neuropsychiatr. Dis. Treat.* **2007**, *3*, 687–693. [PubMed]

41. Vriezinga, S.L.; Schweizer, J.J.; Koning, F.; Mearin, M.L. Coeliac disease and gluten-related disorders in childhood. *Nat. Rev. Gastroenterol. Hepatol.* **2015**, *12*, 527–536. [CrossRef] [PubMed]

42. Hadjivassiliou, M.; Grünewald, R.A.; Davies-Jones, G.A. Gluten sensitivity as a neurological illness. *J. Neurol. Neurosurg. Psychiatry* **2002**, *72*, 560–563. [CrossRef] [PubMed]

43. Hadjivassiliou, M.; Sanders, D.S.; Grünewald, R.A.; Woodroofe, N.; Boscolo, S.; Aeschlimann, D. Gluten sensitivity: From gut to brain. *Lancet Neurol.* **2010**, *9*, 318–330. [CrossRef]

44. Mitoma, H.; Adhikari, K.; Aeschlimann, D.; Chattopadhyay, P.; Hadjivassiliou, M.; Hampe, C.S.; Honnorat, J.; Joubert, B.; Kakei, S.; Lee, J.; et al. Consensus Paper: Neuroimmune Mechanisms of Cerebellar Ataxias. *Cerebellum* **2016**, *15*, 213–232. [CrossRef] [PubMed]

45. Lionetti, E.; Francavilla, R.; Pavone, P.; Pavone, L.; Francavilla, T.; Pulvirenti, A.; Giugno, R.; Ruggieri, M. The neurology of coeliac disease in childhood: What is the evidence? A systematic review and meta-analysis. *Dev. Med. Child Neurol.* **2010**, *52*, 700–707. [CrossRef] [PubMed]

46. Szakács, Z.; Mátrai, P.; Hegyi, P.; Szabó, I.; Vincze, Á.; Balaskó, M.; Mosdósi, B.; Sarlós, P.; Simon, M.; Márta, K.; et al. Younger age at diagnosis predisposes to mucosal recovery in celiac disease on a gluten-free diet: A meta-analysis. *PLoS ONE* **2017**, *12*, e0187526. [CrossRef] [PubMed]

47. Khalifa, N.; von Knorring, A.L. Tourette syndrome and other tic disorders in a total population of children: Clinical assessment and background. *Acta Paediatr.* **2005**, *94*, 1608–1614. [CrossRef] [PubMed]

48. Subcommittee on Attention-Deficit/Hyperactivity Disorder; Steering Committee on Quality Improvement and Management; Wolraich, M.; Brown, L.; Brown, R.T.; DuPaul, G.; Earls, M.; Feldman, H.M.; Ganiats, T.G.; Kaplanek, B.; et al. ADHD: Clinical practice guideline for the diagnosis, evaluation, and treatment of attention-deficit/hyperactivity disorder in children and adolescents. *Pediatrics* **2011**, *128*, 1007–1022. [CrossRef] [PubMed]

49. Ertürk, E.; Wouters, S.; Imeraj, L.; Lampo, A. Association of ADHD and Celiac Disease: What Is the Evidence? A Systematic Review of the Literature. *J. Atten. Disord.* **2016**. [CrossRef] [PubMed]

50. Mulder, C.J.; van Wanrooij, R.L.; Bakker, S.F.; Wierdsma, N.; Bouma, G. Gluten-free diet in gluten-related disorders. *Dig. Dis.* **2013**, *31*, 57–62. [CrossRef] [PubMed]

51. Syage, J.A.; Kelly, C.P.; Dickason, M.A.; Ramirez, A.C.; Leon, F.; Dominguez, R.; Sealey-Voyksner, J.A. Determination of gluten consumption in celiac disease patients on a gluten-free diet. *Am. J. Clin. Nutr.* **2018**, *107*, 201–207. [CrossRef] [PubMed]

52. See, J.A.; Kaukinen, K.; Makharia, G.K.; Gibson, P.R.; Murray, J.A. Practical insights into gluten-free diets. *Nat. Rev. Gastroenterol. Hepatol.* **2015**, *12*, 580–591. [CrossRef] [PubMed]

53. Rostom, A.; Murray, J.A.; Kagnoff, M.F. American Gastroenterological Association (AGA) Institute technical review on the diagnosis and management of celiac disease. *Gastroenterology* **2006**, *131*, 1981–2002. [CrossRef] [PubMed]

54. Newnham, E.D. Coeliac disease in the 21st century: Paradigm shifts in the modern age. *J. Gastroenterol. Hepatol.* **2017**, *32*, 82–85. [CrossRef] [PubMed]
55. Moreno, M.L.; Rodríguez-Herrera, A.; Sousa, C.; Comino, I. Biomarkers to Monitor Gluten-Free Diet Compliance in Celiac Patients. *Nutrients* **2017**, *6*, 1. [CrossRef] [PubMed]

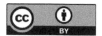

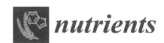

Review

Dermatitis Herpetiformis: A Common Extraintestinal Manifestation of Coeliac Disease

Timo Reunala [1,2,*], Teea T. Salmi [1,2], Kaisa Hervonen [1,2], Katri Kaukinen [1,3] and Pekka Collin [4]

[1] Celiac Disease Research Center, Faculty of Medicine and Life Sciences, University of Tampere, 33014 Tampere, Finland; teea.salmi@staff.uta.fi (T.T.S.); kaisa.hervonen@staff.uta.fi (K.H.); katri.kaukinen@staff.uta.fi (K.K.)

[2] Department of Dermatology, Tampere University Hospital, 33521 Tampere, Finland

[3] Department of Internal Medicine, Tampere University Hospital, 33521 Tampere, Finland

[4] Department of Gastroenterology and Alimentary Tract Surgery, Tampere University Hospital, 33521 Tampere, Finland; pekka.collin@uta.fi

* Correspondence: timo.reunala@uta.fi; Tel.: +358-400-831-805

Received: 13 April 2018; Accepted: 9 May 2018; Published: 12 May 2018

Abstract: Dermatitis herpetiformis (DH) is a common extraintestinal manifestation of coeliac disease presenting with itchy papules and vesicles on the elbows, knees, and buttocks. Overt gastrointestinal symptoms are rare. Diagnosis of DH is easily confirmed by immunofluorescence biopsy showing pathognomonic granular immunoglobulin A (IgA) deposits in the papillary dermis. A valid hypothesis for the immunopathogenesis of DH is that it starts from latent or manifest coeliac disease in the gut and evolves into an immune complex deposition of high avidity IgA epidermal transglutaminase (TG3) antibodies, together with the TG3 enzyme, in the papillary dermis. The mean age at DH diagnosis has increased significantly in recent decades and presently is 40–50 years. The DH to coeliac disease prevalence ratio is 1:8 in Finland and the United Kingdom (U.K.). The annual DH incidence rate, currently 2.7 per 100,000 in Finland and 0.8 per 100,000 in the U.K., is decreasing, whereas the reverse is true for coeliac disease. The long-term prognosis of DH patients on a gluten-free diet is excellent, with the mortality rate being even lower than for the general population.

Keywords: dermatitis herpetiformis; coeliac disease; prevalence; epidermal transglutaminase; gluten-free diet; long-term prognosis

---

1. Introduction

Dermatitis herpetiformis (DH) was described as a clinical entity by Louis Duhring in 1884, four years before Samuel Gee published the symptoms of coeliac disease [1,2]. The hallmark of DH is the symmetrical distribution of small vesicles and papules typically on the elbows, knees, and buttocks [3]. An intense itch is common, meaning that patients often scratch the vesicles. A breakthrough in the accurate diagnosis of DH was the discovery of granular immunoglobulin A (IgA) deposits in the skin in 1969 [4]. Though patients with DH rarely presented with overt gastro-intestinal symptoms, small bowel biopsies taken in the 1960s showed villous atrophy identical to that found in coeliac disease [5]. However, a quarter of the patients had normal small bowel villous architecture. Subsequently, it became evident that these patients also had coeliac-type minor enteropathy, i.e., an increased density of gamma/delta intraepithelial lymphocytes [6].

The rash in DH responds to a strict a gluten-free diet (GFD), albeit slowly, and the symptoms recur on gluten challenge [7–9]. Therefore, a life-long GFD is the treatment of choice for all patients with DH. Additionally, most patients initially receive dapsone (4,4-diaminodiphenylsulfone) medication, which can be tapered off after a mean of two years' strict adherence to a GFD [10].

Genetic and family studies tie DH and coeliac disease closely together. Almost every patient with DH and coeliac disease has the alleles contributing to the HLA-DQ2 or HLA-DQ8 haplotype [11]. These diseases segregate in the same families [12] and even monozygotic twin pairs can be affected by DH and coeliac disease [13].

Clinical presentation of DH is not easy to recognize correctly by general practitioners and delay of diagnosis for over two years occur in one third of the Finnish patients [14]. The presence of the blistering rash with IgA deposits is the major difference between DH and coeliac disease. However, other differences exist such as gender, age at onset, incidence, and long-term prognosis on a GFD. These points will be discussed in more detail along with the immunopathogenesis of DH.

2. Clinical Presentation and Diagnosis of Dermatitis Herpetiformis

The typical sites of predilection of DH are the extensor surfaces of elbows and knees, and the buttocks (Figure 1A,B). In addition, the upper back, abdomen, scalp and face can be affected, but oral lesions are rare [3]. The rash is polymorphic with small blisters (Figure 1C). These are, however, often eroded and crusted because of intense itch and scratching. Purpuric lesions may also appear on the hands and feet, however, this is rare [3]. The presentation and activity of the rash varies greatly from patient to patient, but complete remission is infrequent on a normal, gluten-containing diet.

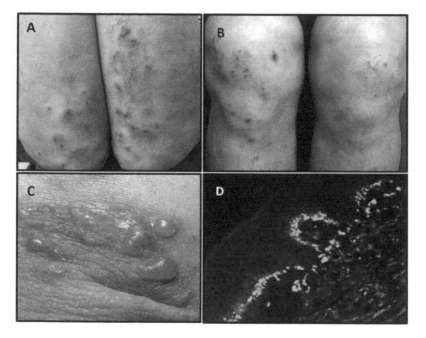

Figure 1. Dermatitis herpetiformis. Typical scratched papules and macules on the elbows (**A**), and on the knees (**B**). Fresh small blisters on the elbow (**C**). Direct immunofluorescence showing granular IgA deposits in the basal membrane zone between epidermis and dermis (**D**).

The clinical picture is often highly suggestive of DH, although, linear IgA bullous disease is always a diagnostic problem [15]. Itchy skin disorders such as urticaria, atopic or nummular dermatitis, and scabies infestation should be considered as a differential diagnosis [3]. The localization and burning itch experienced during the development of blisters is, however, usually severe enough to raise suspicion of DH. The typical histopathological findings in the lesional skin of patients with DH consists of subepidermal vesicles associated with an accumulation of neutrophils at the papillary tips.

The histopathology of a DH skin lesion is not diagnostic since other bullous diseases, such as linear IgA bullous disease and epidermolysis bullosa acquisita, may show similar findings [16]. Moreover, the histopathologic picture of DH is often unspecific revealing only perivascular lymphocytic infiltrate and minimal inflammation in dermal papillae.

The ideal method for diagnosis of DH is a direct immunofluorescence biopsy of unaffected skin in close proximity to an active lesion [17]. This reveals pathognomonic granular IgA deposits at the dermo-epidermal junction (Figure 1D), and the diagnosis of DH should not be made without this finding [16].

3. Gender and Age at Onset

Earlier studies in adults with DH have shown male to female ratios ranging up to 2:1 [3] with two recent large DH studies finding the ratio to be close to 1:1 [18,19]. This is in sharp contrast to coeliac disease, in which females outnumber males [20] (Table 1). This gender imbalance may reduce with increasing age, and it has also been absent in some coeliac disease screening studies [21,22]. These findings suggest that gender differences between DH and coeliac disease are perhaps not as profound as was earlier thought.

Coeliac disease can be diagnosed at any age with the peak incidences being in early childhood and between 40 and 60 years of age [20,23]. Clinical series in adults with DH from Europe and North America have shown that the mean age at diagnosis is between 40 and 50 years [14,24]. Like coeliac disease, the oldest DH patients have been over 80 years of age at diagnosis. In contrast to coeliac disease, DH in childhood seems to be rare; it was found in only 4% of 476 Finnish patients [25]. However, differences may exist. In an Italian series comprising 159 DH patients, 36% were below the age of 20 years [26], and a large series of 127 Hungarian children with DH has been published [27].

A study of 477 patients collected from 1970 onwards in Finland showed a significant increase in the mean age at diagnosis [18]. The increase was from 35 to 51 years in men and from 36 to 46 years in women. A similar increasing trend in the mean age at diagnosis has also been observed in recent decades in adult coeliac disease, both in Finland and elsewhere [28–30]. One explanation for this trend may be changes in dietary habits, such as the consumption of wheat, which in Sweden has changed the appearance of childhood coeliac disease [31]. In Finland, the annual consumption of wheat, rye, and other cereals per person has decreased from 150 kg to 71 kg over the past 50 years [32]. A lower lifetime gluten load might thus explain the increasing age at diagnosis and perhaps also the trend towards less severe small bowel atrophy in DH and coeliac disease [33–35].

Table 1. Differences between dermatitis derpetiformis and coeliac disease.

	Dermatitis Herpetiformis	Coeliac Disease
Gender	Slightly more males	Females predominate
Age at onset	Mainly adults	Children and adults
IgA-TG3 deposits in the skin	100%	0%
Small bowel villous atrophy	75%	100% *
IgA-TG2 deposits in the small bowel mucosa [36,37]	80%	up to 100% **
Prevalence in Finland and United Kingdom [18,19,38]	75 and 30 per 100,000	660 and 240 per 100,000
Incidence	Decreasing	Increasing
Response to a gluten-free diet [7,8,20]	Slow; months, in the beginning most patients need dapsone to control the rash	Rapid; days or weeks until gastro-intestinal symptoms end whereas small bowel villous atrophy may persist for many years
Long-term prognosis on a gluten-free diet [39–41]	Excellent	All-cause and lymphoma mortality may be increased

TG3 = epidermal transglutaminase, TG2 = tissue transglutaminase; * Potential coeliac disease with normal small bowel mucosa architecture, inflammation and positive TG2 serology also exist; ** Data still sparse.

4. Prevalence and Incidence

Two recent large DH studies with a total of 477 and 809 patients found a prevalence of 75.3 per 100,000 in Finland and 30 per 100,000 in the U.K., respectively [18,19] (Table 1). In the U.K. study the prevalence of coeliac disease was 240 per 100,000, i.e., eight times higher than that of DH. The same 8:1 ratio was calculated in the Finnish study, where the national prevalence of coeliac disease was 661 per 100,000 [38]. Nevertheless, DH is evidently the most common extraintestinal manifestation of coeliac disease [42].

The Social Insurance Institution of Finland maintains a nationwide register of adults with coeliac disease and DH. In 2003, it included a total of 18,538 patients, of whom 3121 (17%) had DH [28]. When we compared the annual numbers of new cases in five-year periods from 1980 to 2003, it was evident that in the first period patients with coeliac disease only slightly outnumbered those with DH (Figure 2). After the first period, the annual number of DH patients slowly decreased, whereas the number of coeliac disease patients continuously increased. In the ten-year period of 2005–2014, the proportion of newly diagnosed patients with DH had decreased to only 4% [43] (Figure 2).

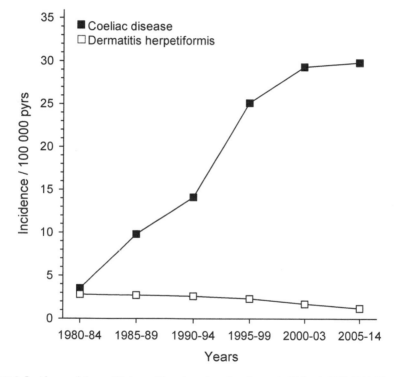

Figure 2. Incidence of dermatitis herpetiformis and coeliac disease in Finland, 1980–2014. The data include 3671 adult patients with Dermatitis herpetiformis and 31,385 adult patients with coeliac disease registered with the Social Insurance Institution of Finland [28,43].

Importantly, a Finnish cohort study [18] and a U.K. register study [19] covering time periods of 30 and 20 years, respectively, showed convincingly that the annual incidence rate of DH has decreased significantly. This decrease was from 5.2 to 2.7 per 100,000 in the Finnish study and from 1.8 to 0.8 per 100,000 in the U.K. study. The opposite was true for coeliac disease; there was a maximum of a fourfold increase in the incidence rate [19]. The reason for this seems to be an increasing awareness of mild symptoms, the development of efficient serological screening tests, and the identification of special risk groups, such as family members [20,23]. Sero-epidemiological studies suggest that in addition to the better recognition of coeliac disease, there has also been a true increase in the incidence in recent decades [44,45].

The decreasing incidence rate of DH in Finland and the U.K., along with a simultaneous rapid increase in coeliac disease, fits our hypothesis that subclinical, undiagnosed coeliac disease is a prerequisite for the development of DH. In support of this hypothesis, we know of patients initially diagnosed with coeliac disease who did not follow or only partially followed a GFD and subsequently developed DH [46]. Moreover, adult patients with DH frequently have coeliac-type dental enamel defects, which develop early in childhood as a result of malabsorption or immune alteration caused by undiagnosed coeliac disease [47].

5. Pathogenesis of Dermatitis Herpetiformis: From Gut to Skin

In DH, pathognomonic granular IgA deposits in the papillary dermis have long been suspected to derive from the gut. In 2002, Sárdy et al. [48] showed that the autoantigen for deposited cutaneous IgA is epidermal transglutaminase (TG3). This is closely related, but not identical, to the tissue transglutaminase (TG2) autoantigen specific for coeliac disease [49]. The TG2 enzyme is a target for IgA class autoantibody deposition in the small bowel mucosa in classical and potential coeliac disease, and in DH [36,37,50]. The TG3 protein has not been detected in the small bowel similarly to the TG2 enzyme, but epitope spreading is a possibility [51]. Recently, DH patients with the active disease have been shown to secrete high levels of TG3 antibodies into the gut organ culture medium, and also have TG3-antibody-positive cells in the small intestinal mucosa [52]. At present, a valid hypothesis is that the immunopathogenesis of DH starts from hidden coeliac disease in the gut with a TG2, and possibly also a TG3, autoantibody response and evolves into an immune complex deposition of high avidity IgA TG3 antibodies together with the TG3 enzyme in the papillary dermis [48]. Further support for this comes from GFD treatment results; TG3 and TG2 antibodies in the blood disappear with the dietary treatment and, at the same time, the rash and small bowel heal [53]. In contrast, the IgA-TG3 aggregates in the skin disappear very slowly with GFD treatment [54]. This seems to be due to the active TG3 enzyme in the aggregates resulting in covalent cross-linking of the complex to dermal structures [55].

6. Long-Term Prognosis on a Gluten-Free Diet Treatment

A GFD is the treatment of choice for all patients with DH regardless of whether they have villous atrophy in the small bowel [7,8,10]. It is important to know the long-term prognosis for DH because, as in coeliac disease, the risk of non-Hodgkin's lymphoma is significantly increased [56]. However, a strict GFD for more than five years seems to protect against lymphoma [57]. In agreement with this, our cohort of 476 patients with DH, where almost all patients adhered to a GFD, showed a significantly increased lymphoma mortality rate during the first five years of follow-up, but not thereafter [39]. Unexpectedly, the same study showed that the standardized mortality rate (SMR 0.70) was statistically significantly reduced in the GFD-treated DH patients compared to the general population. In a previous study of 846 DH patients from the U.K. [40], the adherence to a GFD was only partly known, and the mortality rate was slightly, but non-significantly, reduced (hazard ratio 0.93).

In contrast to the excellent long-term prognosis for DH, a meta-analysis of prospective studies on coeliac disease found a significantly increased risk for all-cause (odds ratio 1.24) and non-Hodgkin's lymphoma (odds ratio 2.61) mortality [41]. A recent large register study from England could only confirm the excess risk of deaths from non-Hodgkin's lymphoma [58]. However, in coeliac disease mortality studies, the adherence to a GFD has not been analyzed or was only partially known [41,59]; therefore, there is a particular need to examine the relationship between mortality rate and dietary compliance.

There are studies suggesting that patients with coeliac disease on a GFD retain a reduced quality of life compared to the general population [60,61]. Recently, we examined long-term GFD-treated patients with DH [62]. Their quality of life was comparable to that of the general population, whereas it was reduced in the coeliac disease controls.

7. Concluding Remarks

DH is the most common extraintestinal clinical manifestation of coeliac disease; at present, the prevalence ratio of the disorders is 1:8. The incidence of DH is decreasing, whereas the opposite is true for coeliac disease. A valid current hypothesis is that subclinical coeliac disease is a prerequisite for the development of DH. The reason why only some undiagnosed coeliac individuals develop an itchy blistering rash with dermal IgA-TG3 deposits remains unknown. The markedly increased age at diagnosis and less severe small bowel damage both in DH and coeliac disease suggests changes in environmental factors, such as a lowered lifetime gluten load. The long-term prognosis of DH patients on a GFD is excellent, which seems to be due to a strict adherence to the diet.

Author Contributions: T.R. and P.C. wrote the paper; T.T.S., K.H., and K.K. commented on the paper, and all authors reviewed the paper.

Acknowledgments: This work was supported by the Academy of Finland; the Sigrid Juselius Foundation; the Finnish Medical Foundation; and the Competitive State Research Financing of the Expert Responsibility area of Tampere University Hospital under Grants 9U019, 9T018, 9T004, and 9U053.

Conflicts of Interest: The authors declare no conflict of interest.

References

1. Duhring, L.A. Landmark article, Aug 30, 1884: Dermatitis herpetiformis. By Louis A. Duhring. *JAMA* **1983**, *250*, 212–216. [CrossRef] [PubMed]
2. Losowsky, M.S. A history of coeliac disease. *Dig. Dis.* **2008**, *26*, 112–120. [CrossRef] [PubMed]
3. Bolotin, D.; Petronic-Rosic, V. Dermatitis herpetiformis. Part I. Epidemiology, pathogenesis, and clinical presentation. *J. Am. Acad. Dermatol.* **2011**, *64*, 1017–1024. [CrossRef] [PubMed]
4. Van der Meer, J.B. Granular deposits of immunoglobulins in the skin of patients with dermatitis herpetiformis. An immunofluorescent study. *Br. J. Dermatol.* **1969**, *81*, 493–503. [CrossRef] [PubMed]
5. Marks, J.; Shuster, S.; Watson, A.J. Small-bowel changes in dermatitis herpetiformis. *Lancet* **1966**, *2*, 1280–1282. [CrossRef]
6. Savilahti, E.; Reunala, T.; Mäki, M. Increase of lymphocytes bearing the gamma/delta T cell receptor in the jejunum of patients with dermatitis herpetiformis. *Gut* **1992**, *33*, 206–211. [CrossRef] [PubMed]
7   Fry, L.; Seah, P.P.; Riches, D.J.; Riches, D.J.; Hoffbrand, A.V. Clearance of skin lesions in dermatitis herpetiformis after gluten withdrawal. *Lancet* **1973**, *1*, 288–291. [CrossRef]
8. Reunala, T.; Blomqvist, K.; Tarpila, S.; Halme, H.; Kangas, K. Gluten-free diet in dermatitis herpetiformis. I. Clinical response of skin lesions in 81 patients. *Br. J. Dermatol.* **1977**, *97*, 473–480. [CrossRef] [PubMed]
9. Leonard, J.; Haffenden, G.; Tucker, W.; Unsworth, J.; Swain, F.; McMinn, R.; Holborow, J.; Fry, L. Gluten challenge in dermatitis herpetiformis. *N. Engl. J. Med.* **1983**, *308*, 816–819. [CrossRef] [PubMed]
10. Garioch, J.J.; Lewis, H.M.; Sargent, S.A.; Leonard, J.N.; Fry, L. 25 years' experience of a gluten-free diet in the treatment of dermatitis herpetiformis. *Br. J. Dermatol.* **1994**, *131*, 541–545. [CrossRef] [PubMed]
11. Balas, A.; Vicario, J.L.; Zambrano, A.; Acuna, D.; Garcia-Novo, D. Absolute linkage of celiac disease and dermatitis herpetiformis to HLA-DQ. *Tissue Antigens* **1997**, *50*, 52–56. [CrossRef] [PubMed]
12. Hervonen, K.; Hakanen, M.; Kaukinen, K.; Collin, P.; Reunala, T. First-degree relatives are frequently affected in coeliac disease and dermatitis herpetiformis. *Scand. J. Gastroenterol.* **2002**, *37*, 51–55. [CrossRef] [PubMed]
13. Hervonen, K.; Karell, K.; Holopainen, P.; Collin, P.; Partanen, J.; Reunala, T. Concordance of dermatitis herpetiformis and celiac disease in monozygous twins. *J. Investig. Dermatol.* **2000**, *115*, 990–993. [CrossRef] [PubMed]
14. Mansikka, E.; Salmi, T.; Kaukinen, K.; Collin, P.; Huhtala, H.; Reunala, T.; Hervonen, K. Diagnostic delay in dermatitis herpetiformis in a high-prevalence area. *Acta Derm. Venereol.* **2018**, *98*, 195–199. [CrossRef] [PubMed]

15. Chanal, J.; Ingen-Housz-Oro, S.; Ortonne, N.; Duong, T.A.; Thomas, M.; Valeyrie-Allanore, L.; Lebrun-Vignes, B.; André, C.; Roujeau, J.C.; Chosidow, O.; et al. Linear IgA bullous dermatosis: Comparison between the drug-induced and spontaneous forms. *Br. J. Dermatol.* **2013**, *169*, 1041–1048. [CrossRef] [PubMed]
16. Caproni, M.; Antiga, E.; Melani, L.; Fabbri, P. Guidelines for the diagnosis and treatment of dermatitis herpetiformis. *J. Eur. Acad. Dermatol. Venereol.* **2009**, *23*, 633–638. [CrossRef] [PubMed]
17. Zone, J.J.; Meyer, L.J.; Petersen, M.J. Deposition of granular IgA relative to clinical lesions in dermatitis herpetiformis. *Arch. Dermatol.* **1996**, *132*, 912–918. [CrossRef] [PubMed]
18. Salmi, T.T.; Hervonen, K.; Kautiainen, H.; Collin, P.; Reunala, T. Prevalence and incidence of dermatitis herpetiformis: A 40-year prospective study from Finland. *Br. J. Dermatol.* **2011**, *165*, 354–359. [CrossRef] [PubMed]
19. West, J.; Fleming, K.M.; Tata, L.J.; Card, T.R.; Crooks, C.J. Incidence and prevalence of celiac disease and dermatitis herpetiformis in the UK over two decades: Population-based study. *Am. J. Gastroenterol.* **2014**, *109*, 757–768. [CrossRef] [PubMed]
20. Green, P.H.; Cellier, C. Celiac disease. *N. Engl. J. Med.* **2007**, *357*, 1731–1743. [CrossRef] [PubMed]
21. Vilppula, A.; Kaukinen, K.; Luostarinen, L.; Krekelä, I.; Patrikainen, H.; Valve, R.; Mäki, M.; Collin, P. Increasing prevalence and high incidence of celiac disease in elderly people: A population-based study. *BMC. Gastroenterol.* **2009**, *9*, 49. [CrossRef] [PubMed]
22. Fasano, A.; Berti, I.; Gerarduzzi, T.; Not, T.; Colletti, R.B.; Drago, S.; Elitsur, Y.; Green, P.H.; Guandalini, S.; Hill, I.D.; et al. Prevalence of celiac disease in at-risk and not-at-risk groups in the United States: A large multicenter study. *Arch. Intern. Med.* **2003**, *163*, 286–292. [CrossRef] [PubMed]
23. Tack, G.J.; Verbeek, W.H.; Schreurs, M.W.; Mulder, C.J. The spectrum of celiac disease: Epidemiology, clinical aspects and treatment. *Nat. Rev. Gastroenterol. Hepatol.* **2010**, *7*, 204–213. [CrossRef] [PubMed]
24. Alonso-Llamazares, J.; Gibson, L.E.; Rogers, R.S., 3rd. Clinical, pathologic, and immunopathologic features of dermatitis herpetiformis: Review of the Mayo Clinic experience. *Int. J. Dermatol.* **2007**, *46*, 910–919. [CrossRef] [PubMed]
25. Hervonen, K.; Salmi, T.T.; Kurppa, K.; Kaukinen, K.; Collin, P.; Reunala, T. Dermatitis herpetiformis in children: A long-term follow-up study. *Br. J. Dermatol.* **2014**, *171*, 1242–1243. [CrossRef] [PubMed]
26. Antiga, E.; Verdelli, A.; Calabri, A.; Fabbri, P.; Caproni, M. Clinical and immunopathological features of 159 patients with dermatitis herpetiformis: An Italian experience. *G. Ital. Dermatol. Venereol.* **2013**, *148*, 163–169. [PubMed]
27. Dahlbom, I.; Korponay-Szabó, I.R.; Kovács, J.B.; Szalai, Z.; Mäki, M.; Hansson, T. Prediction of clinical and mucosal severity of coeliac disease and dermatitis herpetiformis by quantification of IgA/IgG serum antibodies to tissue transglutaminase. *J. Pediatr. Gastroenterol. Nutr.* **2010**, *50*, 140–146. [CrossRef] [PubMed]
28. Collin, P.; Huhtala, H.; Virta, L.; Kekkonen, L.; Reunala, T. Diagnosis of celiac disease in clinical practice: Physician's alertness to the condition essential. *J. Clin. Gastroenterol.* **2007**, *41*, 152–156. [CrossRef] [PubMed]
29. Rampertab, S.D.; Pooran, N.; Brar, P.; Singh, P.; Green, P.H. Trends in the presentation of celiac disease. *Am. J. Med.* **2006**, *119*, 355.e9–355.e14. [CrossRef] [PubMed]
30. Dominguez Castro, P.; Harkin, G.; Hussey, M.; Christopher, B.; Kiat, C.; Liong Chin, J.; Trimble, V.; McNamara, D.; MacMathuna, P.; Egan, B.; et al. Changes in presentation of celiac disease in Ireland from the 1960s to 2015. *Clin. Gastroenterol. Hepatol.* **2017**, *15*, 864–871. [CrossRef] [PubMed]
31. Carlsson, A.; Agardh, D.; Borulf, S.; Grodzinsky, E.; Axelsson, I.; Ivarsson, S.A. Prevalence of celiac disease: Before and after a national change in feeding recommendations. *Scand. J. Gastroenterol.* **2006**, *41*, 553–558. [CrossRef] [PubMed]
32. Finnish National Nutrition Council. *Action Programme for Implementing National Nutrition Recommendations*; Edita Prima: Helsinki, Finland, 2003. (In Finnish)
33. Mansikka, E.; Hervonen, K.; Salmi, T.T.; Kautiainen, H.; Kaukinen, K.; Collin, P.; Reunala, T. The decreasing prevalence of severe villousa atrophy in Dermatitis herpetiformis: A 45-year experience in 393 patients. *J. Clin. Gastroenterol.* **2017**, *51*, 235–239. [PubMed]
34. Brar, P.; Kwon, G.Y.; Egbuna, I.I.; Holleran, S.; Ramakrishnan, R.; Bhagat, G.; Green, P.H. Lack of correlation of degree of villous atrophy with severity of clinical presentation of coeliac disease. *Dig. Liver Dis.* **2007**, *39*, 26–29. [CrossRef] [PubMed]

35. Green, P.H.R.; Stavropoulos, S.N.; Panagi, S.G.; Goldstein, S.L.; Mcmahon, D.J.; Absan, H.; Neugut, A.I. Characteristics of adult celiac disease in the USA: Results of a national survey. *Am. J. Gastroenterol.* **2001**, *96*, 126–131. [CrossRef] [PubMed]

36. Koskinen, O.; Collin, P.; Korponay-Szabo, I.; Salmi, T.; Iltanen, S.; Haimila, K.; Partanen, J.; Mäki, M.; Kaukinen, K. Gluten-dependent small bowel mucosal transglutaminase 2-specific IgA deposits in overt and mild enteropathy coeliac disease. *J. Pediatr. Gastroenterol. Nutr.* **2008**, *47*, 436–442. [CrossRef] [PubMed]

37. Salmi, T.T.; Hervonen, K.; Laurila, K.; Collin, P.; Mäki, M.; Koskinen, O.; Huhtala, H.; Kaukinen, K.; Reunala, T. Small bowel transglutaminase 2-specific IgA deposits in dermatitis herpetiformis. *Acta Derm. Venereol.* **2014**, *94*, 393–397. [CrossRef] [PubMed]

38. Virta, L.; Kaukinen, K.; Collin, P. Incidence and prevalence of diagnosed coeliac disease in Finland: Results of effective case finding in adults. *Scand. J. Gastroenterol.* **2009**, *44*, 933–938. [CrossRef] [PubMed]

39. Hervonen, K.; Alakoski, A.; Salmi, T.T.; Helakorpi, S.; Kautiainen, H.; Kaukinen, K.; Pukkala, E.; Collin, P.; Reunala, T. Reduced mortality in dermatitis herpetiformis: A population-based study of 476 patients. *Br. J. Dermatol.* **2012**, *167*, 1331–1337. [CrossRef] [PubMed]

40. Lewis, N.R.; Logan, R.F.; Hubbard, R.B.; West, J. No increase in risk of fracture, malignancy or mortality in dermatitis herpetiformis: A cohort study. *Aliment. Pharmacol. Ther.* **2008**, *27*, 1140–1147. [CrossRef] [PubMed]

41. Tio, M.; Cox, M.R.; Eslick, G.D. Meta-analysis: Coeliac disease and the risk of all-cause mortality, any malignancy and lymphoid malignancy. *Aliment. Pharmacol. Ther.* **2012**, *35*, 540–551. [CrossRef] [PubMed]

42. Leffler, D.A.; Green, P.H.; Fasano, A. Extraintestinal manifestations of coeliac disease. *Nat. Rev. Gastroenterol. Hepatol.* **2015**, *12*, 561–571. [CrossRef] [PubMed]

43. Virta, L.J.; Saarinen, M.M.; Kolho, K.L. Declining trend in the incidence of biopsy-verified coeliac disease in the adult population of Finland, 2005–2014. *Aliment. Pharmacol. Ther.* **2017**, *46*, 1085–1093. [CrossRef] [PubMed]

44. Kang, J.Y.; Kang, A.H.; Green, A.; Gwee, K.A.; Ho, K.Y. Systematic review: Worldwide variation in the frequency of coeliac disease and changes over time. *Aliment. Pharmacol. Ther.* **2013**, *38*, 226–245. [CrossRef] [PubMed]

45. Lohi, S.; Mustalahti, K.; Kaukinen, K.; Laurila, K.; Collin, P.; Rissanen, H.; Lohi, O.; Bravi, E.; Gasparin, M.; Reunanen, A.; et al. Increasing prevalence of coeliac disease over time. *Aliment. Pharmacol. Ther.* **2007**, *26*, 1217–1225. [CrossRef] [PubMed]

46. Salmi, T.T.; Hervonen, K.; Kurppa, K.; Collin, P.; Kaukinen, K.; Reunala, T. Coeliac disease evolving into dermatitis herpetiformis in patients adhering to normal or gluten-free diet. *Scand. J. Gastroenterol.* **2015**, *50*, 387–392. [CrossRef] [PubMed]

47. Aine, L.; Mäki, M.; Reunala, T. Coeliac-type dental enamel defects in patients with dermatitis herpetiformis. *Acta Derm. Venereol.* **1992**, *72*, 25–27. [PubMed]

48. Sárdy, M.; Kárpáti, S.; Merkl, B.; Paulsson, M.; Smyth, N. Epidermal transglutaminase (TGase 3) is the autoantigen of dermatitis herpetiformis. *J. Exp. Med.* **2002**, *195*, 747–757. [CrossRef] [PubMed]

49. Dieterich, W.; Ehnis, T.; Bauer, M.; Donner, P.; Volta, U.; Riecken, E.O.; Schuppan, D. Identification of tissue transglutaminase as the autoantigen of celiac disease. *Nat. Med.* **1997**, *3*, 797–801. [CrossRef] [PubMed]

50. Korponay-Szabó, I.R.; Halttunen, T.; Szalai, Z.; Laurila, K.; Király, R.; Kovács, J.B.; Király, R.; Kovács, J.B.; Fésüs, L.; Mäki, M. In vivo targeting of intestinal and extraintestinal transglutaminase 2 by coeliac autoantibodies. *Gut* **2004**, *53*, 641–648. [CrossRef] [PubMed]

51. Kárpáti, S.; Sárdy, M.; Németh, K.; Mayer, B.; Smyth, N.; Paulsson, M.; Traupe, H. Transglutaminases in autoimmune and inherited skin diseases: The phenomena of epitope spreading and functional compensation. *Exp. Dermatol.* **2018**, 1–8. [CrossRef] [PubMed]

52. Hietikko, M.; Hervonen, K.; Ilus, T.; Salmi, T.; Huhtala, H.; Laurila, K.; Rauhavirta, T.; Reunala, T.; Kaukinen, K.; Lindfors, K. Ex vivo culture of duodenal biopsies from patients with Dermatitis herpetiformis indicates that transglutaminase 3 antibody production occurs in the gut. *Acta Derm. Venereol.* **2018**, *98*, 366–372. [CrossRef] [PubMed]

53. Reunala, T.; Salmi, T.T.; Hervonen, K.; Laurila, K.; Kautiainen, H.; Collin, P.; Kaukinen, K. IgA anti-epidermal transglutaminase antibodies in dermatitis herpetiformis: A significant but not complete response to a gluten-free diet treatment. *Br. J. Dermatol.* **2015**, *172*, 1139–1141. [CrossRef] [PubMed]

54. Hietikko, M.; Hervonen, K.; Salmi, T.; Ilus, T.; Zone, J.J.; Kaukinen, K.; Reunala, T.; Lindfors, K. Disappearance of epidermal transglutaminase and IgA deposits from the papillary dermis of dermatitis herpetiformis patients after a long-term gluten-free diet. *Br. J. Dermatol.* **2018**, *178*, e198–e201. [CrossRef] [PubMed]

55. Taylor, T.B.; Schmidt, L.A.; Meyer, L.J.; Zone, J.J. Transglutaminase 3 present in the IgA aggregates in dermatitis herpetiformis skin is enzymatically active and binds soluble fibrinogen. *J. Investig. Dermatol.* **2015**, *135*, 623–625. [CrossRef] [PubMed]

56. Grainge, M.J.; West, J.; Solaymani-Dodaran, M.; Card, T.R.; Logan, R.F. The long-term risk of malignancy following a diagnosis of coeliac disease or dermatitis herpetiformis: A cohort study. *Aliment. Pharmacol. Ther.* **2012**, *35*, 730–739. [CrossRef] [PubMed]

57. Lewis, H.M.; Reunala, T.L.; Garioch, J.J.; Leonard, J.N.; Fry, J.S.; Collin, P.; Evans, D.; Fry, L. Protective effect of gluten-free diet against development of lymphoma in dermatitis herpetiformis. *Br. J. Dermatol.* **1996**, *135*, 363–367. [CrossRef] [PubMed]

58. Abdul Sultan, A.; Crooks, C.J.; Card, T.; Tata, L.J.; Fleming, K.M.; West, J. Causes of death in people with coeliac disease in England compared with the general population: A competing risk analysis. *Gut* **2015**, *64*, 1220–1226. [CrossRef] [PubMed]

59. Corrao, G.; Corazza, G.R.; Bagnardi, V.; Brusco, G.; Ciacci, C.; Cottone, M.; Sategna Guidetti, C.; Usai, P.; Cesari, P.; Pelli, M.A.; et al. Mortality in patients with coeliac disease and their relatives: A cohort study. *Lancet* **2001**, *358*, 356–361. [CrossRef]

60. Paarlahti, P.; Kurppa, K.; Ukkola, A.; Collin, P.; Huhtala, H.; Mäki, M.; Kaukinen, K. Predictors of persistent symptoms and reduced quality of life in treated coeliac disease patients: A large cross-sectional study. *BMC Gastroenterol.* **2013**, *13*, 75. [CrossRef] [PubMed]

61. Burger, J.P.W.; de Brouwer, B.; IntHout, J.; Wahab, P.J.; Tummers, M.; Drenth, J.P.H. Systematic review with meta-analysis: Dietary adherence influences normalization of health-related quality of life in coeliac disease. *Clin. Nutr.* **2017**, *36*, 399–406. [CrossRef] [PubMed]

62. Pasternack, C.; Kaukinen, K.; Kurppa, K.; Mäki, M.; Collin, P.; Reunala, T.; Huhtala, H.; Salmi, T. Quality of life and gastrointestinal symptoms in long-term treated Dermatitis herpetiformis patients: A cross-sectional study in Finland. *Am. J. Clin. Dermatol.* **2015**, *16*, 545–552. [CrossRef] [PubMed]

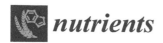

Article

Prognosis of Dermatitis Herpetiformis Patients with and without Villous Atrophy at Diagnosis

Eriika Mansikka [1,2], Kaisa Hervonen [1,2], Katri Kaukinen [2,3], Pekka Collin [4], Heini Huhtala [5], Timo Reunala [1,2] and Teea Salmi [1,2,*]

1   Department of Dermatology, Tampere University Hospital, 33521 Tampere, Finland;
    mansikka.eriika.k@student.uta.fi (E.M.); kaisa.hervonen@staff.uta.fi (K.H.); timo.reunala@uta.fi (T.R.)
2   Celiac Disease Research Center, Faculty of Medicine and Life Sciences, University of Tampere,
    33014 Tampere, Finland; katri.kaukinen@staff.uta.fi
3   Department of Internal Medicine, Tampere University Hospital, 33521 Tampere, Finland
4   Department of Gastroenterology and Alimentary Tract Surgery, Tampere University Hospital,
    33521 Tampere, Finland; pekka.collin@uta.fi
5   Faculty of Social Sciences, University of Tampere, 33014 Tampere, Finland; heini.huhtala@staff.uta.fi
*   Correspondence: Teea.Salmi@staff.uta.fi; Tel.: +358-03-311-611

Received: 18 April 2018; Accepted: 15 May 2018; Published: 19 May 2018

Abstract: Dermatitis herpetiformis (DH) is a cutaneous manifestation of coeliac disease. At diagnosis, the majority of patients have villous atrophy in the small bowel mucosa. The objective of this study was to investigate whether the presence or absence of villous atrophy at diagnosis affects the long-term prognosis of DH. Data were gathered from the patient records of 352 DH and 248 coeliac disease patients, and follow-up data via questionnaires from 181 DH and 128 coeliac disease patients on a gluten-free diet (GFD). Of the DH patients, 72% had villous atrophy when DH was diagnosed, and these patients were significantly younger at diagnosis compared to those with normal small bowel mucosa (37 vs. 54 years, $p < 0.001$). Clinical recovery on a GFD did not differ significantly between the DH groups, nor did current adherence to a GFD, the presence of long-term illnesses, coeliac disease-related complications or gastrointestinal symptoms, or quality of life. By contrast, the coeliac disease controls had more often osteopenia/osteoporosis, thyroid diseases, malignancies and current gastrointestinal symptoms compared to the DH patients. In conclusion, villous atrophy at the time of DH diagnosis does not have an impact on the clinical recovery or long-term general health of DH patients.

Keywords: dermatitis herpetiformis; coeliac disease; gluten-free diet; small bowel; villous atrophy; prognosis

1. Introduction

Dermatitis herpetiformis (DH) is an extraintestinal manifestation of coeliac disease currently affecting approximately 13% of coeliac disease patients [1,2]. DH induces intense pruritus and a symmetrical papulovesicular rash typically on the elbows, knees, and buttocks [3]. Coeliac disease and DH are genetically predisposed by the human leukocyte antigen (HLA) *DQ2* or *DQ8* haplotypes, and exogenous gluten causes an immune response and small bowel mucosal injury in both [4,5]. Furthermore, autoantibodies against endogenous enzyme tissue transglutaminase (TG2) are characteristically present in the serum and the intestine in both conditions [6–9].

Diagnosis of DH is verified with the detection of pathognomonic granular immunoglobulin A (IgA) deposits in the uninvolved skin by direct immunofluorescence (IF) examination [10]. This IgA is known to target epidermal transglutaminase (TG3) [11], which is considered the autoantigen in DH, while in coeliac disease it is TG2 [6]. In addition to the skin, TG3 antibody response is often present in the sera of DH patients, although TG3 antibodies are occasionally also found in the serum of some coeliac disease patients without DH [12–14].

At the time of the DH diagnosis, some degree of small bowel mucosal villous atrophy is known to exist in approximately 75% of patients, but the remainder have normal villous architecture with only coeliac-type inflammation [15,16]. Regardless of the small bowel mucosal alterations, DH patients only rarely present with obvious gastrointestinal symptoms [17,18].

A strict life-long gluten-free diet (GFD) is the mainstay of treatment in both DH and coeliac disease. However, resolution of DH rash can take months or even longer on the dietary treatment, and therefore, DH patients with severe skin symptoms are additionally treated with dapsone medication to control the rash more quickly [3,19]. Coeliac disease and DH both carry an increased risk of concomitant autoimmune conditions such as thyroid diseases and type 1-diabetes; furthermore, the risk of developing non-Hodgkin lymphoma is increased [20–22]. Mortality in coeliac disease, but not in DH, has shown to be increased [23]. A GFD is known to have a preventive effect against the development of lymphoma in DH [24], but other than that, previous research about the factors influencing the prognosis of DH is lacking. Currently, it is not known whether DH patients with small bowel villous atrophy at diagnosis have a worse outcome compared to those with normal small bowel mucosa, and furthermore, whether the prognosis of DH patients with villous atrophy is corresponding to that of classical coeliac disease patients. This issue is of importance when necessary investigations, at the time of DH diagnosis, are assessed.

The aim of the current study was to assess whether the presence of villous atrophy at DH diagnosis would affect clinical recovery on a GFD or the long-term prognosis of DH. In addition, DH patients were compared to classical coeliac disease controls with abdominal symptoms at diagnosis and a histologically confirmed diagnosis. The hypothesis of this study was that the presence or absence of villous atrophy at diagnosis would not be an influential factor in the prognosis of DH.

2. Materials and Methods

Between 1970 and 2014, a total of 526 DH patients were diagnosed at the Department of Dermatology, Tampere University Hospital. During the study period, all patients with DH living in a defined area around Tampere were diagnosed at this dermatology unit since IF biopsies required for the diagnosis were not performed elsewhere. Each DH patient's diagnosis was based on the typical clinical picture and the demonstration of granular IgA deposits in skin biopsies [10]. In addition, all diagnosed patients were routinely suggested to undergo gastroscopy and small bowel biopsy obtainment at the time of the diagnosis while on a gluten-containing diet. After diagnosis, a strict GFD was advised to all patients and dapsone was instituted in those with severe skin symptoms. According to routine treatment policies, all patients were followed up at a DH outpatient clinic until the rash had cleared and the dapsone medication could be discontinued. In this study, all DH patients without prior coeliac disease diagnosis (made ≥2 years earlier) diagnosed between 1970 and 2014 and having an available small bowel biopsy result and commencing on a GFD after diagnosis, were included as study patients. Altogether, 352 DH patients fulfilled the inclusion criteria and were included as DH study patients. Further, 248 classical coeliac disease patients with abdominal symptoms at diagnosis and a histologically confirmed diagnosis at Tampere University Hospital during the same time period served as controls.

Data on demographic characteristics, the severity of clinical symptoms and small bowel mucosal histology, and the results of coeliac autoantibodies and hemoglobin values at the time of DH or coeliac disease diagnosis were gathered from the patient records of Tampere University Hospital between March and October 2016. The small bowel biopsy results were graded as subtotal villous atrophy (SVA), partial villous atrophy (PVA), or normal mucosa according to the analysis of the routine pathologist as previously described [16]. In DH patients, the skin symptoms at the time of the diagnosis were graded as mild, moderate, or severe according to the presence of a few, several or many blisters, macular eruptions and erosions. The grading was performed by one dermatologist. In addition, the commencement and duration of dapsone medication after diagnosis was recorded.

Follow-up data were collected using questionnaires (see below for more detail) mailed to all 294 living DH patients fulfilling the inclusion criteria of this study (on December 2015) and the 222 living coeliac disease controls (on May 2016). The final response rate was 62% for the DH patients and 58% for the coeliac disease patients; hence, the follow-up study included 181 DH and 128 coeliac disease patients.

The study protocol and usage of the register-based data were approved by the Regional Ethics Committee of Tampere University Hospital (R15143), and furthermore, informed consent was obtained from each patient participating in the follow-up study.

2.1. Questionnaires

The disease-specific questionnaire designed for this study, the Psychological General Well-Being (PGWB) [25] and Gastrointestinal Symptom Rating Scale (GSRS) [26] questionnaires were mailed to the DH and coeliac disease study patients. PGWB and GSRS questionnaires are validated questionnaires, which have been widely applied in previous coeliac disease studies [27–31]. In addition, the DH patients received the Dermatology Life Quality Index (DLQI) questionnaire [32].

The disease-specific questionnaire included both open and multiple-choice questions. The patients were asked about the presence and duration of DH and coeliac disease-related symptoms before and after the diagnosis, the strictness of the GFD, smoking and other lifestyle characteristics, the number of children born, the family history of coeliac disease or DH, and the patient's current height and weight. Compliance with a GFD was reported as strict diet without dietary lapses, dietary lapses once per month, dietary lapses one to five times per month, or dietary lapses once per week. In addition, the questionnaire included questions about the presence of coeliac disease complications and associated diseases, malignancies, other long-term illnesses, and the regular usage of physician-prescribed medications and over-the-counter (OTC) medications. In the malignancy analysis, non-melanoma skin cancers were excluded, as were excessive trauma fractures in bone fracture analyses.

As previously described, the validated 22-item PGWB questionnaire evaluates self-perceived health-related well-being and distress and includes six dimensions: Anxiety, depressed mood, positive well-being, self-control, vitality, and general health [25]. The total score ranges from 22 to 132, with a higher score indicating better quality of life. The 15-item GSRS questionnaire assesses the severity and existence of gastrointestinal symptoms in five categories: Diarrhea, indigestion, constipation, abdominal pain, and reflux [26]. It uses a seven-point Likert scale for each question: One indicates an absence of symptoms and seven indicates severe symptoms. The DLQI is a 10-item dermatology-specific quality of life instrument. The questionnaire includes six different sections: Symptoms and feelings, daily activities, leisure, work and school, personal relationships, and treatment unit. The scores of all ten questions are calculated together, and the total score varies from a minimum of 0 to a maximum of 30, with a higher score indicating a more impaired life quality [32].

2.2. Statistical Analysis

A Two-sided chi-squared test was used to compare the categorical variables and a Kruskall–Wallis test was performed to assess differences between the continuous variables. Logistic regression analysis was used to standardize the study groups according to age at the time of the study. Statistical significance was set at $p < 0.05$. The analyses were performed using IBM SPSS Statistics for Windows (Version 23.0., IBM Corp., Armonk, NY, USA).

3. Results

3.1. DH Patients with Normal Villous Architecture Compared to DH Patients with Villous Atrophy at Diagnosis

Of the 352 DH patients, 98 (28%) had normal villous architecture, and 254 (72%) had small bowel mucosal villous atrophy (PVA or SVA) at the time of the DH diagnosis (Table 1). GFD was not initiated before the diagnosis in study participants. Mean time since the year of DH diagnosis, was 20 years in the DH patients with normal villous architecture and 23 years in the DH patients with villous atrophy, and the difference was not statistically significant. The median age at diagnosis was significantly higher in the DH patients with normal villous architecture compared to the DH patients with villous atrophy ($p < 0.001$, Table 1). At diagnosis, the DH patients with villous atrophy were significantly more often serum coeliac autoantibody-positive compared to the DH patients with normal villous architecture (73% vs. 39%, $p < 0.001$, Table 1). The severity of the DH rash at diagnosis did not differ significantly between the DH groups ($p = 0.862$). Eighty percent of all DH patients used dapsone after the diagnosis. The duration of dapsone usage was longer in the DH patients with normal villous architecture compared to the DH patients with villous atrophy at diagnosis (median 36 vs. 24 months), but the difference was not statistically significant ($p = 0.097$, Table 1).

Table 1. Demographic data and disease-related characteristics of 98 dermatitis herpetiformis (DH) patients with normal small bowel villous architecture and 254 DH patients with villous atrophy at diagnosis, and 248 coeliac disease (CD) control patients.

	DH Patients		CD Controls ($n = 248$)	p-Value *
	With Normal Villous Architecture ($n = 98$)	With Villous Atrophy ($n = 254$)		
Females; n (%)	50 (51)	125 (49)	193 (78)	<0.001
Age at diagnosis; median (range)	52 (3–84)	37 (4–78)	42 (7–75)	<0.001 [a]
Coeliac autoantibodies [1] present in the serum at diagnosis; n (%)	28/72 (39)	139/191 (73)	124/148 (84)	<0.001 [a]
Haemoglobin level at diagnosis [2], g/L; median (Q_1–Q_3) [3]	138 (128–148)	136 (129–146)	130 (121–140)	0.057
Dapsone treatment used; n (%)	75/93 (81)	191/243 (79)	-	-
Duration of dapsone treatment, months; median (range)	36 (5–324)	24 (2–384)	-	-

* p-value measured across the three study groups; [1] Transglutaminase 2-, endomysium-, or antireticulin IgA antibodies; [2] Statistical analysis was further performed for patients $\geq$16 years of age and for females and males separately—there were no statistically significant differences between the three groups; [3] Interquartile range; [a] Statistically significant difference ($p < 0.001$) between DH patients with normal villous architecture and DH patients with villous atrophy.

Of the 181 DH patients with available follow-up data, 39 (22%) had normal villous architecture, and 142 (78%) had villous atrophy at the time of DH diagnosis. The median follow-up time was 20 years in patients with normal villous architecture and 23 years in the DH patients with villous atrophy at diagnosis (Table 2). The presence of gastrointestinal symptoms at diagnosis did not differ between the DH study groups according to the follow-up study questionnaire ($p = 0.170$). At the time of the follow-up study, DH patients with normal villous architecture were significantly older compared to those DH patients who had villous atrophy at diagnosis (Table 2).

The strictness of the GFD and BMI did not differ between the DH study groups at the time of the study (Table 2). Similarly, no significant differences were detected in smoking habits or physical activity: 3% of DH patients without villous atrophy and 13% of patients with villous atrophy at diagnosis were current smokers, and 49% and 69% exercised at least three times a week, respectively.

Table 2. Follow-up data of 39 dermatitis herpetiformis (DH) patients with normal villous architecture and 142 DH patients with small bowel mucosal villous atrophy at diagnosis, and 128 coeliac disease (CD) control patients.

	DH Patients		CD Controls ($n = 128$)	p-Value *
	With Normal Villous Architecture ($n = 39$)	With Villous Atrophy ($n = 142$)		
Females; n (%)	18 (46)	67 (47)	104 (81)	<0.001
Follow-up time, years; median (range)	20 (1–44)	23 (1–42)	18 (6–43)	0.003
Age; median (range)	68 (52–85)	61 (18–96)	65 (34–85)	<0.001 [a]
BMI, kg/m² ; median (range)	25 (19–37)	25 (16–38)	26 (15–46)	0.772
Strict adherence to GFD, no dietary lapses; n (%)	30 (77)	101 (71)	107 (84)	0.170 [b]
Number of long-term illnesses; median (range)	1 (0–7)	1 (0–14)	2 (0–9)	<0.001
Number of prescription medications used; median (range)	2 (0–11)	1 (0–18)	3 (0–16)	0.078

Table 2. *Cont.*

	DH Patients		CD Controls (n = 128)	p-Value *
	With Normal Villous Architecture (n = 39)	With Villous Atrophy (n = 142)		
Uses statin medication; n (%)	14 (36)	21 (15)	15 (12)	0.001 c
Uses antihypertensive medication; n (%)	20 (51)	50 (35)	49 (38)	0.188
Uses proton pump inhibitor medication; n (%)	5 (13)	16 (11)	16 (13)	0.938
Number of over-the-counter medications used; median (range)	0 (0–5)	1 (0–7)	2 (0–7)	<0.001
Number of children born; median (range)	2 (0–5)	2 (0–6)	2 (0–5)	0.497
First-degree relatives with DH or CD; n (%)	13 (33)	53 (37)	55 (43)	0.464

BMI: Body mass index; GFD: Gluten-free diet. * p-value measured across the three study groups; a Statistically significant difference (p < 0.001) between DH patients with normal villous architecture and DH patients with villous atrophy at diagnosis; b p-value was tested for categorical variables including categories: strict diet, dietary lapses once per month, dietary lapses 1–5 times/month, dietary lapses once per week; c Statistically significant difference (p = 0.003) between DH patients with normal villous architecture and DH patients with villous atrophy at diagnosis.

At the time of the follow-up study, coronary heart disease and hypertension were significantly more common among the DH patients with normal villous architecture compared to the DH patients with villous atrophy at diagnosis (Figure 1); however, after adjustment for the current age, significant differences disappeared (p = 0.198, OR = 0.482 and p = 0.273, OR = 0.653, respectively). Significant differences were not detected in the presence of type 1- or 2-diabetes, thyroid diseases, cerebrovascular diseases, osteopenia or osteoporosis, or malignancies between the DH study groups (Figure 1). Patients with self-reported bone fractures were slightly more numerous among the DH patients with villous atrophy than among those with normal villous architecture at diagnosis, but the difference was not statistically significant (p = 0.321, Figure 1).

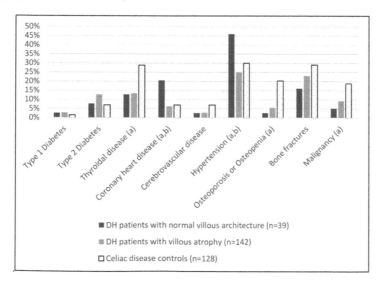

Figure 1. Percentages of dermatitis herpetiformis (DH) patients with normal small bowel mucosal villous architecture and with villous atrophy at diagnosis, and coeliac disease control patients with long-term illnesses or complications at the time of the follow-up study. (a) Statistically significant difference (p < 0.05) between the three study groups; (b) statistically significant difference (p < 0.05) between DH patients with normal villous architecture and DH patients with villous atrophy at diagnosis.

Statistically significant differences were not detected in the use of physician-prescribed regular medications between the DH study groups; even the significant difference in the use of statin medication disappeared after adjustment for the current age (OR = 0.479, p = 0.88, Table 2). Furthermore, the total amount of used OTC medications was similar in the DH groups; only the usage of vitamin D was more frequent among DH patients with villous atrophy at diagnosis compared to those without villous atrophy (40% vs. 23%, p = 0.050).

The presence of gastrointestinal symptoms or the quality of life according to the total or the subscores of the GSRS, PGWB (Table 3) and DLQI questionnaires at the time of the study did not differ between the DH study groups

Table 3. The Psychological General Well-Being (PGWB) and Gastrointestinal Symptom Rating Scale (GSRS) questionnaires' median and interquartile range (Q1–Q3) results for the gluten-free diet-treated dermatitis herpetiformis (DH) patients with normal villous architecture and with villous atrophy at diagnosis, and the coeliac disease (CD) controls at the time of the follow-up study.

		DH Patients				CD Controls (n = 128)		p-Value *
		With Normal Villous Architecture (n = 39)		With Villous Atrophy (n = 142)				
PGWB		median	(Q1–Q3)	median	(Q1–Q3)	median	(Q1–Q3)	
	Total	110	(99–116)	110	(101–117)	106	(96–117)	0.200
	Anxiety	26	(23–27)	26	(23–27)	25	(23–28)	0.891
	Depression	17	(16–18)	17	(16–18)	17	(15–18)	0.587
	Well-being	18	(16–20)	18	(16–20)	18	(16–20)	0.279
	Self-control	16	(15–17)	16	(15–17)	16	(14–17)	0.295
	General health	13	(12–15)	14	(12–16)	13	(11–15)	0.022
	Vitality	20	(17–21)	19	(17–21)	18	(16–20)	0.104
GSRS		median	(Q1–Q3)	median	(Q1–Q3)	median	(Q1–Q3)	
	Total	1.6	(1.3–2.0)	1.7	(1.3–2.3)	2.1	(1.5–4.2)	<0.001
	Diarrhoea	1.0	(1.0–1.7)	1.3	(1.0–2.3)	1.7	(1.0–2.7)	0.006
	Indigestion	1.8	(1.5–2.5)	2.0	(1.5–2.5)	2.0	(1.5–3.0)	0.227
	Constipation	1.7	(1.0–2.3)	1.7	(1.0–2.3)	1.7	(1.0–2.4)	0.482
	Pain	1.3	(1.0–1.7)	1.7	(1.0–2.0)	1.7	(1.3–2.3)	0.007
	Reflux	1.0	(1.0–1.5)	1.0	(1.0–2.0)	1.5	(1.0–2.0)	0.084

* p-value measured across the three study groups.

3.2. Comparisons between the DH Patients and the Classical Coeliac Disease Controls

Compared to the DH patients, the coeliac disease controls were more often female (Tables 1 and 2), and their median diagnostic age was significantly lower compared to DH patients with normal villous architecture at diagnosis (Table 1).

In the long-term follow-up data, there were no observed differences in current smoking habits or physical activity between the DH patients and the coeliac disease controls. By contrast, the total number of long-term illnesses was found to be higher among the coeliac disease controls compared to the DH patients (Table 2). More specifically, after adjustment for the current age, thyroid diseases (OR = 3.443, p = 0.019) and osteopenia or osteoporosis (OR = 14.132, p = 0.012) were more common among the coeliac disease controls than among the DH patients (Figure 1). However, the presence of self-reported bone fractures did not differ significantly between the DH study groups and the coeliac disease controls. In the malignancy analysis, the coeliac disease controls outnumbered the DH patients after adjustment for the current age (OR = 6.527, p = 0.016) (Figure 1).

In the analysis of regularly used physician-prescribed medications and after adjustment for the current age, the coeliac disease controls were found to use less statin medication compared to the DH patients with normal villous architecture (OR = 0.319, p = 0.01). In turn, the total number of regularly used OTCs was higher among the coeliac disease patients compared to the DH patients (p = 0.003, Table 2), and specifically the use of calcium (p = 0.011) and vitamin D (p < 0.001) was more common.

Quality of life measured with the PGWB did not differ between the coeliac disease controls and the DH patients with normal villous architecture at diagnosis, but the coeliac disease controls had significantly lower PGWB general health scores compared to the DH patients with villous atrophy at diagnosis (Table 3). In the GSRS questionnaire, the coeliac disease controls had significantly higher total symptoms gastrointestinal pain and diarrhea scores compared to both DH groups.

4. Discussion

This study demonstrated that the disease severity and the clinical response to a GFD does not differ between DH patients with normal villous architecture and those with villous atrophy at diagnosis. Furthermore, the long-term general health and well-being of DH patients are not influenced by the severity of small bowel mucosal damage at the time of DH diagnosis. The outcomes of the current study were obtained from a large, prospectively collected series of DH patients, all of whom adhered to a GFD treatment. Furthermore, in the present study, the proportions of DH patients with villous atrophy and normal villous architecture were consistent with the findings in earlier DH studies [15,33].

In our previous study, the presence of villous atrophy at DH diagnosis was found to be associated with a delayed diagnosis, i.e., the presence of the rash for two years or more before the diagnosis, suggesting that prolonged diagnosis might enable the small bowel mucosal damage to progress [34]. In the current study, the occurrence of villous atrophy did not associate with the severity of the rash or with the presence of gastrointestinal symptoms at diagnosis. The duration of dapsone medication was considered the most reliable method of determining the active period of rash after adherence to a GFD since the majority of patients used dapsone medication, and the medicine was discontinued as early as possible without a relapse in skin symptoms. The median duration of dapsone usage in DH study groups corresponded well with previous GFD treatment studies [35,36], and even though the duration was longer in DH patients with normal small bowel mucosa than in those with villous atrophy at diagnosis, the difference was not statistically significant. Therefore, presence or absence of small bowel villous atrophy at diagnosis seems not to influence the clinical recovery of the DH rash.

The long-term follow-up performed in the present DH patients further demonstrated that small bowel villous atrophy at diagnosis did not have any impact on the presence of long-term illnesses and complications, or long-term quality of life or the presence of persistent gastrointestinal symptoms. Additionally, our previous study showed that the mortality of DH patients with villous atrophy at diagnosis does not differ from that of DH patients with normal villous architecture, and in fact, the mortality of DH patients was shown to be lower than in the general population [37]. Therefore, all these results show that DH patients with and without villous atrophy at diagnosis have a similar good long-term prognosis when they adhere to a GFD.

In contrast to DH, the mortality rate of the patients with coeliac disease are known to be increased compared to the general population [23,38]. Moreover, when the GFD-treated coeliac disease patients in the current study were compared to the DH patient groups, they had significantly more malignancies and long-term illnesses, especially thyroid diseases and osteopenia or osteoporosis. A previous comparison between DH and coeliac disease also showed a higher frequency of diseases of autoimmune origin in patients with coeliac disease [39], but then another study demonstrated that autoimmune diseases were as common among DH patients without classical coeliac disease symptoms than in those DH patients with preceding coeliac disease diagnosis [40]. In the present study, the coeliac disease controls were further found to have worse self-reported general health, and they had more gastrointestinal symptoms at the time of the study compared to the DH patients. These results fit with our recent study that likewise found a better quality of life and fewer gastrointestinal symptoms among long-term treated DH patients compared to treated coeliac disease patients [41].

The results of the present study thus suggest that the prognosis of different phenotypes of coeliac disease diverge and villous atrophy is not the determinative factor in the outcome of DH. Different adherence rates to GFD or varying lifestyle habits did not explain the outcome differences between coeliac disease and DH study patients in this study. One explanation for the different prognosis between coeliac disease and DH might be slightly diverse autoimmune reactions, but this remains to be elucidated in future studies.

In the current study, the median age at diagnosis in DH patients with normal villous architecture was significantly higher compared to DH patients with villous atrophy. We were aware from our earlier long-term DH studies that the age at diagnosis had increased significantly from 1970 onwards [1], and further, that there was a significant trend towards milder villous atrophy [16]. However, in the present study, the time period of DH diagnosis did not differ significantly between DH study groups. Therefore, the divergence in diagnostic periods does not explain the difference in the diagnostic age between DH patients with and without villous atrophy at diagnosis. One explanation might be, however, that older patients are more prone to develop milder small bowel mucosal alterations, e.g., due to divergent immune responses. Previous research shows that older coeliac disease patients are more likely to remain seronegative and further, a trend toward less severe histopathology has been observed with increasing age at the time of coeliac disease diagnosis [42,43]. Nonetheless, these age-related findings detected in coeliac disease and DH should be examined in more detail in further studies.

As a possible limitation of the current study, it must be recognized that the follow-up data were obtained from questionnaires, which might cause selection bias. Recall bias is always a possibility when requiring data from several decades ago. The disease-specific questionnaire used in the study was designed for this particular study and for comparing the results of the study groups, and it has not been used in other disease studies, and it has not been validated. GSRS is not optimized for coeliac disease, but it has been the most commonly used generic questionnaire in coeliac disease studies [28]. PGWB is not a disease-specific instrument, and therefore, it is possible that it might not assess all of the issues that are having an impact on life in DH and coeliac disease patients. GSRS and PGWB questionnaires have not been validated specifically for coeliac disease. Furthermore, all study patients were recruited from the same hospital, and in the future, results from a more comprehensive geographical distribution would be of value. In turn, the major strengths of the study are: A well-defined, prospectively collected DH cohort from a high prevalence area with excellent dietary adherence rates, and the long follow-up time [1]. Moreover, similar large DH studies with knowledge about the diagnostic small bowel mucosal findings and long-term follow-up data consisting of GFD adherence rates have not been performed previously to our knowledge.

5. Conclusions

The major outcome of this study is that skin IgA-IF proven DH patients evincing coeliac-type small bowel mucosal villous atrophy at diagnosis does not differ from DH patients with non-atrophic small bowel mucosa with regard to GFD treatment response, long-term quality of life, or the presence of chronic illnesses or coeliac disease-associated complications.

Author Contributions: E.M., T.S., K.H., T.R., K.K., and P.C. conceived and designed the experiments and wrote the paper; E.M., T.S., and K.H. performed the experiments; and H.H. analyzed the data.

Acknowledgments: This work was supported by the Academy of Finland; the Sigrid Juselius Foundation; the Competitive State Research Financing of the Expert Responsibility area of Tampere University Hospital under Grants 9U019, 9T018, 9V017, 9T058, and 9U053; the Finnish Cultural Foundation; and the Finnish Medical Foundation.

Conflicts of Interest: The authors report no conflicts of interest.

References

1. Salmi, T.; Hervonen, K.; Kautiainen, H.; Collin, P.; Reunala, T. Prevalence and incidence of dermatitis herpetiformis: A 40-year prospective study from Finland. *Br. J. Dermatol.* **2011**, *165*, 354–359. [CrossRef] [PubMed]

2. West, J.; Fleming, K.M.; Tata, L.J.; Card, T.R.; Crooks, C.J. Incidence and prevalence of celiac disease and dermatitis herpetiformis in the UK over two decades: Population-based study. *Am. J. Gastroenterol.* **2014**, *109*, 757–768. [CrossRef] [PubMed]

3. Bolotin, D.; Petronic-Rosic, V. Dermatitis herpetiformis: Part I. Epidemiology, pathogenesis, and clinical presentation. *J. Am. Acad. Dermatol.* **2011**, *64*, 1017–1024. [CrossRef] [PubMed]

4. Spurkland, A.; Ingvarsson, G.; Falk, E.; Knutsen, I.; Sollid, L.; Thorsby, E. Dermatitis herpetiformis and celiac disease are both primarily associated with the HLA-DQ (α1* 0501,(β1* 02) or the HLA-DQ (α1* 03,(β1* 0302) heterodimers. *HLA* **1997**, *49*, 29–34. [CrossRef]
5. Collin, P.; Salmi, T.T.; Hervonen, K.; Kaukinen, K.; Reunala, T. Dermatitis herpetiformis: A cutaneous manifestation of coeliac disease. *Ann. Med.* **2017**, *49*, 23–31. [CrossRef] [PubMed]
6. Dieterich, W.; Ehnis, T.; Bauer, M.; Donner, P.; Volta, U.; Riecken, E.O.; Schuppan, D. Identification of tissue transglutaminase as the autoantigen of celiac disease. *Nat. Med.* **1997**, *3*, 797–801. [CrossRef] [PubMed]
7. Korponay-Szabó, I.R.; Halttunen, T.; Szalai, Z.; Laurila, K.; Kiraly, R.; Kovacs, J.; Fésüs, L.; Mäki, M. In vivo targeting of intestinal and extraintestinal transglutaminase 2 by coeliac autoantibodies. *Gut* **2004**, *53*, 641–648. [CrossRef] [PubMed]
8. Salmi, T.T.; Hervonen, K.; Laurila, K.; Collin, P.; Mäki, M.; Koskinen, O.; Huhtala, H.; Kaukinen, K.; Reunala, T. Small bowel transglutaminase 2-specific IgA deposits in dermatitis herpetiformis. *Acta Derm. Veneorol.* **2014**, *94*, 393–397. [CrossRef] [PubMed]
9. Dieterich, W.; Schuppan, D.; Laag, E.; Bruckner-Tuderman, L.; Reunala, T.; Kárpáti, S.; Zágoni, T.; Riecken, E.O. Antibodies to tissue transglutaminase as serologic markers in patients with dermatitis herpetiformis. *J. Investig. Dermatol.* **1999**, *113*, 133–136. [CrossRef] [PubMed]
10. Zone, J.J.; Meyer, L.J.; Petersen, M.J. Deposition of granular IgA relative to clinical lesions in dermatitis herpetiformis. *Arch. Dermatol.* **1996**, *132*, 912–918. [CrossRef] [PubMed]
11. Sárdy, M.; Kárpáti, S.; Merkl, B.; Paulsson, M.; Smyth, N. Epidermal transglutaminase (TGase3) is the autoantigen of dermatitis herpetiformis. *J. Exp. Med.* **2002**, *195*, 747–757. [CrossRef] [PubMed]
12. Marietta, E.V.; Camilleri, M.J.; Castro, L.A.; Krause, P.K.; Pittelkow, M.R.; Murray, J.A. Transglutaminase autoantibodies in dermatitis herpetiformis and celiac sprue. *J. Investig. Dermatol.* **2008**, *128*, 332–335. [CrossRef] [PubMed]
13. Hull, C.M.; Liddle, M.; Hansen, N.; Meyer, L.; Schmidt, L.; Taylor, T.; Jaskowski, T.; Hill, H.; Zone, J. Elevation of IgA anti-epidermal transglutaminase antibodies in dermatitis herpetiformis. *Br. J. Dermatol.* **2008**, *159*, 120–124. [CrossRef] [PubMed]
14. Salmi, T.T.; Kurppa, K.; Hervonen, K.; Laurila, K.; Collin, P.; Huhtala, H.; Saavalainen, P.; Sievänen, H.; Reunala, T.; Kaukinen, K. Serum transglutaminase 3 antibodies correlate with age at celiac disease diagnosis. *Dig. Liver Dis.* **2016**, *48*, 632–637. [CrossRef] [PubMed]
15. Marks, J.; Shuster, S.; Watson, A. Small-bowel changes in dermatitis herpetiformis. *Lancet* **1966**, *288*, 1280–1282. [CrossRef]
16. Mansikka, E.; Hervonen, K.; Salmi, T.T.; Kautiainen, H.; Kaukinen, K.; Collin, P.; Reunala, T. The decreasing prevalence of severe villous atrophy in dermatitis herpetiformis: A 45-year experience in 393 patients. *J. Clin. Gastroenterol.* **2017**, *51*, 235–239. [CrossRef] [PubMed]
17. Kárpáti, S. Dermatitis herpetiformis: Close to unravelling a disease. *J. Dermatol. Sci.* **2004**, *34*, 83–90. [CrossRef] [PubMed]
18. Zone, J.J. Skin manifestations of celiac disease. *Gastroenterology* **2005**, *128*, S87–S91. [CrossRef] [PubMed]
19. Fry, L.; Riches, D.; Seah, P.; Hoffbrand, A. Clearance of skin lesions in dermatitis herpetiformis after gluten withdrawal. *Lancet* **1973**, *301*, 288–291. [CrossRef]
20. Kaplan, R.P.; Callen, J.P. Dermatitis herpetiformis: Autoimmune disease associations. *Clin. Dermatol.* **1991**, *9*, 347–360. [CrossRef]
21. Hervonen, K.; Viljamaa, M.; Collin, P.; Knip, M.; Reunala, T. The occurrence of type 1 diabetes in patients with dermatitis herpetiformis and their first-degree relatives. *Br. J. Dermatol.* **2004**, *150*, 136–138. [CrossRef] [PubMed]
22. Ventura, A.; Magazzù, G.; Greco, L. Duration of exposure to gluten and risk for autoimmune disorders in patients with celiac disease. *Gastroenterology* **1999**, *117*, 297–303. [CrossRef] [PubMed]
23. Viljamaa, M.; Kaukinen, K.; Pukkala, E.; Hervonen, K.; Reunala, T.; Collin, P. Malignancies and mortality in patients with coeliac disease and dermatitis herpetiformis: 30-year population-based study. *Dig. Liver Dis.* **2006**, *38*, 374–380. [CrossRef] [PubMed]
24. Hervonen, K.; Vornanen, M.; Kautiainen, H.; Collin, P.; Reunala, T. Lymphoma in patients with dermatitis herpetiformis and their first-degree relatives. *Br. J. Dermatol.* **2005**, *152*, 82–86. [CrossRef] [PubMed]

25. Dimenäs, E.; Carlsson, G.; Glise, H.; Israelsson, B.; Wiklund, I. Relevance of norm values as part of the documentation of quality of life instruments for use in upper gastrointestinal disease. *Scand. J. Gastroenterol.* **1996**, *31*, 8–13. [CrossRef]

26. Svedlund, J.; Sjödin, I.; Dotevall, G. GSRS—A clinical rating scale for gastrointestinal symptoms in patients with irritable bowel syndrome and peptic ulcer disease. *Dig. Dis. Sci.* **1988**, *33*, 129–134. [CrossRef] [PubMed]

27. Ludvigsson, J.F.; Ciacci, C.; Green, P.H.; Kaukinen, K.; Korponay-Szabo, I.R.; Kurppa, K.; Murray, J.A.; Lundin, K.E.A.; Maki, M.J.; Popp, A. Outcome measures in coeliac disease trials: The Tampere recommendations. *Gut* **2018**. [CrossRef] [PubMed]

28. Hindryckx, P.; Levesque, B.G.; Holvoet, T.; Durand, S.; Tang, C.-M.; Parker, C.; Khanna, R.; Shackelton, L.M.; D'haens, G.; Sandborn, W.J. Disease activity indices in coeliac disease: Systematic review and recommendations for clinical trials. *Gut* **2016**, *67*, 61–69. [CrossRef] [PubMed]

29. Roos, S.; Kärner, A.; Hallert, C. Psychological well-being of adult coeliac patients treated for 10 years. *Dig. Liver Dis.* **2006**, *38*, 177–180. [CrossRef] [PubMed]

30. Viljamaa, M.; Collin, P.; Huhtala, H.; Sievänen, H.; Mäki, M.; Kaukinen, K. Is coeliac disease screening in risk groups justified? A fourteen-year follow-up with special focus on compliance and quality of life. *Aliment. Pharmacol. Ther.* **2005**, *22*, 317–324. [CrossRef] [PubMed]

31. Hallert, C.; Svensson, M.; Tholstrup, J.; Hultberg, B. Clinical trial: B vitamins improve health in patients with coeliac disease living on a gluten-free diet. *Aliment. Pharmacol. Ther.* **2009**, *29*, 811–816. [CrossRef] [PubMed]

32. Finlay, A.Y.; Khan, G. Dermatology life quality index (DLQI)—A simple practical measure for routine clinical use. *Clin. Exp. Dermatol.* **1994**, *19*, 210–216. [CrossRef] [PubMed]

33. Fry, L.; Keir, P.; McMinn, R.; Cowan, J.; Hoffbrand, A. Small-intestinal structure and function and haematological changes in dermatitis herpetiformis. *Lancet* **1967**, *290*, 729–734. [CrossRef]

34. Mansikka, E.; Salmi, T.; Kaukinen, K.; Collin, P.; Huhtala, H.; Reunala, T.; Hervonen, K. Diagnostic delay in dermatitis herpetiformis in a high-prevalence area. *Acta Derm. Venereol.* **2018**, *98*, 195–199. [CrossRef] [PubMed]

35. Fry, L.; Leonard, J.; Swain, F.; Tucker, W.; Haffenden, G.; Ring, N.; McMinn, R. Long term follow-up of dermatitis herpetiformis with and without dietary gluten withdrawal. *Br. J. Dermatol.* **1982**, *107*, 631–640. [CrossRef] [PubMed]

36. Gawkrodger, D.; Blackwell, J.; Gilmour, H.; Rifkind, E.; Heading, R.; Barnetson, R. Dermatitis herpetiformis: Diagnosis, diet and demography. *Gut* **1984**, *25*, 151–157. [CrossRef] [PubMed]

37. Hervonen, K.; Alakoski, A.; Salmi, T.; Helakorpi, S.; Kautiainen, H.; Kaukinen, K.; Pukkala, E.; Collin, P.; Reunala, T. Reduced mortality in dermatitis herpetiformis: A population-based study of 476 patients. *Br. J. Dermatol.* **2012**, *167*, 1331–1337. [CrossRef] [PubMed]

38. Tio, M.; Cox, M.; Eslick, G. Meta-analysis: Coeliac disease and the risk of all-cause mortality, any malignancy and lymphoid malignancy. *Aliment. Pharmacol. Ther.* **2012**, *35*, 540–551. [CrossRef] [PubMed]

39. Reunala, T.; Collin, P. Diseases associated with dermatitis herpetiformis. *Br. J. Dermatol.* **1997**, *136*, 315–318. [CrossRef] [PubMed]

40. Krishnareddy, S.; Lewis, S.K.; Green, P.H. Dermatitis herpetiformis: Clinical presentations are independent of manifestations of celiac disease. *Am. J. Clin. Dermatol.* **2014**, *15*, 51–56. [CrossRef] [PubMed]

41. Pasternack, C.; Kaukinen, K.; Kurppa, K.; Mäki, M.; Collin, P.; Reunala, T.; Huhtala, H.; Salmi, T. Quality of life and gastrointestinal symptoms in long-term treated dermatitis herpetiformis patients: A cross-sectional study in Finland. *Am. J. Clin. Dermatol.* **2015**, *16*, 545–552. [CrossRef] [PubMed]

42. Salmi, T.T.; Collin, P.; Korponay-Szabo, I.R.; Laurila, K.; Partanen, J.; Huhtala, H.; Kiraly, R.; Lorand, L.; Reunala, T.; Mäki, M. Endomysial antibody-negative coeliac disease: Clinical characteristics and intestinal autoantibody deposits. *Gut* **2006**, *55*, 1746–1753. [CrossRef] [PubMed]

43. Vivas, S.; De Morales, J.M.R.; Fernandez, M.; Hernando, M.; Herrero, B.; Casqueiro, J.; Gutierrez, S. Age-related clinical, serological, and histopathological features of celiac disease. *Am. J. Gastroenterol.* **2008**, *103*, 2360. [CrossRef] [PubMed]

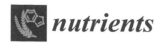

Article

Quality of Life in Patients with Gluten Neuropathy: A Case-Controlled Study

Panagiotis Zis *, Ptolemaios Georgios Sarrigiannis, Dasappaiah Ganesh Rao and Marios Hadjivassiliou

Academic Department of Neurosciences, Sheffield Teaching Hospitals NHS Foundation Trust, Sheffield S10 2JF, South Yorkshire, UK; Ptolemaios.Sarrigiannis@sth.nhs.uk (P.G.S.); Ganesh.Rao@sth.nhs.uk (D.G.R.); m.hadjivassiliou@sheffield.ac.uk (M.H.)
* Correspondence: takiszis@gmail.com

Received: 15 April 2018; Accepted: 15 May 2018; Published: 23 May 2018

Abstract: Background: Gluten neuropathy (GN) is defined as an otherwise idiopathic peripheral neuropathy in the presence of serological evidence of gluten sensitivity (positive native gliadin antibodies and/or transglutaminase or endomysium antibodies). We aimed to compare the quality of life (QoL) of GN patients with that of control subjects and to investigate the effects of a gluten-free diet (GFD) on the QoL. Methods: All consecutive patients with GN attending a specialist neuropathy clinic were invited to participate. The Overall Neuropathy Limitations Scale (ONLS) was used to assess the severity of the neuropathy. The 36-Item Short Form Survey (SF-36) questionnaire was used to measure participants' QoL. A strict GFD was defined as effectively being able to eliminate all circulating gluten sensitivity-related antibodies. Results: Fifty-three patients with GN and 53 age- and gender-matched controls were recruited. Compared to controls, GN patients showed significantly worse scores in the physical functioning, role limitations due to physical health, energy/fatigue, and general health subdomains of the SF-36. After adjusting for age, gender, and disease severity, being on a strict GFD correlated with better SF-36 scores in the pain domain of the SF-36 (beta 0.317, $p = 0.019$) and in the overall health change domain of the SF-36 (beta 0.306, $p = 0.017$). Conclusion: In GN patients, physical dysfunctioning is the major determinant of poor QoL compared to controls. Routine checking of the elimination of gluten sensitivity-related antibodies that results from a strict GFD should be encouraged, as such elimination ameliorates the overall pain and health scores, indicating a better QoL.

Keywords: gluten neuropathy; coeliac disease; gluten free diet; quality of life; male

1. Introduction

Gluten neuropathy (GN) is one of the commonest neurological manifestations of gluten sensitivity [1] and it is defined as an otherwise idiopathic peripheral neuropathy (PN) [2] in the presence of serological evidence of gluten sensitivity (positive native gliadin antibodies, and/or transglutaminase or endomysium antibodies) [1,3]. Some patients with GN have evidence of enteropathy revealed by duodenal biopsy and are diagnosed with coeliac disease (CD), whereas the majority of patients with GN do not have enteropathy.

The main type of gluten neuropathy is symmetrical sensorimotor axonal peripheral neuropathy [1], however sensory ganglionopathy (SG) and, rarely, mononeuritis multiplex (MMX) may also occur [1,4,5]. A gluten-free diet (GFD) has been shown to be effective in treating GN, irrespective of the presence or not of enteropathy [6].

As in all axonal neuropathies, symptoms can be divided into sensory and motor. Incoordination and gait disturbance are symptoms usually attributed to damage of the sensory nerves (sensory ataxia) [2]. Other sensory symptoms include tingling, pins and needles, numbness, tightness, burning, and pain. Motor symptoms include muscle cramps, stiffness, weakness, and wasting [2]. The clinical diagnosis is confirmed with nerve conduction studies.

Robust epidemiological data on the prevalence of GN neuropathy are lacking, however it is known that PN of any etiology can affect between 2.4% and 8% of the general population [2] and that CD is associated with a 2.5-fold increased risk of later neuropathy [5].

As in all chronic diseases, patients with GN are expected to have an impaired quality of life (QoL) for reasons that are either directly or indirectly related to the disease. It has been shown that patients with advanced peripheral neuropathy, for example, show worse scores in questionnaires measuring QoL when compared to less impaired patients [7]. Such impairment, refers not only to motor symptoms (i.e., weakness) but also to sensory symptoms, in particular pain [8–13]. Indirectly, however, GN might cause an additional burden by having to adhere to a strict GFD. It has been shown that the degree of difficulty in adhering to a GFD is associated with reductions in patient wellbeing and psychological distress that the dietician is critically placed to address [14].

The purpose of this study was twofold. We wanted to compare the QoL of GN patients with that of controls (subjects without peripheral neuropathy or gluten sensitivity) and to investigate the effect of being on a GFD on the QoL in these patients.

2. Methods

2.1. Procedure and Participants

This was a cross-sectional study conducted at the Sheffield Institute of Gluten-Related Diseases (SIGReD). Patients were recruited during their regular visits to the gluten/neurology clinic based at the Royal Hallamshire Hospital, Sheffield, UK. Individuals (i.e., carers or relatives) without a diagnosis of PN or risk factors for developing PN participated as controls.

To be enrolled, the patients had to meet the following inclusion criteria: (1) diagnosis of PN, as confirmed by nerve conduction studies, (2) serological evidence of gluten sensitivity (positive for native gliadin IgG and/or IgA antibodies with or without positivity for endomysial and transgultaminase antibodies) at diagnosis prior to commencing a gluten-free diet, (3) absence of other risk factors for developing PN (i.e., diabetes, vitamin deficiencies, exposure to neurotoxic agents) (4) age equal to or greater than 18 years, (5) able to provide a written informed consent.

The study protocol was approved by the local ethics committee.

2.2. Measures

The demographic characteristics included age and gender. All patients went through extensive investigations for possible causes of PN [2]. Patients with a family history of neuropathy were excluded.

The type of neuropathy (sensorimotor length-dependent PN, sensory ganglionopathy [15,16], mononeuritis multiplex) for all patients was determined on the basis of nerve conduction studies, which were performed by the same clinician on the day of the recruitment.

All patients were referred for an endoscopy and duodenal biopsy to establish the presence of enteropathy. All biopsies were histologically assessed by an experienced pathologist for evidence of enteropathy (triad of villous atrophy, crypt hyperplasia, and increase in intraepithelial lymphocytes).

The severity of neuropathy was assessed by the Overall Neuropathy Limitations Scale (ONLS), which is a validated scale that measures limitations in the everyday activities of the upper and lower limbs [17].

Biagi score was used to document adherence to a gluten-free diet [18]. Patients with a Biagi score of equal to or above 3 were considered as being on a gluten-free diet. Furthermore, patients with negative serology at the time of recruitment were considered to be on a strict gluten-free diet.

The 36-Item Short Form Survey (SF-36), a self-reported measure of health status and quality of life [19], was used to determine patient health-related quality of life. SF-36 covers nine health and QoL domains. These domains include physical functioning, role limitations due to physical health, role limitations due to emotional problems, energy/fatigue, emotional well-being, social functioning, pain, general health and health change. Each item is measured using a Likert-type scale. The scores were converted and analysed according to the marking guidelines for the SF-36, such that higher scores (out of a total of 100 for each domain) constitute better health-related quality of life in this domain.

2.3. Statistical Analyses

A database was developed using the Statistical Package for Social Science (version 23.0 for Mac; SPSS). Frequencies and descriptive statistics were examined for each variable. Comparisons between patients on a gluten-free diet and patients not on a gluten-free diet were made using Student's t-tests for normally distributed continuous data, Mann–Whitney's U test for non-normally distributed, and chi-square test or Fischer's exact test for categorical data.

Where differences with a p value lower than 0.10 were found, these variables were entered into linear regression models, with the QoL domain score being the dependent variable. All accuracy and generalization assumptions for the model were checked.

The level of statistical significance was set at the 0.05 level.

3. Results

3.1. Study Population

Fifty-three patients with GN were recruited (73.6% male, mean age 68.2 ± 9.3 years) and were age- and gender-matched with 53 control subjects without a history of peripheral neuropathy or gluten sensitivity. Thirty-six patients (67.9%) had a symmetrical length-dependent sensorimotor axonal PN, 16 (30.2%) had a sensory ganglionopathy, and 1 patient had mononeuritis multiplex (1.9%). The mean disease duration was 12.6 ± 9.5 years (ranging from 0 to 37 years), suggesting that the GN is a late extra-intestinal manifestation of serologically confirmed gluten sensitivity (occurring usually in the sixth decade of life). Overall ONLS scores ranged from 1 to 7 (mean 3.1 ± 1.8).

Not all of the patients agreed to a duodenal biopsy. Of 32 patients who underwent duodenal biopsy, nine (28.1%) had enteropathy (eight coeliac disease—Marsh type 3, one increased intraepithelial lymphocytes—Marsh type 2).

3.2. QoL Compared to Controls

Table 1 summarizes the scores in all SF-36 subdomains in patients with GN and in controls. Patients with GN showed significantly worse scores compared to controls in the following quality of life modalities: physical functioning ($p < 0.001$), role limitations due to physical health ($p < 0.001$), energy/fatigue ($p = 0.045$), and general health ($p = 0.029$). A trend of statistical significance ($p = 0.094$) was observed in the pain modality of the SF-36 questionnaire.

Table 1. Demopgraphics and quality of life (QoL) parameters of patients with gluten neuropathy (GN).

	GN (*n* = 53)	Controls (*n* = 53)	*p* Value
Demographics			
Age, in years (SD)	68.2 (9.3)	66.8 (10.0)	0.440
Male gender (%)	39 (73.6)	38 (71.7)	0.828
Quality of life modalities			
Physical functioning	50.8 (32.8)	78.0 (23.0)	<0.001 *
Role limitations due to physical health	53.9 (34.0)	77.4 (25.8)	<0.001 *
Role limitations due to emotional problems	76.7 (29.4)	83.3 (25.5)	0.219
Energy/Fatigue	48.0 (21.8)	56.3 (20.1)	0.045 **
Emotional well-being	75.5 (15.9)	74.2 (16.7)	0.677
Social functioning	70.2 (30.5)	79.2 (25.9)	0.104
Pain	59.4 (27.9)	68.5 (27.3)	0.094
General Health	54.8 (23.6)	64.3 (20.1)	0.029 **
Health change	42.9 (19.8)	49.1 (18.3)	0.101

* *p* < 0.001; ** *p* < 0.05.

3.3. The Role of GFD (Self-Reported) on QoL

On the basis of the self-reported adherence to GFD (Biagi score equal to or greater than 3), 31 patients (58.5%) were on a GFD. Table 2 summarizes the demographic, clinical, and quality-of-life-related characteristics of patients with GN reporting being on GFD versus patients with GN reporting being on a gluten-containing diet. The two groups did not differ significantly in age, gender, disease duration, neuropathy severity, or neuropathy type. A trend of statistical significance (*p* = 0.094) was observed on the overall health change subdomain of the SF-36.

Table 2. Demographic, clinical, and quality-of-life-related characteristics of patients with gluten neuropathy reporting being on a gluten-free diet (GFD) compared to patients with gluten neuropathy reporting being on a gluten-containing diet.

	Gluten-Free Diet (*n* = 31)	Gluten-Containing Diet (*n* = 22)	*p* Value
Demographics			
Age, in years (SD)	68.6 (8.3)	67.6 (10.8)	0.702
Male gender (%)	20 (64.5)	19 (86.4)	0.115
Clinical characteristics			
Disease duration, in years (SD)	13.8 (8.0)	11.0 (10.2)	0.259
Type of neuropathy			0.690
Symmetrical length-dependent PN (%)	21 (67.8)	15 (68.2)	
Sensory ganglionopathy (%)	9 (29.0)	7 (31.8)	
Mononeuritis multiplex (%)	1 (3.2)	0 (0.0)	
Neuropathy severity			
Total ONLS score (SD)	3.1 (1.7)	3.2 (1.8)	0.814
Quality of life modalities			
Physical functioning	53.5 (34.3)	47.0 (31.0)	0.482
Role limitations due to physical health	56.0 (32.6)	50.9 (36.5)	0.589
Role limitations due to emotional problems	79.6 (25.2)	72.7 (34.7)	0.409
Energy/Fatigue	49.2 (23.5)	46.3 (19.5)	0.640
Emotional well-being	76.5 (16.1)	74.1 (15.9)	0.599
Social functioning	70.4 (27.4)	69.9 (35.1)	0.951
Pain	63.6 (28.0)	53.5 (27.3)	0.197
General Health	56.5 (22.9)	52.7 (24.9)	0.576
Health change	46.8 (19.1)	37.5 (20.0)	0.094

PN: peripheral neuropathy; ONLS: overall neuropathy limitations scale; SD: standard deviation.

After adjusting for age, gender, and disease severity, being on GFD (self-reported) was positively correlated with better SF-36 scores on the overall health change domain of the SF-36 (beta 0.258, $p = 0.047$).

3.4. The Role of Strict GFD on QoL

Twenty-two patients managed to eliminate antigliadin, endomysial, and transglutaminase antibodies by adopting the GFD. This population, which accounted for 41.5% of the total GN study group and 71% of those GN patients self-reporting as being on a GFD, was considered to be on a strict GFD.

Table 3 summarizes the demographic, clinical, and quality-of-life-related characteristics of patients with GN being on a strict GFD versus patients with GN not on a strict GFD. The two groups did not differ significantly in age, gender, disease duration, neuropathy severity, or neuropathy type. Patients on a strict GFD had significantly higher scores (indicating better QoL) on the pain sub-domain of the SF-36 ($p = 0.03$). A trend of statistical significance ($p = 0.066$) was also observed on the overall health change subdomain of the SF-36.

Table 3. Demographic, clinical, and quality-of-life-related characteristics of patients with gluten neuropathy being on a strict gluten-free diet versus patients not being on a strict gluten-free diet (serologically confirmed by the elimination of anti-gliadin antibodies).

	On Strict GFD (n = 22)	Not on Strict GFD (n = 31)	p Value
Demographics			
Age, in years (SD)	69.7 (8.5)	67.2 (9.9)	0.329
Male gender (%)	14 (63.6)	25 (80.6)	0.166
Clinical characteristics			
Disease duration, in years (SD)	13.9 (8.1)	11.7 (9.6)	0.385
Type of neuropathy			0.462
Symmetrical length-dependent PN (%)	14 (63.6)	22 (71.0)	
Sensory ganglionopathy (%)	7 (31.8)	9 (29.0)	
Mononeuritis multiplex (%)	1 (4.5)	0 (0.0)	
Neuropathy severity			
Total ONLS score (SD)	3.2 (1.8)	3.0 (1.7)	0.695
Quality of life modalities			
Physical functioning	58.4 (35.7)	45.5 (30.0)	0.160
Role limitations due to physical health	58.5 (33.9)	50.6 (34.2)	0.409
Role limitations due to emotional problems	81.8 (23.7)	73.1 (32.8)	0.293
Energy/Fatigue	50.0 (26.1)	46.6 (18.5)	0.578
Emotional well-being	76.8 (18.2)	74.5 (14.2)	0.608
Social functioning	69.6 (28.4)	70.6 (32.4)	0.916
Pain	69.2 (26.6)	52.5 (27.1)	0.030*
General Health	56.4 (23.9)	53.9 (23.7)	0.708
Health change	48.9 (21.1)	38.7 (18.1)	0.066

GFD: gluten free diet; PN: peripheral neuropathy; ONLS: overall neuropathy limitations scale; SD: standard deviation.

After adjusting for age, gender, and disease severity, being on a strict GFD (serologically proven) was positive correlated with better SF-36 scores on the pain domain of the SF-36 (beta 0.317, $p = 0.019$) and the overall health change domain of the SF-36 (beta 0.306, $p = 0.017$).

4. Discussion

This case-controlled study demonstrates that patients with GN have significantly worse QoL compared to age- and gender-matched controls on the basis of the SF-36 modalities of physical functioning, role limitations due to physical health, energy/fatigue, and general health. This finding adds to the existing literature that the main impact of peripheral neuropathy on patients' QoL is on the modalities affecting their dysfunctioning (i.e., impaired activities of daily living) [7]. To our knowledge, this is the first study investigating the QoL of patients with GN.

Another novelty of the current study is the examination of the role of GFD on QoL. For this, we conducted two separate analyses, one based on the patients' reports and the other based on the evidence of the elimination of all gluten sensitivity-related antibodies.

In their study, Lee et al. found that patients with coeliac disease reported that GFD had a negative impact on their quality of life, as it restricted their social activities such as travelling or dining out [20]. In our study, patients on a GFD had higher scores in the sub-domains of SF-36 (Table 2), though not statistically significant. There was, however, a trend for a statistically significant difference in the scores of the overall health change subdomain of the SF-36. There are possible explanations for such disparity. Firstly, awareness of gluten sensitivity and coeliac disease has increased over the last decade with improved availability and a better range of gluten-free products. Furthermore, dining out or travelling is much easier, as many restaurants and hotels do have gluten-free menus. Secondly, the heterogeneity of the study populations may have affected the results, as Lee et al. included patients with different gender distribution (female predominance), different age (younger), and a different clinical picture (coeliac disease with gastrointestinal symptoms), whereas our cohort of patients presented a neuropathy.

When comparing patients who strictly adhered to the GFD (as evidenced by the elimination of all circulating gluten sensitivity-related antibodies) with patients either not being on the GFD or not being strictly on the GFD, we showed that the former had significantly better scores in the pain and the overall health change domain. This is in keeping with the current literature, which shows that patients with GN benefit from a GFD with evidence of improvement of the neuropathy usually after one year on strict GFD, associated with the elimination of gluten sensitivity-related antibodies [6,20]. Moreover, this finding highlights the importance of serological monitoring in an attempt to improve adherence to a GFD. Interestingly, in our cohort, 29% of patients on the GFD still had positive serology.

Our study population comprised predominantly males (male to female ratio 3:1). As we recruited patients in succession, this might indicate that GN is commoner in males, which is in contrast with what Thawani et al. reported in their epidemiological study where they assessed the risk of neuropathy among patients with CD and found no difference in the risk of developing neuropathy between the two genders [5]. This difference in findings might be due to the fact that the majority of patients with GN do not have enteropathy and, therefore, the male predominance possibly reflects this. Our observation, however, is important, as male patients perceive illness and quality of life differently, and adherence to a GFD has a different emotional impact in males compared to females [21].

Our results should be interpreted with some caution, given the limitations of our design. This is a cross-sectional study based on patients attending a specialized clinic, and the results may not be generalizable to other settings. Furthermore, our cohort included patients with large fiber axonal peripheral neuropathies only. Pure small fiber neuropathy associated with gluten sensitivity is another area that merits further consideration, as it is a particularly painful condition and therefore can affect patients' QoL.

In conclusion, in patients with GN, physical dysfunctioning is the major determinant of QoL compared to control subjects. Contrary to previous observations in patients with classical CD, being on a GFD does not have a negative effect on social functioning in patients with GN. Clinicians are advised to regularly monitor the adherence to the GFD diet by serological testing for gluten sensitivity-related antibodies, because a strict GFD ameliorates the overall pain and health change scores, indicating better QoL.

Author Contributions: P.Z. and M.H.: drafting/revising the manuscript, study concept and design, data collection, statistical analysis. P.G.S. and D.G.R.: drafting/revising the manuscript, data collection.

Funding: Zis is sincerely thankful to the Ryder Briggs Fund.

Acknowledgments: This is a summary of independent research carried out at the NIHR Sheffield Biomedical Research Centre (Translational Neuroscience). The views expressed are those of the authors and not necessarily those of the NHS, the NIHR or the Department of Health.

Conflicts of Interest: The authors declare no conflict of interest.

References

1. Hadjivassiliou, M.; Sanders, D.S.; Grünewald, R.A.; Woodroofe, N.; Boscolo, S.; Aeschlimann, D. Gluten sensitivity: From gut to brain. *Lancet Neurol.* **2010**, *9*, 318–330. [CrossRef]
2. Zis, P.; Sarrigiannis, P.G.; Rao, D.G.; Hewamadduma, C.; Hadjivassiliou, M. Chronic idiopathic axonal polyneuropathy: A systematic review. *J. Neurol.* **2016**, *263*, 1903–1910. [CrossRef] [PubMed]
3. Zis, P.; Rao, D.G.; Sarrigiannis, P.G.; Aeschlimann, P.; Aeschlimann, D.P.; Sanders, D.; Grünewald, R.A.; Hadjivassiliou, M. Transglutaminase 6 antibodies in gluten neuropathy. *Dig. Liver Dis.* **2017**, *49*, 1196–1200. [CrossRef] [PubMed]
4. Kelkar, P.; Ross, M.A.; Murray, J. Mononeuropathy multiplex associated with celiac sprue. *Muscle Nerve* **1996**, *19*, 234–236. [CrossRef]
5. Thawani, S.P.; Brannagan, T.H., 3rd; Lebwohl, B.; Green, P.H.; Ludvigsson, J.F. Risk of Neuropathy among 28,232 Patients with Biopsy-Verified Celiac Disease. *JAMA Neurol.* **2015**, *72*, 806–811. [CrossRef] [PubMed]
6. Hadjivassiliou, M.; Kandler, R.H.; Chattopadhyay, A.K.; Davies-Jones, A.G.; Jarratt, J.A.; Sanders, D.S.; Sharrack, B.; Grünewald, R.A. Dietary treatment of gluten neuropathy. *Muscle Nerve* **2006**, *34*, 762–766. [CrossRef] [PubMed]
7. Teunissen, L.L.; Eurelings, M.; Notermans, N.C.; Hop, J.W.; van Gijn, J. Quality of life in patients with axonal polyneuropathy. *J. Neurol.* **2000**, *247*, 195–199. [CrossRef] [PubMed]
8. Zis, P.; Varrassi, G. Painful Peripheral Neuropathy and Cancer. *Pain Ther.* **2017**, *6*, 115–116. [CrossRef] [PubMed]
9. Zis, P.; Paladini, A.; Piroli, A.; McHugh, P.C.; Varrassi, G.; Hadjivassiliou, M. Pain as a First Manifestation of Paraneoplastic Neuropathies: A Systematic Review and Meta-Analysis. *Pain Ther.* **2017**, *6*, 143–151. [CrossRef] [PubMed]
10. Vadalouca, A.; Raptis, E.; Moka, E.; Zis, P.; Sykioti, P.; Siafaka, I. Pharmacological treatment of neuropathic cancer pain: A comprehensive review of the current literature. *Pain Pract.* **2012**, *12*, 219–251. [CrossRef] [PubMed]
11. Zis, P.; Grünewald, R.A.; Chaudhuri, R.K.; Hadjivassiliou, M. Peripheral neuropathy in idiopathic Parkinson's disease: A systematic review. *J. Neurol. Sci.* **2017**, *378*, 204–209. [CrossRef] [PubMed]
12. Brozou, V.; Vadalouca, A.; Zis, P. Pain in Platin-Induced Neuropathies: A Systematic Review and Meta-Analysis. *Pain Ther.* **2017**. [CrossRef] [PubMed]
13. Zis, P.; Daskalaki, A.; Bountouni, I.; Sykioti, P.; Varrassi, G.; Paladini, A. Depression and chronic pain in the elderly: Links and management challenges. *Clin. Interv. Aging* **2017**, *12*, 709–720. [CrossRef] [PubMed]
14. Barratt, S.M.; Leeds, J.S.; Sanders, D.S. Quality of life in Coeliac Disease is determined by perceived degree of difficulty adhering to a gluten-free diet, not the level of dietary adherence ultimately achieved. *J. Gastrointest. Liver Dis.* **2011**, *20*, 241–245.
15. Camdessanché, J.P.; Jousserand, G.; Ferraud, K.; Vial, C.; Petiot, P.; Honnorat, J.; Antoine, J.C. The pattern and diagnostic criteria of sensory neuronopathy: A case-control study. *Brain* **2009**, *132*, 1723–1733. [CrossRef] [PubMed]
16. Zis, P.; Hadjivassiliou, M.; Sarrigiannis, P.G.; Barker, A.S.J.E.; Rao, D.G. Rapid neurophysiological screening for sensory ganglionopathy: A novel approach. *Brain Behav.* **2017**, *7*, e00880. [CrossRef] [PubMed]
17. Graham, R.C.; Hughes, R.A. A modified peripheral neuropathy scale: The Overall Neuropathy Limitations Scale. *J. Neurol. Neurosurg. Psychiatry* **2006**, *77*, 973–976. [CrossRef] [PubMed]
18. Biagi, F.; Andrealli, A.; Bianchi, P.I.; Marchese, A.; Klersy, C.; Corazza, G.R. A gluten-free diet score to evaluate dietary compliance in patients with coeliac disease. *Br. J. Nutr.* **2009**, *102*, 882–887. [CrossRef] [PubMed]

19. Ware, J.E., Jr.; Sherbourne, C.D. The MOS 36-item short-form health survey (SF-36). I. Conceptual framework and item selection. *Med. Care* **1992**, *30*, 473–483. [CrossRef] [PubMed]

20. Hadjivassiliou, M.; Rao, D.G.; Wharton, S.B.; Sanders, D.S.; Grünewald, R.A.; Davies-Jones, A.G. Sensory ganglionopathy due to gluten sensitivity. *Neurology* **2010**, *75*, 1003–1008. [CrossRef] [PubMed]

21. Zarkadas, M.; Dubois, S.; MacIsaac, K.; Cantin, I.; Rashid, M.; Roberts, K.C.; La Vieille, S.; Godefroy, S.; Pulido, O.M. Living with coeliac disease and a gluten-free diet: A Canadian perspective. *J. Hum. Nutr. Diet.* **2013**, *26*, 10–23. [CrossRef] [PubMed]

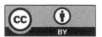

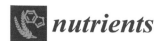

Review

Extra-Intestinal Manifestation of Celiac Disease in Children

Hilary Jericho * and Stefano Guandalini

Department of Pediatrics, Section of Gastroenterology, Hepatology and Nutrition, University of Chicago Celiac Disease Center-Comer Children's Hospital, Chicago, IL 60637, USA; guandalini@peds.bsd.uchicago.edu
* Correspondence: hjericho@peds.bsd.uchicago.edu; Tel.: +1-773-702-8646

Received: 23 May 2018; Accepted: 8 June 2018; Published: 12 June 2018

Abstract: The aim of this literature review is to discuss the extra-intestinal manifestations of celiac disease within the pediatric celiac population.

Keywords: extra-intestinal; gastrointestinal; celiac disease

1. Overview

Celiac disease (CD) is a complex autoimmune disease that is triggered by the ingestion of gluten (the major storage protein in wheat, rye, and barley) in genetically predisposed individuals, leading to elevated titers of celiac-specific autoantibodies and resulting in a variable degree of small intestinal inflammation and a wide range of gastrointestinal and extra-intestinal manifestations.

The extra-intestinal manifestations of CD seen most often in the pediatric population include, but are not limited to, short stature, delayed puberty, dental enamel hypoplasia, osteopenia/osteoporosis, iron-deficiency anemia refractory to oral iron supplementation, recurrent stomatitis, liver and biliary disease, dermatitis herpetaformis, arthralgia/arthritis, headaches, ataxia, peripheral neuropathy, epilepsy, behavioral changes, and psychiatric disorders and alopecia.

While the prevalence of extra-intestinal manifestations of CD is similar between the pediatric and adult populations (60% and 62%, respectively), specific extra-intestinal manifestations and rates of improvement differ. While short stature is the most common extra-intestinal manifestation of CD in children, iron deficiency anemia is most common in adults. The other more commonly encountered extra-intestinal manifestations in both children and adults include fatigue and headaches. Additionally, on average, children appear to have much greater and faster rates of improvement as compared to adults [1,2].

It has been shown that children with extra-intestinal manifestations of CD as the main presenting symptom have a more severe degree of villous atrophy than those that are presenting with gastrointestinal manifestations or asymptomatic patients that were detected through screening [2]. The exact etiology for this finding is uncertain. It is not then surprising, though, that at 24 months after starting a strict gluten free diet (GFD), both children and adults with CD show greater and faster rates of improvements in gastrointestinal (90% and 86%, respectively) versus extra-intestinal manifestations of CD (87% and 80%, respectively), which is possibly owing to the more severe histologic findings and more complex mechanism involved with extra-intestinal manifestations. Overall children show greater rates of extra-intestinal symptom resolution as compared to adults and males show greater rates of improvement as compared to females. Factors that appear to predict better rates of symptom resolution after the initiation of a strict GFD include a strong family history of CD, shorter durations of symptoms prior to the diagnosis of CD (those with longer duration of symptoms have greater risk of an altered gut-brain axis setting off a cycle of amplified pain [3]), and strict adherence to the GFD [4].

2. Short Stature and Delayed Puberty

Short stature is the most commonly encountered extra-intestinal manifestation of CD in children, being found in roughly one-third of all new pediatric celiac diagnoses. While it can be directly related to malabsorption of nutrients, it should completely reverse once a child is strictly adherent to a GFD. In fact, within 24 months of starting a strict GFD, celiac children should attain appropriate catch up growth and return to their expected trajectory for height. However, if a child is diagnosed post-puberty, their chances for catch up growth are much decreased as the child has likely missed their window. Thus, for post-pubertal patients with short stature, a bone age determination is important to best predict the child's capacity for additional height growth [1]. If short stature in a prepuberal patient persists beyond 24 months on a strict GFD, it is imperative that the physician start an additional investigation for other missed comorbidities.

In the 2017 study by Jericho et al. [1], 28% of children with persistent short stature despite strict adherence to the GFD had another missed comorbidity (inflammatory bowel disease, food aversion, Turner Syndrome, or growth hormone deficiency) requiring alternate treatments. Therefore, one must never continue to attribute ongoing short stature to CD, once it appears that the CD has been adequately treated [1].

Delayed puberty is another common manifestation of CD affecting roughly 10% of new pediatric celiac patients [1]. Delayed puberty is defined by a lack of physical or hormonal signs of puberty at the age of usual onset. Visible secondary sexual development usually begins when girls achieve a bone age of 11 years and boys achieve a bone age of 12 years. In girls, a lack of breast development by 13 years, or a lack of menarche within three years after breast development or by 16 years is considered to be abnormal. For boys, no testicular enlargement by 14 years or a delay in development for five years or more after onset of genitalia enlargement is considered abnormal. In the case of CD, this delay in puberty is directly related to malabsorption and malnutrition, and should resolve on a GFD, which should prevent any long-term complications and restore normal maturation. If the delay in puberty fails to improve within 12–24 months of starting a GFD, it is imperative that the patient be referred to endocrinology for further evaluation of other underlying defects within the reproductive system [5].

3. Dental Enamel Hypoplasia and Recurrent Stomatitis

Dental Enamel Hypoplasia can be seen in as many as 40–50% of new pediatric celiac patients as compared to 6% of the healthy population and it leads to the appearance of white, yellow, or brown spots on the teeth with a mottled or translucent-looking appearance [6]. While there is no consensus as to the exact mechanism by which CD leads to dental enamel hypoplasia it is hypothesized that it is secondary to malabsorption of calcium in addition to genetic and immunological factors disturbing the normal process of amelogenesis [7]. Dental enamel hypoplasia occurring in deciduous teeth, within a symmetrical and chronological manner, and detectable in all quadrants of the dentition is most suggestive of an underlying chronic malabsorptive disease, such as CD, as opposed to non-symmetric defects, which are considered to be non-specific [8]. When dental enamel hypoplasia occurs in a child's permanent teeth, this is most often permanent and will not improve after adopting a strict GFD [9].

Roughly 46% of children with CD also suffer from aphthous stomatitis as compared to 20% of the healthy population. It is not yet established whether aphthous ulcers are a direct manifestation of CD or if they occur due to the indirect effects of malabsorption [10]. It is speculated that systemic CD leads to an imbalance in the oral ecosystem that impairs oral health conditions, leading to both dental enamel hypoplasia and aphthous stomatitis. The impact of oral ecosystem alterations, including a change to salivary flow rate and alterations of the hard and soft oral tissues, and its impact on the development of dental enamel defects and aphthous ulcers are being closely evaluated. In a study by Mida et al. in 2011, there did not appear to be significant differences in salivary factors between celiac patients and healthy controls [11], but there were significant differences in the quantity of leukocytes that are present in patients with infectious processes and/or other systemic diseases involving the immune system as compared to healthy controls. They showed that 80% of celiac children who complied with a strict GFD had the complete resolution of leukocyte presence in oral smears as compared to patients with poor adherence to the diet. These non-adherent patients continued to show elevated leukocyte levels and it was hypothesized that these leukocytes in oral smears are what contribute to the formation of the recurrent aphthous ulcers [12] when the appropriate genetic predisposition is present [13]. Others speculate that the direct presence of gluten within the oral cavity may stimulate lymphocyte activity directly into the oral mucosa [11]. Aphthous stomatitis in celiac patients show high rates of resolution on a strict GFD [1].

4. Osteopenia/Osteoporosis

Osteopenia (reduced bone density) and osteoporosis (reduced bone density leading to weak and brittle bones) are the most frequent bone related complications of CD, and can ultimately lead to bone fragility and a high prevalence of bone fractures if CD is left untreated. Roughly 75% of pediatric celiac patients at the time of diagnosis will have osteopenia, while only 30% have osteoporosis.

Osteoblasts, which are derived from mesenchymal stem cells, are responsible for new bone formation, while osteoclasts, which are differentiated monocyte-derived cells, are involved in bone matrix removal. Through complicated mechanisms, bones are constantly remodeled through the process of resorption and formation, and in a balanced manner, to limit ultimate bone loss. Nutrition plays a very important role in this bone homeostasis, with the main players being vitamin D, calcium, and minerals, which are predominantly absorbed in the proximal small bowel [14]. While our bodies strive to produce strong bones, the ultimate goal of the human body is to maintain adequate serum calcium levels. When calcium levels are adequate the body favors bone formation. Reduced serum calcium levels, though, leads to parathyroid gland stimulation, increased production of parathyroid hormone (PTH), subsequent bone resorption, and the release of stored calcium to bring the serum calcium levels back into equilibrium.

Untreated CD to leads to inflammation and villous atrophy in the proximal small bowel, malabsorption of calcium, and low serum levels. This, in turn, leads to secondary hyperparathyroidism, the release of calcium and phosphate from the bone matrix, and the thinning of bones [15]. There is also now evidence to suggest that, in addition to low calcium levels leading to thinning of bones, the chronic release of proinflammatory cytokines, hormonal components, and other misbalanced bone remodeling factors can also predispose celiac patients, on or off the GFD, to mineral metabolism derangements. Specifically, cytokines interleukin 1 beta (IL-1β), interleukin 6 (IL-6), tumor necrosis factor alpha (TNF-α), and interferon gamma (IFN-γ) has been implicated in bone loss during CD [16–19]. Lastly, there have also been recent advances in the identification of receptor activators of nuclear factor kappa B/receptor activator of nuclear factor kappa B-ligand (RANK/RANKL) signaling system, in addition to the discovery of osteoprotegerin (OPG), a protein that may protect from excessive bone reabsorption. Bone homeostasis is maintained through the balance of the reabsorbing activity of RANKL and the decoy receptor OPG. It has been shown that the OPG/RANKL ratio is significantly lower in celiac patients with recovery of intestinal mucosa as compared to healthy controls that are positively correlating with their lower bone mass density [20].

Strict adherence to the GFD is the first-choice therapy for the treatment of osteopenia and osteoporosis in children as it leads to healing of the small bowel and the reversal of intestinal malabsorption. By 12 months on a strict and balanced GFD, most children will have near complete re-mineralization of the bones, even without additional vitamin D and calcium supplementation [21,22]. A greater improvement at 12 months is seen in pediatric celiac patients with GI symptoms as compared to non-GI symptoms, which is likely explained by a delay in the diagnosis of patients lacking GI symptoms leading to more extensive disturbances in bone metabolism at the time of celiac diagnosis [23].

5. Iron-Deficiency Anemia

While iron-deficiency anemia is one of the most common extra-intestinal manifestations at diagnosis in adult CD patients (50%), and it is only found in roughly 10–15% of new pediatric celiac patients [1,2,24]. This discrepancy can be attributed to delayed diagnoses of CD in adults given the propensity for less typical gastrointestinal celiac symptoms than that seen in children. Iron is predominantly absorbed in the first portion of the small bowel, the duodenum, which is the main portion of the bowel affected by CD. CD induced duodenal inflammation subsequently leads to the malabsorption of iron and resultant iron-deficiency anemia. This anemia will often temporarily improve with iron supplementation only to recur when discontinued given the ongoing iron malabsorption from the untreated CD. Eighty-four percent of celiac children receiving iron supplementation and with strict adherence to a GFD had the complete recovery of their iron stores by 12–24 months [1].

6. Liver and Biliary Disease

Liver disease is seen in up to 50% of new pediatric celiac patients [25]. While is it possible for celiac patients to have more severe liver disease, such as autoimmune hepatitis, primary biliary cirrhosis, and sclerosing cholangitis, the majority develop a benign hypertransaminasemia or "celiac hepatitis". While it is not clear why damage to the liver occurs in CD, it is felt to be likely secondary to damaged gut mucosa with resulting increased gut permeability allowing for endotoxins from gut bacteria to reach the portal vein. Once in the liver, these endotoxins trigger a toll-like receptor-mediated inflammatory response from immune cells, ultimately leading to inflammation and liver damage [26]. Patients with "celiac hepatitis" have excellent response rates to a strict GFD, with a 75–95% rate of complete liver enzyme normalization by 12–24 months [1,27].

7. Dermatitis Herpetiformis

Dermatitis Herpetiformis (DH) is rather rare in pediatric celiac patients with rates of roughly 5% or less. DH is a bilateral, itching, blistering skin disease that typically presents as a rash on the elbows, knees, and buttocks. The diagnosis is confirmed by a skin biopsy with direct immunofluorescence demonstrating granular immunoglobulin A (IgA) deposits in the papillary dermis. The majority (but not all) of these patients will also have celiac specific enteropathy in the small intestine at diagnosis as well. The rash responds well to a strict GFD with near 100% rates or resolution in children [1,28]. While some may receive additional medical therapy with diamino-diphenyl sulfone (dapsone) at diagnosis, most celiac patients can be successfully weaned off the medication with time and remain well controlled on a gluten free diet alone [28].

8. Arthralgia/Arthritis

Musculoskeletal manifestations, including arthralgia and arthritis, are seen in roughly 5–10% of new celiac pediatric patients [1]. In a paper by Garg et al. in 2017, the authors investigated the prevalence of early joint involvement in children with CD through the use of musculoskeletal ultrasound, which is felt to be superior to conventional radiology in detecting a wide array of early inflammatory and structural abnormalities in joints. They compared children aged 2–18 with newly diagnosed CD on a strict GFD as compared to children with CD who had been on a GFD for at least six months. Ultrasonographic assessment showed the presence of at least one abnormality in the joints of 32% of newly diagnosed celiac patients as compared to only 3% of those on the diet for at least six months. The most frequently involved joint was the knee with findings, including joint effusion, synovial hypertrophy, and joint effusion with synovitis. Other joints, less often affected, included the hip and ankle. Interestingly, the majority of patients with ultrasonographic evidence of joint abnormalities were asymptomatic, suggesting a subclinical synovitis. The lower rates of joint involvement found in children on a GFD for more than six months is suggestive that the GFD may lead to improvements in the joint abnormalities associated with CD [29]. Limitations of this study included the small sample size and lack of healthy controls for comparison, though. To better understand the rates of subclinical synovitis in the healthy population, Breton et al. in 2011 assessed 41 healthy control pediatric patients, none of whom showed signs of subclinical synovitis evaluated by musculoskeletal ultrasonography [30]. The children studied, however, were French with a mean age of nine years old as compared to Indian children with a mean age of 6 in Garg, et al.'s study, thus making this healthy control group not well suited for such a comparison.

9. Headaches, Peripheral Neuropathy, Ataxia and Epilepsy

While headaches can be seen in up to 20–30% of children with new CD, rates of peripheral neuropathy and epilepsy are rarer. While these diseases may occur simultaneously by chance, there are several reports demonstrating neurological improvement following the introduction of a strict gluten free diet supporting a causative association.

Headaches are the most common neurological symptoms seen in pediatric CD. The exact mechanism by which CD leads to headaches in is unclear, but it is speculated that it may be secondary to a lack of vitamins, macro elements, such as magnesium [31], low levels of serotonin [32], which are the direct result of the celiac associated malabsorption. An alternate hypothesis is that the impaired immune response results in an imbalance of pro-inflammatory cytokines in response to ingested gluten, leading to altered vascular tone, and subsequently, the onset of the headache [33]. Most pediatric patients show excellent rates of headache improvement on a strict GFD, approaching 100% [1,34,35].

The most common neuropathy noted in CD is chronic, symmetric distal neuropathy, but autonomic neuropathy, chronic inflammatory demyelinating neuropathy, acute inflammatory demyelinating neuropathy (Guillain-Barre syndrome), and mononeuritis multiplex have also been described [36]. Rates of peripheral neuropathy in pediatric CD range form 0.1–7.4% [37–39]. It is speculated there may be an autoimmune cause for the neuropathy as many studies have located anti-ganglioside antibodies in these patients [40]. It is also possible that the nutritional deficiencies common to CD patients may account for the neuropathy. There has been great discrepancy as to the effectiveness of the GFD on resolution of peripheral neuropathies in celiac disease, ranging from findings of great symptom improvement [41], to only subjective improvements [42], to little to no improvements at all [43]. Intravenous immunoglobulin, plasmapheresis and etanercept do not appear to be effective in celiac related peripheral neuropathies [42].

While cerebellar ataxia is a well-recognized extra-intestinal manifestation of CD in adults occurring in as many as 40% of adult CD patients, it is far less common in children with rates that are closer to 0.068–1.79% [44–46]. The clinical presentation is indistinguishable from other forms of cerebellar ataxia with progressive unsteadiness of the gait and limbs. Both sexes appear to be affected equally, the mean age of onset is 53 years, and cerebellar atrophy can be detected by brain magnetic resonance imaging (MRI) in a vast number of adult patients as well [47]. On the contrary cerebellar atrophy appears to be exceptionally rare in children. While children are more prone to developing unilateral or bilateral focal hyper-intense white matter lesions, actual cerebellar atrophy is very uncommon [45,46]. The severity of cerebellar atrophy appears to correlate with the duration of exposure to gluten likely explaining the decreased rates and severity of cerebellar atrophy seen in children [48]. Similar to other neurologic manifestations in celiac patients, the effects of the GFD on recovery are highly variable [49], and if there have been no improvements on the diet within a year or the ataxia is rapidly progressive, the use of intravenous immunoglobulins has been reported to provide possible benefits [50].

Most pediatric studies have failed to find and increase the prevalence of epilepsy in CD as compared with the general population [37]. Epilepsy specifically associated with cerebral calcifications, though, has been associated with CD. It was first reported in the pediatric literature in 1994 by Pascotto, et al. who described four separate patients with epilepsy with cerebral calcifications refractory to medical management, followed between 1980 and 1990 at the Clinic of Child Neuropsychiatry of

Naples University. Despite extensive testing, an origin for the calcifications was not discovered. These patients later underwent celiac testing, 1 for failure to thrive (FTT), while the other three had no obvious gastrointestinal complaints. Two of the four patients, including the patient with FTT, had elevated titers of immunoglobulin A (IgA) and Immunoglobulin G (IgG) antigliadin antibodies and also demonstrated histologic findings of crypt hyperplasia, alterations of superficial epithelium with picnotic, cubic cells, and remarkable lymphoplasmacellular infiltration, as is consistent with the diagnosis of celiac disease. Following diagnosis, these two patients started a strict GFD with reverse of the FTT and initial improvements in the seizure frequency, but worsened again roughly six months later [51]. A subsequent, similar case report was published in 2012. In this case, the child was positive for endomysial (EMA) immunoglobulin IgA, gliadin (DGP) IgA, and IgG and transglutaminase (tTG) two IgA and IgG antibodies. Endoscopic biopsies showed subtotal villous atrophy in the duodenum confirming the diagnosis. Additionally, high levels of antibodies to tTG six IgA and EMA (IgA) were also found in the cerebrospinal fluid. The child was placed on a GFD and was seizure free for 18 months at the time of the publication of the paper [52].

10. Behavioral Changes and Psychiatric Disorders

A wide range of psychiatric symptoms and disorders have been associated with CD, including anxiety disorders, depressive disorders, attention deficit hyperactivity disorders (ADHD), and autism spectrum disorders (ASD). While psychiatric disorders that occur after the diagnosis of celiac disease has been made are more often associated with an impaired quality of life and difficulty adapting to the chronic nature of the disease [53], psychiatric disorders that occur prior to the diagnosis of celiac disease have been hypothesized to be related to disease related cerebral hypoperfusion [54], proinflammatory cytokines [55], and low folate levels [56]. We will focus on anxiety and depressive disorders within this review as to date, no greater rates of ADHD and ASD have been found in the celiac population as compared to the general population [57–59].

Rates of psychiatric disorders, including anxiety and depression, in pediatric celiac patients range from 5–10% [1,60], substantially lower than those found in adults [61]. A recent study by Smith et al. in 2018 examined maternal reports of their children's psychological functioning over 3.5 years in celiac children aged 2–3 years who were persistently positive for tTG IgA as compared to children with normalized tTG IgA. These serology results were obtained in a retrospective manner by sampling of stored blood. The mothers were blinded to the results of the serological testing. Mothers completed the Achenbach Child Behavior Checklist, a well-validate questionnaire to measure behavioral and emotional function in preschoolers aged 1.5–5 years old. There was a statistically significant difference in the scores from mothers of celiac children with persistently elevated tTG IgA as compared to those with normalized tTG IgA. Celiac children with persistently elevated tTG IgA scored significantly higher for anxiety, depression, aggressive behaviors, and sleep problems. Initiation of the GFD did not appear to have an impact on the psychological functioning of the patients in this study (though very young children) [62]. Another study by Simsek et al. in 2015 assessed the rates of psychiatric symptoms in newly diagnosed celiac pediatric patients aged 9 to 16 years old as compared to age and sex matched healthy controls that had presented for routine checkup. On the contrary to the previous study, this study showed no statistically significant differences between depression scores in newly diagnosed CD patients and controls, though there were statistically lower scores on emotional well within the CD patients as compared to the controls. Patients on a strict GFD showed significant reductions in follow up depression scores as compared to patients that were non-compliant with the diet [63]. There have been very mixed results, though, on improvements in depression once on a GFD ranging from no change in depression [53], to moderate improvements in depression [1], to complete resolution of depression [64].

11. Alopecia

While alopecia has an association with pediatric CD, it is one of the less common extra-intestinal manifestations seen, occurring in roughly 1% of patients [1]. It is presumed to occur through an autoimmune reaction involving T-cell dysregulation and can lead to patchy loss of skull hair (alopecia areata), total loss of skull and facial hair (alopecia totalis), and total loss of full body hair (alopecia universalis). It is speculated that there are autoantibodies directed against anagen-stage hair follicle structures and a direct association with the human leukocyte antigen (HLA)-DQB1*0201 allele. A number of studies have assessed the involvement of alopecia areata in CD patients. Rates of alopecia areata appear to be equally distributed between male and female celiac patients, roughly 40% have a coinciding alternate autoimmune disorder, 70% had gastrointestinal symptoms in addition to the alopecia, and 100% of patients had positive celiac serologies (tTG IgA or EMA IgA) with subtotal or total villous atrophy on duodenal biopsies. Trials of oral zinc and other topical treatments were attempted with minimal response. Of the patients who started a strict GFD, 26% had no regrowth, 22% had a partial regrowth, and 52% had the complete regrowth of hair by 12–24 months (most within the first 2–3 months). All of the patients had a normalization of their celiac serologies and duodenal biopsies by 24 months, despite the growth or lack of growth of hair. Younger patients and shorter lag times between the onset of alopecia areata and initiation of the GFD led to a more favorable hair growth response. Sex, lack of GI symptoms, and the severity of biopsy results did not appear to impact whether a patient would or would not have regrowth of hair [65–71].

12. Treatment of the Extra-Intestinal Manifestations of CD

Strict, lifelong adherence to a GFD remains the only available treatment for patients that are diagnosed with CD, and, as stated previously, should result in a complete return to health in the majority of patients, especially pediatric. Other pharmacological therapies are being evaluated for the treatment of CD, including enzymes, to inactivate immunogenic gluten peptides in the human gastrointestinal tract [72], agents that sequester gluten in the lumen [73], modulators of gut permeability [74], and of antigen presentation and immune responses, including those that block tTG [75] and HLA [76], IL-15 inhibitors [77], and the development of vaccines that are able to induce oral tolerance to gluten [78]. Of these treatment options, the only one that is currently on the market is the gluten-specific enzyme, GliadinX (AN-PEP). Unfortunately, it is only capable of detoxifying 0.2 g of gluten or roughly that of 1/8 of a slice of gluten-containing bread. For this reason, it should only be used as an adjunct to the GFD when there are concerns for accidental gluten contamination and in an effort to ameliorate symptoms, not as a replacement for the GFD.

While these pharmacological options are promising, it is still unclear how well they will work to minimize gut inflammation and alleviate gastrointestinal, and, the even more complex extra-intestinal manifestations of CD. While it is likely that some of the alternatives may come to fruition in the next year or two, a true "cure", although certainly possible, might take much longer [79].

Conflicts of Interest: The authors declare no conflict of interest.

References

1. Jericho, H.; Sansotta, N.; Guandalini, S. Extraintestinal Manifestations of Celiac Disease: Effectiveness of the Gluten-Free Diet. *J. Pediatr. Gastroenterol. Nutr.* **2017**, *65*, 75–79. [CrossRef] [PubMed]
2. Nurminen, S.; Kivela, L.; Huhtala, H.; Kaukinen, K.; Kurppa, K. Extraintestinal manifestations were common in children with coeliac disease and were more prevalent in patients with more severe clinical and histological presentation. *Acta Paediatr.* **2018**. [CrossRef] [PubMed]
3. Knowles, C.H.; Aziz, Q. Basic and clinical aspects of gastrointestinal pain. *Pain* **2009**, *141*, 191–209. [CrossRef] [PubMed]
4. Sansotta, N.; Amirikian, K.; Guandalini, S.; Jericho, H. Celiac Disease Symptom Resolution: Effectiveness of the Gluten-free Diet. *J. Pediatr. Gastroenterol. Nutr.* **2018**, *66*, 48–52. [CrossRef] [PubMed]

5. Traggiai, C.; Stanhope, R. Disorders of pubertal development. *Best Pract. Res. Clin. Obstet. Gynaecol.* **2003**, *17*, 41–56. [CrossRef] [PubMed]
6. Majorana, A.; Bardellini, E.; Ravelli, A.; Plebani, A.; Polimeni, A.; Campus, G. Implications of gluten exposure period, CD clinical forms, and HLA typing in the association between celiac disease and dental enamel defects in children. A case-control study. *Int. J. Paediatr. Dent.* **2010**, *20*, 119–124. [CrossRef] [PubMed]
7. Pastore, L.; Carroccio, A.; Compilato, D.; Panzarella, V.; Serpico, R.; Lo Muzio, L. Oral manifestations of celiac disease. *J. Clin. Gastroenterol.* **2008**, *42*, 224–232. [CrossRef] [PubMed]
8. Aine, L. Dental enamel defects and dental maturity in children and adolescents with coeliac disease. *Proc. Finn. Dent. Soc.* **1986**, *82* (Suppl. 3), 1–71. [PubMed]
9. Campisi, G.; Di Liberto, C.; Iacono, G.; Compilato, D.; Di Prima, L.; Calvino, F.; Di Marco, V.; Lo Muzio, L.; Sferrazza, C.; Scalici, C.; et al. Oral pathology in untreated coeliac [corrected] disease. *Aliment. Pharmacol. Ther.* **2007**, *26*, 1529–1536. [CrossRef] [PubMed]
10. Krzywicka, B.; Herman, K.; Kowalczyk-Zajac, M.; Pytrus, T. Celiac disease and its impact on the oral health status—Review of the literature. *Adv. Clin. Exp. Med.* **2014**, *23*, 675–681. [CrossRef] [PubMed]
11. Mina, S.; Riga, C.; Azcurra, A.I.; Brunotto, M. Oral ecosystem alterations in celiac children: A follow-up study. *Arch. Oral Biol.* **2012**, *57*, 154–160. [CrossRef] [PubMed]
12. Sedghizadeh, P.P.; Shuler, C.F.; Allen, C.M.; Beck, F.M.; Kalmar, J.R. Celiac disease and recurrent aphthous stomatitis: A report and review of the literature. *Oral Surg. Oral Med. Oral Pathol. Oral Radiol. Endod.* **2002**, *94*, 474–478. [CrossRef] [PubMed]
13. Eguia-del Valle, A.; Martinez-Conde-Llamasas, R.; Lopez-Vicente, J.; Uribarri-Etxebarria, A.; Aguirre-Urizar, J.M. Salivary levels of Tumour Necrosis Factor-alpha in patients with recurrent aphthous stomatitis. *Med. Oral Patol. Oral Cir. Bucal* **2011**, *16*, e33–e36. [CrossRef] [PubMed]
14. Teitelbaum, S.L. Bone resorption by osteoclasts. *Science* **2000**, *289*, 1504–1508. [CrossRef] [PubMed]
15. Selby, P.L.; Davies, M.; Adams, J.E.; Mawer, E.B. Bone loss in celiac disease is related to secondary hyperparathyroidism. *J. Bone Miner. Res.* **1999**, *14*, 652–657. [CrossRef] [PubMed]
16. Fornari, M.C.; Pedreira, S.; Niveloni, S.; Gonzalez, D.; Diez, R.A.; Vazquez, H.; Mazure, R.; Sugai, E.; Smecuol, E.; Boerr, L.; et al. Pre- and post-treatment serum levels of cytokines IL-1beta, IL-6, and IL-1 receptor antagonist in celiac disease. Are they related to the associated osteopenia? *Am. J. Gastroenterol.* **1998**, *93*, 413–418. [CrossRef] [PubMed]
17. Tilg, H.; Moschen, A.R.; Kaser, A.; Pines, A.; Dotan, I. Gut, inflammation and osteoporosis: Basic and clinical concepts. *Gut* **2008**, *57*, 684–694. [CrossRef] [PubMed]
18. Garrote, J.A.; Gomez-Gonzalez, E.; Bernardo, D.; Arranz, E.; Chirdo, F. Celiac disease pathogenesis: The proinflammatory cytokine network. *J. Pediatr. Gastroenterol. Nutr.* **2008**, *47* (Suppl. 1), S27–S32. [CrossRef] [PubMed]
19. Mora, S. Celiac disease in children: Impact on bone health. *Rev. Endocr. Metab. Disord.* **2008**, *9*, 123–130. [CrossRef] [PubMed]
20. Fiore, C.E.; Pennisi, P.; Ferro, G.; Ximenes, B.; Privitelli, L.; Mangiafico, R.A.; Santoro, F.; Parisi, N.; Lombardo, T. Altered osteoprotegerin/RANKL ratio and low bone mineral density in celiac patients on long-term treatment with gluten-free diet. *Horm. Metab. Res.* **2006**, *38*, 417–422. [CrossRef] [PubMed]
21. Choudhary, G.; Gupta, R.K.; Beniwal, J. Bone Mineral Density in Celiac Disease. *Indian J. Pediatr.* **2017**, *84*, 344–348. [CrossRef] [PubMed]
22. Caraceni, M.P.; Molteni, N.; Bardella, M.T.; Ortolani, S.; Nogara, A.; Bianchi, P.A. Bone and mineral metabolism in adult celiac disease. *Am. J. Gastroenterol.* **1988**, *83*, 274–277. [PubMed]
23. Kalayci, A.G.; Kansu, A.; Girgin, N.; Kucuk, O.; Aras, G. Bone mineral density and importance of a gluten-free diet in patients with celiac disease in childhood. *Pediatrics* **2001**, *108*, E89. [CrossRef] [PubMed]
24. Deora, V.; Aylward, N.; Sokoro, A.; El-Matary, W. Serum Vitamins and Minerals at Diagnosis and Follow-up in Children With Celiac Disease. *J. Pediatr. Gastroenterol. Nutr.* **2017**, *65*, 185–189. [CrossRef] [PubMed]
25. Bonamico, M.; Pitzalis, G.; Culasso, F.; Vania, A.; Monti, S.; Benedetti, C.; Mariani, P.; Signoretti, A. Hepatic damage in celiac disease in children. *Miner. Pediatr.* **1986**, *38*, 959–962.
26. Schwabe, R.F.; Seki, E.; Brenner, D.A. Toll-like receptor signaling in the liver. *Gastroenterology* **2006**, *130*, 1886–1900. [CrossRef] [PubMed]

27. Novacek, G.; Miehsler, W.; Wrba, F.; Ferenci, P.; Penner, E.; Vogelsang, H. Prevalence and clinical importance of hypertransaminasaemia in coeliac disease. *Eur. J. Gastroenterol. Hepatol.* **1999**, *11*, 283–288. [CrossRef] [PubMed]

28. Fry, L.; Seah, P.P.; Riches, D.J.; Hoffbrand, A.V. Clearance of skin lesions in dermatitis herpetiformis after gluten withdrawal. *Lancet* **1973**, *1*, 288–291. [CrossRef]

29. Garg, K.; Agarwal, P.; Gupta, R.K.; Sitaraman, S. Joint Involvement in Children with Celiac Disease. *Indian Pediatr.* **2017**, *54*, 946–948. [CrossRef] [PubMed]

30. Breton, S.; Jousse-Joulin, S.; Cangemi, C.; de Parscau, L.; Colin, D.; Bressolette, L.; Saraux, A.; Devauchelle-Pensec, V. Comparison of clinical and ultrasonographic evaluations for peripheral synovitis in juvenile idiopathic arthritis. *Semin. Arthritis Rheum.* **2011**, *41*, 272–278. [CrossRef] [PubMed]

31. Lionetti, V.; Bianchi, G.; Recchia, F.A.; Ventura, C. Control of autocrine and paracrine myocardial signals: An emerging therapeutic strategy in heart failure. *Heart Fail. Rev.* **2010**, *15*, 531–542. [CrossRef] [PubMed]

32. Jernej, B.; Vladic, A.; Cicin-Sain, L.; Hranilovic, D.; Banovic, M.; Balija, M.; Bilic, E.; Sucic, Z.; Vukadin, S.; Grgicevic, D. Platelet serotonin measures in migraine. *Headache* **2002**, *42*, 588–595. [CrossRef] [PubMed]

33. Gabrielli, M.; Cremonini, F.; Fiore, G.; Addolorato, G.; Padalino, C.; Candelli, M.; De Leo, M.E.; Santarelli, L.; Giacovazzo, M.; Gasbarrini, A.; et al. Association between migraine and Celiac disease: Results from a preliminary case-control and therapeutic study. *Am. J. Gastroenterol.* **2003**, *98*, 625–629. [CrossRef] [PubMed]

34. Zelnik, N.; Pacht, A.; Obeid, R.; Lerner, A. Range of neurologic disorders in patients with celiac disease. *Pediatrics* **2004**, *113*, 1672–1676. [CrossRef] [PubMed]

35. Nenna, R.; Petrarca, L.; Verdecchia, P.; Florio, M.; Pietropaoli, N.; Mastrogiorgio, G.; Bavastrelli, M.; Bonamico, M.; Cucchiara, S. Celiac disease in a large cohort of children and adolescents with recurrent headache: A retrospective study. *Dig. Liver Dis.* **2016**, *48*, 495–498. [CrossRef] [PubMed]

36. Thawani, S.P.; Brannagan, T.H., 3rd; Lebwohl, B.; Green, P.H.; Ludvigsson, J.F. Risk of Neuropathy Among 28,232 Patients With Biopsy-Verified Celiac Disease. *JAMA Neurol.* **2015**, *72*, 806–811. [CrossRef] [PubMed]

37. Cakir, D.; Tosun, A.; Polat, M.; Celebisoy, N.; Gokben, S.; Aydogdu, S.; Yagci, R.V.; Tekgul, H. Subclinical neurological abnormalities in children with celiac disease receiving a gluten-free diet. *J. Pediatr. Gastroenterol. Nutr.* **2007**, *45*, 366–369. [CrossRef] [PubMed]

38. Ruggieri, M.; Incorpora, G.; Polizzi, A.; Parano, E.; Spina, M.; Pavone, P. Low prevalence of neurologic and psychiatric manifestations in children with gluten sensitivity. *J. Pediatr.* **2008**, *152*, 244–249. [CrossRef] [PubMed]

39. Lionetti, E.; Francavilla, R.; Pavone, P.; Pavone, L.; Francavilla, T.; Pulvirenti, A.; Giugno, R.; Ruggieri, M. The neurology of coeliac disease in childhood: What is the evidence? A systematic review and meta-analysis. *Dev. Med. Child Neurol.* **2010**, *52*, 700–707. [CrossRef] [PubMed]

40. Alaedini, A.; Green, P.H.; Sander, H.W.; Hays, A.P.; Gamboa, E.T.; Fasano, A.; Sonnenberg, M.; Lewis, L.D.; Latov, N. Ganglioside reactive antibodies in the neuropathy associated with celiac disease. *J. Neuroimmunol.* **2002**, *127*, 145–148. [CrossRef]

41. Polizzi, A.; Finocchiaro, M.; Parano, E.; Pavone, P.; Musumeci, S.; Polizzi, A. Recurrent peripheral neuropathy in a girl with celiac disease. *J. Neurol. Neurosurg. Psychiatry* **2000**, *68*, 104–105. [CrossRef] [PubMed]

42. Chin, R.L.; Sander, H.W.; Brannagan, T.H.; Green, P.H.; Hays, A.P.; Alaedini, A.; Latov, N. Celiac neuropathy. *Neurology* **2003**, *60*, 1581–1585. [CrossRef] [PubMed]

43. Simonati, A.; Battistella, P.A.; Guariso, G.; Clementi, M.; Rizzuto, N. Coeliac disease associated with peripheral neuropathy in a child: A case report. *Neuropediatrics* **1998**, *29*, 155–158. [CrossRef] [PubMed]

44. Chin, R.L.; Latov, N.; Green, P.H.; Brannagan, T.H., 3rd; Alaedini, A.; Sander, H.W. Neurologic complications of celiac disease. *J. Clin. Neuromuscul. Dis.* **2004**, *5*, 129–137. [CrossRef] [PubMed]

45. Hadjivassiliou, M.; Grunewald, R.A.; Chattopadhyay, A.K.; Davies-Jones, G.A.; Gibson, A.; Jarratt, J.A.; Kandler, R.H.; Lobo, A.; Powell, T.; Smith, C.M. Clinical, radiological, neurophysiological, and neuropathological characteristics of gluten ataxia. *Lancet* **1998**, *352*, 1582–1585. [CrossRef]

46. Gobbi, G. Coeliac disease, epilepsy and cerebral calcifications. *Brain Dev.* **2005**, *27*, 189–200. [CrossRef] [PubMed]

47. Green, P.H.; Alaedini, A.; Sander, H.W.; Brannagan, T.H., 3rd; Latov, N.; Chin, R.L. Mechanisms underlying celiac disease and its neurologic manifestations. *Cell. Mol. Life Sci. CMLS* **2005**, *62*, 791–799. [CrossRef] [PubMed]

48. Collin, P.; Pirttila, T.; Nurmikko, T.; Somer, H.; Erila, T.; Keyrilainen, O. Celiac disease, brain atrophy, and dementia. *Neurology* **1991**, *41*, 372–375. [CrossRef] [PubMed]

49. Bushara, K.O. Neurologic presentation of celiac disease. *Gastroenterology* **2005**, *128*, S92–S97. [CrossRef] [PubMed]

50. Burk, K.; Melms, A.; Schulz, J.B.; Dichgans, J. Effectiveness of intravenous immunoglobin therapy in cerebellar ataxia associated with gluten sensitivity. *Ann. Neurol.* **2001**, *50*, 827–828. [CrossRef] [PubMed]

51. Pascotto, A.; Coppola, G.; Ecuba, P.; Liguori, G.; Guandalini, S. Epilepsy and Occipital Calcifications with or without celiac disease: Report of four cases. *J. Epilepsy* **1994**, *7*, 130–136. [CrossRef]

52. Johnson, A.M.; Dale, R.C.; Wienholt, L.; Hadjivassiliou, M.; Aeschlimann, D.; Lawson, J.A. Coeliac disease, epilepsy, and cerebral calcifications: Association with TG6 autoantibodies. *Dev. Med. Child Neurol.* **2013**, *55*, 90–93. [CrossRef] [PubMed]

53. Fera, T.; Cascio, B.; Angelini, G.; Martini, S.; Guidetti, C.S. Affective disorders and quality of life in adult coeliac disease patients on a gluten-free diet. *Eur. J. Gastroenterol. Hepatol.* **2003**, *15*, 1287–1292. [CrossRef] [PubMed]

54. Addolorato, G.; Di Giuda, D.; De Rossi, G.; Valenza, V.; Domenicali, M.; Caputo, F.; Gasbarrini, A.; Capristo, E.; Gasbarrini, G. Regional cerebral hypoperfusion in patients with celiac disease. *Am. J. Med.* **2004**, *116*, 312–317. [CrossRef] [PubMed]

55. Manavalan, J.S.; Hernandez, L.; Shah, J.G.; Konikkara, J.; Naiyer, A.J.; Lee, A.R.; Ciaccio, E.; Minaya, M.T.; Green, P.H.; Bhagat, G. Serum cytokine elevations in celiac disease: Association with disease presentation. *Hum. Immunol.* **2010**, *71*, 50–57. [CrossRef] [PubMed]

56. Saibeni, S.; Lecchi, A.; Meucci, G.; Cattaneo, M.; Tagliabue, L.; Rondonotti, E.; Formenti, S.; De Franchis, R.; Vecchi, M. Prevalence of hyperhomocysteinemia in adult gluten-sensitive enteropathy at diagnosis: Role of B12, folate, and genetics. *Clin. Gastroenterol. Hepatol.* **2005**, *3*, 574–580. [CrossRef]

57. Ludvigsson, J.F.; Reichenberg, A.; Hultman, C.M.; Murray, J.A. A nationwide study of the association between celiac disease and the risk of autistic spectrum disorders. *JAMA Psychiatry* **2013**, *70*, 1224–1230. [CrossRef] [PubMed]

58. Jozefczuk, J.; Konopka, E.; Bierla, J.B.; Trojanowska, I.; Sowinska, A.; Czarnecki, R.; Sobol, L.; Jozefczuk, P.; Surdy, W.; Cukrowska, B. The Occurrence of Antibodies Against Gluten in Children with Autism Spectrum Disorders Does Not Correlate with Serological Markers of Impaired Intestinal Permeability. *J. Med. Food* **2018**, *21*, 181–187. [CrossRef] [PubMed]

59. Kumperscak, H.G.; Rebec, Z.K.; Sobocan, S.; Fras, V.T.; Dolinsek, J. Prevalence of Celiac Disease Is Not Increased in ADHD Sample. *J. Atten. Disord.* **2016**. [CrossRef] [PubMed]

60. Butwicka, A.; Lichtenstein, P.; Frisen, L.; Almqvist, C.; Larsson, H.; Ludvigsson, J.F. Celiac Disease Is Associated with Childhood Psychiatric Disorders: A Population-Based Study. *J. Pediatr.* **2017**, *184*, 87–93. [CrossRef] [PubMed]

61. Ciacci, C.; Iovino, P.; Amoruso, D.; Siniscalchi, M.; Tortora, R.; Di Gilio, A.; Fusco, M.; Mazzacca, G. Grown-up coeliac children: The effects of only a few years on a gluten-free diet in childhood. *Aliment. Pharmacol. Ther.* **2005**, *21*, 421–429. [CrossRef] [PubMed]

62. Smith, L.B.; Lynch, K.F.; Kurppa, K.; Koletzko, S.; Krischer, J.; Liu, E.; Johnson, S.B.; Agardh, D.; TEDDY Study Group. Psychological Manifestations of Celiac Disease Autoimmunity in Young Children. *Pediatrics* **2017**, *139*. [CrossRef] [PubMed]

63. Simsek, S.; Baysoy, G.; Gencoglan, S.; Uluca, U. Effects of Gluten-Free Diet on Quality of Life and Depression in Children With Celiac Disease. *J. Pediatr. Gastroenterol. Nutr.* **2015**, *61*, 303–306. [CrossRef] [PubMed]

64. Pynnonen, P.A.; Isometsa, E.T.; Verkasalo, M.A.; Kahkonen, S.A.; Sipila, I.; Savilahti, E.; Aalberg, V.A. Gluten-free diet may alleviate depressive and behavioural symptoms in adolescents with coeliac disease: A prospective follow-up case-series study. *BMC Psychiatry* **2005**, *5*, 14. [CrossRef] [PubMed]

65. Ertekin, V.; Tosun, M.S.; Erdem, T. Screening of celiac disease in children with alopecia areata. *Indian J. Dermatol.* **2014**, *59*, 317. [CrossRef] [PubMed]

66. Corazza, G.R.; Andreani, M.L.; Venturo, N.; Bernardi, M.; Tosti, A.; Gasbarrini, G. Celiac disease and alopecia areata: Report of a new association. *Gastroenterology* **1995**, *109*, 1333–1337. [CrossRef]

67. Volta, U.; Bardazzi, F.; Zauli, D.; DeFranceschi, L.; Tosti, A.; Molinaro, N.; Ghetti, S.; Tetta, C.; Grassi, A.; Bianchi, F.B. Serological screening for coeliac disease in vitiligo and alopecia areata. *Br. J. Dermatol.* **1997**, *136*, 801–802. [CrossRef] [PubMed]

68. Barbato, M.; Viola, F.; Grillo, R.; Franchin, L.; Lo Russo, L.; Lucarelli, S.; Frediani, T.; Mazzilli, M.C.; Cardi, E. Alopecia and coeliac disease: Report of two patients showing response to gluten-free diet. *Clin. Exp. Dermatol.* **1998**, *23*, 236–237. [CrossRef] [PubMed]

69. Storm, W. Celiac disease and alopecia areata in a child with Down's syndrome. *J. Intellect. Disabil. Res. JIDR* **2000**, *44*, 621–623. [CrossRef] [PubMed]

70. Bardella, M.T.; Marino, R.; Barbareschi, M.; Bianchi, F.; Faglia, G.; Bianchi, P. Alopecia areata and coeliac disease: No effect of a gluten-free diet on hair growth. *Dermatology* **2000**, *200*, 108–110. [CrossRef] [PubMed]

71. Fessatou, S.; Kostaki, M.; Karpathios, T. Coeliac disease and alopecia areata in childhood. *J. Paediatr. Child Health* **2003**, *39*, 152–154. [CrossRef] [PubMed]

72. Shan, L.; Molberg, O.; Parrot, I.; Hausch, F.; Filiz, F.; Gray, G.M.; Sollid, L.M.; Khosla, C. Structural basis for gluten intolerance in celiac sprue. *Science* **2002**, *297*, 2275–2279. [CrossRef] [PubMed]

73. Dickey, W.; Kearney, N. Overweight in celiac disease: Prevalence, clinical characteristics, and effect of a gluten-free diet. *Am. J. Gastroenterol.* **2006**, *101*, 2356–2359. [CrossRef] [PubMed]

74. Pinier, M.; Verdu, E.F.; Nasser-Eddine, M.; David, C.S.; Vezina, A.; Rivard, N.; Leroux, J.C. Polymeric binders suppress gliadin-induced toxicity in the intestinal epithelium. *Gastroenterology* **2009**, *136*, 288–298. [CrossRef] [PubMed]

75. Rauhavirta, T.; Oittinen, M.; Kivisto, R.; Mannisto, P.T.; Garcia-Horsman, J.A.; Wang, Z.; Griffin, M.; Maki, M.; Kaukinen, K.; Lindfors, K. Are transglutaminase 2 inhibitors able to reduce gliadin-induced toxicity related to celiac disease? A proof-of-concept study. *J. Clin. Immunol.* **2013**, *33*, 134–142. [CrossRef] [PubMed]

76. Kapoerchan, V.V.; Wiesner, M.; Overhand, M.; van der Marel, G.A.; Koning, F.; Overkleeft, H.S. Design of azidoproline containing gluten peptides to suppress CD4+ T-cell responses associated with celiac disease. *Bioorg. Med. Chem.* **2008**, *16*, 2053–2062. [CrossRef] [PubMed]

77. Waldmann, T.A.; Conlon, K.C.; Stewart, D.M.; Worthy, T.A.; Janik, J.E.; Fleisher, T.A.; Albert, P.S.; Figg, W.D.; Spencer, S.D.; Raffeld, M.; et al. Phase 1 trial of IL-15 trans presentation blockade using humanized Mikbeta1 mAb in patients with T-cell large granular lymphocytic leukemia. *Blood* **2013**, *121*, 476–484. [CrossRef] [PubMed]

78. Tye-Din, J.A.; Stewart, J.A.; Dromey, J.A.; Beissbarth, T.; van Heel, D.A.; Tatham, A.; Henderson, K.; Mannering, S.I.; Gianfrani, C.; Jewell, D.P.; et al. Comprehensive, quantitative mapping of T cell epitopes in gluten in celiac disease. *Sci. Transl. Med.* **2010**, *2*, 41ra51. [CrossRef] [PubMed]

79. McCarville, J.L.; Caminero, A.; Verdu, E.F. Pharmacological approaches in celiac disease. *Curr. Opin. Pharmacol.* **2015**, *25*, 7–12. [CrossRef] [PubMed]

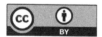

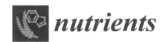

Review

Cutaneous and Mucosal Manifestations Associated with Celiac Disease

Luis Rodrigo [1,*], Valia Beteta-Gorriti [2], Nuria Alvarez [1], Celia Gómez de Castro [2], Alvaro de Dios [2], Laura Palacios [2] and Jorge Santos-Juanes [2,3,*]

[1] Gastroenterology Unit, Hospital Universitario Central de Asturias (HUCA), Avda. de Roma s/n, 33011 Oviedo, Asturias, Spain; nuriaalvarezh@gmail.com

[2] Dermatology Unit, Hospital Universitario Central de Asturias (HUCA), Avda. de Roma s/n, 33011 Oviedo, Asturias, Spain; valita_bg@hotmail.com (V.B.-G.); celiagomez_88@hotmail.com (C.G.d.C.); aldedivel@gmail.com (A.d.D.); llaurinapalacios@hotmail.com (L.P.)

[3] Facultad de Medicina, Universidad de Oviedo, 33003 Oviedo, Asturias, Spain

* Correspondence: lrrodrigo@uniovi.es (L.R.); santosjjorge@uniovi.es (J.S.-J.); Tel.: +34-985-23-44-16 (L.R.)

Received: 9 May 2018; Accepted: 18 June 2018; Published: 21 June 2018

Abstract: Celiac disease (CD) is an immune-mediated, gluten-induced enteropathy that affects predisposed individuals of all ages. Many patients with CD do not report gastrointestinal symptoms making it difficult to reach an early diagnosis. On the other hand, CD is related to a wide spectrum of extra-intestinal manifestations, with dermatitis herpetiformis (DH) being the best characterized. These associated conditions may be the clue to reaching the diagnosis of CD. Over the last few years, there have been multiple reports of the association between CD and several cutaneous manifestations that may improve with a gluten-free diet (GFD). The presence of some of these skin diseases, even in the absence of gastrointestinal symptoms, should give rise to an appropriate screening method for CD. The aim of this paper is to describe the different cutaneous manifestations that have been associated with CD and the possible mechanisms involved.

Keywords: celiac disease; dermatitis herpetiformis; urticaria; atopic dermatitis; psoriasis; recurrent aphtous ulceration; rosacea; alopecia areata; cutaneous vasculitis; gluten-free diet

1. Introduction

Celiac disease (CD) is a chronic autoimmune systemic disease associated with an enteropathy triggered by gluten intake which affects genetically predisposed individuals of both sexes and can develop at any age. Gluten and its major protein fractions, gliadin and glutenin, are present in wheat, rye, barley, oats, related species and hybrids, and processed foods [1]. Almost all patients with CD present the human leukocyte antigen (HLA) DQ2 (>90%) or HLA DQ8 (5–10%); nevertheless, up to 40% of people in the Americas, Europe, and Southeast Asia also carry these alleles, indicating that these genes are necessary but not sufficient for CD development [2]. The findings of inflammatory changes in intestinal biopsies, ranging from lymphocytic enteritis to various degrees of villous atrophy, are the gold standard for CD diagnosis, even in the presence of a negative serology for CD. IgA anti-tissue transglutaminases are the most sensitive and cost-effective antibodies for the diagnosis of CD, although deamidated gliadin peptide IgG antibodies might be useful in seronegative patients with innate IgA deficiency. A life-long gluten-free diet (GFD) is mandatory, achieving clinical and histological recovery in most patients [1].

In past decades, CD was considered to be an uncommon disease affecting mainly children and limited to individuals of European ancestry. Currently, we know that this disorder may be detected at any age and is regarded as one of the most common chronic diseases encountered worldwide with a prevalence of about 1–2% [3]. The mean age of adult CD diagnosis is 45 years, although up to 20% of patients are diagnosed at the age of 60 years or above. CD is probably an under-diagnosed entity in adulthood partly because many patients in this age group lack the classical symptoms, such as diarrhea or signs of malabsorption. In fact, in most adult patients, gastrointestinal symptoms are subtle or even absent, and clinical suspicion arises from extra-intestinal manifestations (non-classic or atypical CD), such as anemia, cutaneous disorders, neurological disease, osteoporosis, and abnormal liver function tests [2,4]. We emphasize the importance of considering non-typical symptoms to diagnose adult CD and actively searching extra-intestinal associated manifestations in order to start an early GFD and prevent the onset of long-term complications.

CD patients are more frequently affected by other immune-mediated disorders (ID) compared to the general population, as reported in previous studies, mainly thyroid and skin diseases and type 1 diabetes mellitus [5,6]. This observation may be partially explained by a possible spread of the adaptive immune response, initially triggered in the gastrointestinal tract, to other tissues [4,6]. Hashimoto's thyroiditis is the most frequently associated ID, followed by several skin disorders, such as psoriasis, atopic dermatitis (AD), vitiligo, systemic lupus erythematosus (SLE), alopecia areata (AA), and oral lichen planus (OLP) [6]. Interestingly, 60% of CD patients with associated thyroid disease that develop a third ID are skin related. These data suggest a relationship among the immunological systems of the thyroid, skin, and small bowel, which seem to be more susceptible to developing aberrant immunological responses against auto-antigens. [6–12].

Cutaneous manifestations associated with CD, other than dermatitis herpetiformis (DH), are poorly known. It is currently recognized that DH is an undoubted extra-intestinal manifestation of CD. In addition, there is growing evidence that supports the link between CD and several skin disorders. In 2006, Humbert et al. proposed a classification of skin diseases associated with CD, dividing them into four categories: autoimmune, allergic, inflammatory, and miscellaneous (Table 1) [9–19]. Recently, Bonciolini et al. described 17 patients affected by non-celiac gluten sensitivity with skin manifestations similar to eczema, psoriasis, and DH who did not show a specific histological pattern [20]. The only common findings in most of these patients were severe itching, the presence of C3 at the dermo–epidermal junction and rapid resolution after adopting a GFD. The authors emphasized the importance of close collaboration between gastroenterologists and dermatologists due to the multiple associations between gastrointestinal and skin disorders. In the present paper, we aim to describe the multiple skin disorders associated with CD and the possible mechanisms involved.

Table 1. Strength of evidence for the association between celiac disease and skin diseases.

Type of Mechanism	Diseases Found in Association with Celiac Disease	Relative Risk in Celiac Disease Compared to the General or Control Population [Reference]	Fortuitous Association (Sporadic Cases)
Allergic	Urticaria Chronic urticaria Atopic dermatitis	HR: 1.51 (CI = 1.36–1.68) [12] HR: 1.92 (CI = 1.48–2.48) [12] OR:3.17 (CI = 1.02–9.82) [13]	Prurigo nodularis
Inflammatory			Pityriasis rubra pilaris Erythroderma Erythema elevatum diutinum Necrolytic migratory erythema Pityriasis lichenoides Erythema nodosum
Immune-mediated	Psoriasis	HR: 1.72 (CI = 1.54–1.92) [14] OR: 1.44 (CI = 1.40–1.92) [15] OR: 3.09 (CI = 1.92–4.97) [16] IgA anti-gliadin: OR: 2.36 (CI = 1.15–4.83) [17]	

Table 1. *Cont.*

Type of Mechanism	Diseases Found in Association with Celiac Disease	Relative Risk in Celiac Disease Compared to the General or Control Population [Reference]	Fortuitous Association (Sporadic Cases)
Autoimmune			Alopecia areata Cutaneous vasculitis Ig A linear dermatosis Dermatomyositis Vitiligo Lupus erythematous Lichen sclerosus
Miscellaneous	Aphthous stomatitis Rosacea	OR: 3.79 (CI = 2.67–5.39) [18] HR: 1.46 (CI = 1.11–1.93) [19]	Cutaneous amyloidosis Annular erythema Partial lipodystrophy Generalized acquired cutis laxa Icthyosis Transverse leukonychia Porphyria Hypertricosis lanuginosa

GFD: gluten-free diet; CD: celiac disease; HR: hazard ratio; OR: odds ratio; CI: 95% confidence interval; IgA: immunoglobulin A.

2. Immunopathogenesis of Skin and Oral Lesions Associated with CD

The immune responses in CD are very wide. A probable explanation lies in the presence of an increase in intestinal permeability in both groups of patients, in relation to the direct toxic effect of gliadin on the surface of the intestinal epithelium [21,22]. This enables the passage of gluten peptides and other related peptides to the bloodstream, provoking the appearance of different inflammatory or autoimmune processes that may affect any organ or tissue, which can be the result of aberrant immune responses [21,23,24]. As Hadjivassiliou stated more than 15 years ago, "that gluten sensitivity is regarded as principally a disease of the small bowel is a historical misconception." [22,25].

In the submucosa of the small intestine, starting with the the action of tissue transglutaminase type 2 which unfolds gluten, a cascade of events occurs, causing a Th1 response that stimulates B lymphocytes that release IgE and other immunoglobulins [26] which play a important roles in the appearance of urticaria and AD, and a stimulation of Th2 mediated by T-lymphocytes which produces the release of pro-inflammatory cytokines, such as TNF-α and interferon gamma (IFNγ), among others [27], and that play important roles in several types of immune-mediated dermatitis, such as psoriasis. In addition, these immunological responses can also cause the production of circulating immunocomplexes due to antigen–antibody interactions which predominate in vasculitic lesions.

3. Dermatitis Herpetiformis

DH is a common extra-intestinal manifestation of CD. A special review article on this disease was recently published in the May 2018 special issue in Nutrients [28]. In summary, DH presents with itchy vesicles and papules, mainly on the elbows, knees, and buttocks. Overt gastrointestinal symptoms are rare. Although in duodenal biopsies, up to 75% of patients with DH with varying degrees of villous atrophy are observed, predominantly mild to moderate, it should be taking into account that in the remaining 25%, only inflammatory changes of changes of lymphocytic enteritis are observed, in the absence of villous atrophy. A diagnosis of DH is easily confirmed by biopsies showing pathognomonic granular immunoglobulin A (IgA) deposits in the papillary dermis by direct immunofluorescence. A valid hypothesis for the immune pathogenesis of DH is that it starts from latent or manifested CD in the gut and evolves into an immune complex deposition of high avidity IgA epidermal transglutaminase (TG3) antibodies, together with the TG3 enzyme, in the papillary dermis. The DH to CD prevalence ratio is 1:8 in Finland and the United Kingdom (UK). The annual

DH incidence rate, currently 2.7 per 100,000 in Finland and 0.8 per 100,000 in the UK, is decreasing, whereas the reverse is true for CD. The long-term prognosis of DH patients on a GFD is excellent, with the mortality rate being even lower than for the general population [28].

4. Urticaria

Urticaria is characterized by the onset of wheals, angioedema, or both (Figure 1) [29]. Urticaria is a common disorder, occurring in 15–25% of individuals at some point in life [29,30]. Chronic urticaria (CU) (duration ≥6 weeks) is seen in about 0.5–1% of the general population [31,32]. CU is associated with a substantial decrease in quality of life [31]. The etiopathogenesis of CU is thought to be associated with autoimmune mechanisms [33–36]. CU has been shown to have a genetic association with the human leukocyte antigen HLA-DQ8 alleles [37]. Interestingly, HLADQ8 has an association with CD [37,38].

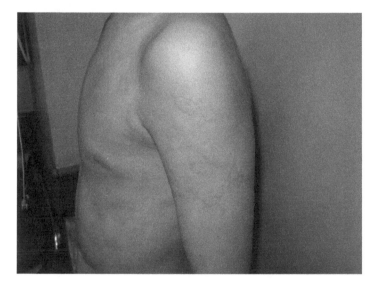

Figure 1. Urticaria. Pale to red, well-demarcated, transient swellings, involving the dermis, mainly at the thorax and the left arm.

In 1987, Hauteke et al. first described the association between CD and chronic urticaria [39], although the relationship between these two diseases is not fully clear. Recently, Kolkhir et al. stated that chronic spontaneous urticaria is strongly linked with various autoimmune diseases, including Hashimoto's thyroiditis, pernicious anemia, vitiligo, diabetes mellitus type 1, Grave's disease, rheumatoid arthritis, and CD [40]. In a large population study, 453 patients with CD and no previous diagnosis of urticaria developed urticaria, and 79 of these 453 patients had chronic urticaria [12]. The corresponding hazard ratios were 1.51 for any urticaria (95%CI = 1.36–1.68) and 1.92 for chronic urticaria (95%CI = 1.48–2.48). These data support an increased prevalence of urticaria and chronic urticaria in patients with CD [12].

In some cases of CU, the adoption of a GFD has proven its effectiveness in controlling skin flares [41,42], further sustaining that CU may be a cutaneous manifestation of CD and not only a fortuitous association [11].

5. Atopic Dermatitis

AD is a chronic inflammatory skin disease that is associated with a heterogeneous group of symptoms and signs. The cutaneous signs of AD include erythema, lichenification, scaling, and prurigo nodules (Figure 2). The symptoms of AD include cutaneous itch and pain [43], sleep disturbance and fatigue [44,45], and mental health symptoms [46–48]. All of these manifestations contribute to diminish the quality of life, limiting the ability to perform activities of daily life and causing psychosocial distress and stigma [49]. AD affects 40 million individuals worldwide [50], and its prevalence is still increasing. Notably, AD appears to be more prevalent among children under five years of age, and its prevalence decreases with advancing age [51]. The onset of AD occurs primarily in childhood and is thought to precede allergic disorders mediated by immunoglobulin E (IgE) sensitization to environmental antigens, namely AD, asthma, and allergic rhino-conjunctivitis, the so-called atopic triade [52–55]. Though extensive recent studies have shed light on the understanding of AD, the exact pathogenesis of the disease is still unknown. The complex interaction between genetics, environmental factors, microbiota, skin barrier deficiency, immunological derangement, and possibly autoimmunity contributes to the development of the disease [56–59].

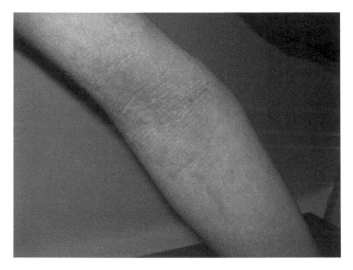

Figure 2. Atopic dermatitis. Excoriated bilateral erythematous scaling papules and plaques on the right flexor elbow surface.

AD has also been linked with CD. Ress et al. analyzed the prevalence of CD in 351 children with AD compared with a general pediatric population and showed a four-fold greater risk of developing CD in patients with AD (OR, 4.18; 95% CI, 1.12–15.64) [60]. This study also emphasizes the need to evaluate the cost-effectiveness of screening patients with AD for CD in time to prevent long-term complications. Moreover, Ciacci et al. conducted a case control study involving 4114 adult patients, with and without CD, and observed that AD was three-fold more frequent in patients with CD and two-fold more frequent in their relatives than in their spouses (OR, 3.17; 95% CI, 1.02–9.82) [13].

6. Psoriasis

Psoriasis is an autoimmune chronic inflammatory skin disease with an estimated prevalence of 2–4% in the adult population [61,62]. It affects over 7.5 million people in the United States and approximately 125 million people worldwide [54]. Psoriasis is considered to be a multifactorial disease, in which the genetic background interacts with environmental factors to define an individual's risk [62–64]. The classical clinical manifestations of psoriasis consist of the presence of red, infiltrated plaques, covered with a coarse, silvery scaling (Figures 3 and 4). Predilection sites include the elbows and knees, scalp, and periumbilical and lumbar regions, although any anatomical site might be affected [65]. The clinical course of psoriasis is marked by frequent relapses with fluctuating rates [62].

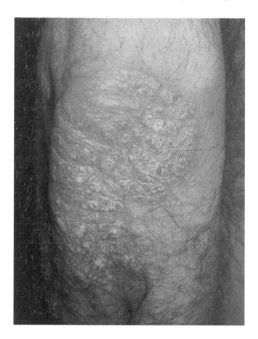

Figure 3. Extense plaque of psoriasis at the left elbow extensor side.

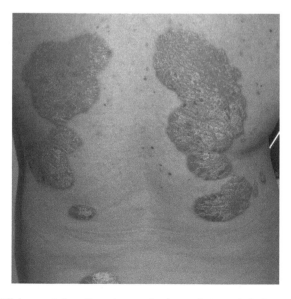

Figure 4. Psoriasis. Well demarcated, erythematous, scaly plaques that are relatively symmetrical on the back.

Psoriasis is known to be associated with an increased risk of several comorbidities, including inflammatory arthritis, metabolic syndrome, and atherosclerotic disease [63]. The association between psoriasis and CD has been of recent interest, but its first recognition was in 1971 by Marks and Shuster [66]. They described, for the first time, a "psoriatic enteropathy" in a small group of patients with severe psoriasis. For many years, the relationship between psoriasis and CD has remained controversial since the few available data were inconclusive. A recent meta-analysis demonstrated a significantly higher risk of CD among patients with psoriasis compared with participants without psoriasis with the OR of 3.09 (95%CI = 1.92–4.97) [16]. Furthermore, seven studies have reported a positive association between psoriasis and CD markers [66–72]. In contrast, other studies did not find evidence of an association between psoriasis and CD markers. However, these studies were of smaller size and some did not employ control groups [73–77]. To resume the evidence for CD antibody positivity in psoriasis, Bhatia et al. performed a meta-analysis of nine studies that reported the frequency of IgA anti-gliadin antibody (IgA AGA) positivity in psoriasis cases and controls [17]. They found a statistically significant higher relative risk of having positive IgA AGA in patients with psoriasis compared to controls (OR = 2.36, 95% CI 1.15–4.83). Other two studies suggested that levels of CD antibodies correlate with psoriasis or psoriatic arthritis severity [78,79]. The use of AGA determination for the diagnosis of CD has low sensitivity, and its use in clinical practice is being abandoned, being replaced by other types of antibodies, such as anti-transglutaminase and deaminated peptides of gliadin [6,21].

The pathophysiologic mechanisms behind the increased risk of CD among patients with psoriasis are not known, but there are different hypotheses that try to explain them [16,80]. The association between CD and several autoimmune diseases, such as type I diabetes mellitus and autoimmune thyroid disease, is well-documented [81,82]. It is believed that shared genes (at-risk HLA haplotypes) might be responsible for this association. The shared genes might play similar roles in the association between psoriasis and CD. Genetic-wide association studies of these two conditions identified genetic susceptibility loci at eight genes that regulate innate and adaptive immune responses: *TNFAIP3*, *RUNX3*, *ELMO1*, *ZMIZ1*, *ETS1*, *SH2B3*, *SOCS1* and *UBE2L3* [80,83–85]. Another possible explanation is that the increased proliferation rate of keratinocytes found in patients with psoriasis is known to produce an excessive amount of interleukin (IL)-1 and IL-18, the essential signals for the induction of Th1 response. Interestingly, mucosal inflammation in patients with CD is also caused by the activation of Th1 in response to dietary gluten [86]. Therefore, it is possible that these ILs might predispose patients to CD. On the other hand, it is possible that intestinal barrier dysfunction associated with undiagnosed or untreated CD may allow the increased passage of immune triggers resulting in an increased risk of autoimmune diseases, including psoriasis [86,87]. Finally, CD-related malabsorption may affect psoriasis by causing a vitamin D deficiency status [9,88]. It is well known that low levels of vitamin D predispose individuals to psoriasis and that exposure to sunlight and topical administration of vitamin D analogues improves psoriatic lesions, probably due to its immunoregulatory properties [88].

Although available data regarding the coexistence of CD and psoriasis are still inconclusive, there is a considerable amount of evidence that suggests that psoriatic patients with concomitant CD may benefit from a GFD [17,21,80,89]. Furthermore, the prevalence of the anti-gliadin IgA antibody is significant higher among patients with psoriasis without a diagnosis of gluten-related disorders. For this reason, anti-gliadin IgA testing can identify patients who are likely to benefit from GFDs [90].

To summarize, the relatively frequent coexistence of CD and psoriasis justifies monitoring of patients with either condition for clinical evidence of the other. This is especially important in the case of psoriasis, as it could be the only manifestation of an undiagnosed CD, even in the absence of obvious digestive symptoms. It is advisable to perform the entire protocol to actively search for CD, including duodenal biopsies, even when serological markers are negative. In the case of negative CD findings, performing a trial with a GFD is currently the recognized diagnostic method [23].

7. Aphthous Stomatitis

Numerous authors have described a wide variety of oral cavity disorders in patients with CD, and some of these manifestations may be considered diagnostic clues in silent, atypical forms of CD [91].

Recurrent aphthous stomatitis (RAS) is a common clinical condition that produces painful ulcerations in the oral cavity. RAS is characterized by multiple recurrent small, round, or ovoid ulcers with circumscribed margins, erythematous haloes, and yellow or gray floors, typically first presenting in childhood or adolescence [92,93] (Figure 5). RAS has been recognized for many years as a symptom of CD (CD) [93–96]. A recent meta-analysis showed that celiac patients have greater frequency of RAS (OR = 3.79, 95%CI = 2.67–5.39). When only the children were considered, the OR was 4.31 (95%CI = 3.03–6.13), while in the adults, the OR of only one study was 47.90 (95%CI 6.29–364.57) [18]. RAS patients should be considered at-risk subjects, even in the absence of any gastrointestinal symptoms and should therefore undergo a diagnostic procedure for CD [97]. RAS may also be present in patients with DH [98]. A study reported non-specific mucosal ulcers in up to 40% of patients with DH [99]. The etiopathology of RAS is obscure; it is not known whether RAS lesions are directly influenced by the gluten sensitivity disorder, or if these are related to hematinic deficiency with low levels of serum iron, folic acid, and vitamin B12 or trace element deficiencies due to malabsorption in patients with untreated CD [96].

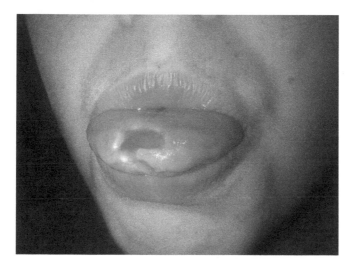

Figure 5. Aphthous lesion on the tip of the tongue, on the upper side.

8. Rosacea

Rosacea is an inflammatory skin condition characterized primarily by persistent or recurrent episodes of centrofacial erythema, with women being more affected than men [100] (Figure 6). The pathophysiology is not completely understood, but dysregulation of the immune system as well as changes in the nervous and vascular systems have been identified [101]. Rosacea can seriously affect a patient's quality of life, and this should prompt clinicians to diagnose it early and start treatment [100]. Rosacea shares genetic risk loci with autoimmune diseases, such as type 1 diabetes mellitus and CD [102]. One study showed that women with rosacea had a significantly increased risk of CD (OR = 2.03, 95%CI 1.35–3.07) [103]. In a nationwide cohort study, the prevalence of CD was higher among patients with rosacea when compared to control subjects (HR = 1.46, 95%CI = 1.11–1.93) [19]. In this study, rosacea was associated with an increased prevalence of Crohn's disease, ulcerative colitis, irritable bowel disease, small intestinal bacterial overgrowth, and *Helicobacter pylori* infection.

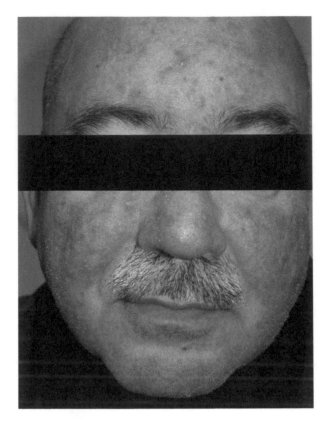

Figure 6. Rosacea. Papule-pustular lesions on the face.

9. Alopecia Areata

AA is an autoimmune disease that presents as a non-scarring type of hair loss. AA affects both sexes equally, affects patients of all ages, and is found in approximately 2% of the general population [104]. Clinical presentation of AA is very heterogeneous, ranging from small and well-circumscribed patches of hair loss to a complete absence of body and scalp hair (Figure 7). Exclamation point hairs, dystrophic hairs, and yellow dots are features of AA that can be identified with trichoscopy. Nail abnormalities, such as pitting, brittleness, or striations are seen in 10% to 20% of patients. The main factors affecting prognosis include age at onset and disease extent; younger age at initial presentation and severity at onset are the most important prognostic indicators [105]. The etiology of AA remains unclear, though it is believed to result from a loss of immune privilege in the hair follicle, autoimmune-mediated hair follicle destruction, and the upregulation of inflammatory pathways [105].

AA is associated with other autoimmune disorders, such as Addison's disease, autoimmune thyroiditis, atrophic gastritis, systemic lupus erythematous, rheumatoid arthritis, myasthenia gravis, and vitiligo [106]. In 1995, Corazza et al. described, for the first time, the association between AA and CD [107]. Since then, there have been other reports of this association. The estimated prevalence rate of CD in patients with AA is from 1:85 to 1:116 [108,109], similar to that found in the general population, so it could be considered to be a random association. However, due to the fact that alopecia improves and even disappears with a GFD, its presence should indicate the possible existence of an undiagnosed CD [11,108–110]. In addition, the prevalence of anti-gliadin antibodies in patients with AA was 18:100

in a study conducted in 2011, occurring more often in severe variants of AA, in particular, alopecia universalis [109]. An active search for CD using serological screening tests has been recommended to diagnose the numerous cases of subclinical CD [9], but a recent study stated that the biological tests to search for CD do not bring enough information and proof to disclose gluten intolerance in AA patients [111].

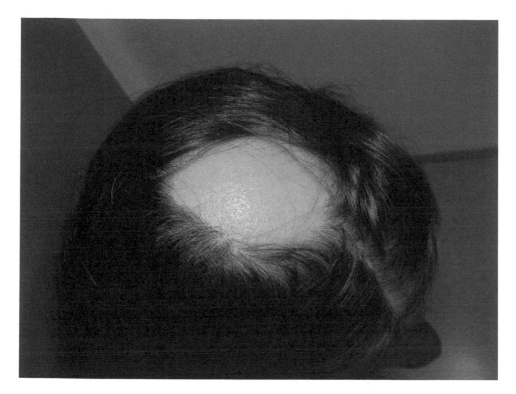

Figure 7. Alopecia areata. Patchy head hair loss.

The positive effects of a GFD on the pattern of autoimmune conditions associated with CD, such as AA, have been attributed to the normalization of the immune response [109]. Although remission and recurrence may be observed during the clinical course of AA, many patients on a GFD have shown complete regrowth of the scalp and other body hair and no further recurrence of AA at follow-up [112].

10. Cutaneous Vasculitis

Leukocytoclastic vasculitis, also known as "hypersensitivity vasculitis", is a histopathologic diagnosis given to cutaneous, small vessel vasculitis, characterized by the inflammation of the walls of postcapillary venules [113]. The clinical features of leukocitoclastic vasculitis include palpable purpura, nodules, hemorrhagic vesicles, bullae, and livedo reticularis, mainly distributed in the lower extremities (Figure 8) [114]. Extracutaneous involvement is seen in approximately 30% of patients. Systemic vasculitis shows a predilection for certain organs, such as the kidneys and lungs. In most cases, leucocytoclastic vasculitis is mediated by immunocomplex deposition, with the antigen being either exogenous or endogenous [115–118].

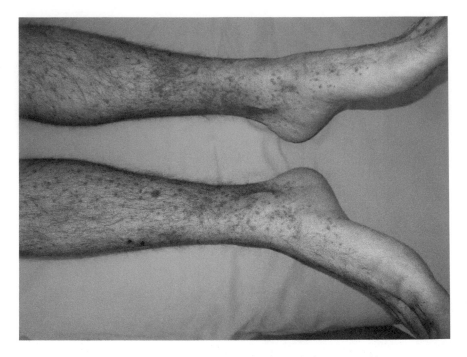

Figure 8. Vasculitis. Palpable purpuric papules on the lower extremities.

When leukocytoclastic vasculitis is suspected, a biopsy should be performed, preferably in the first 24 to 48 h of lesion onset. Additionally, direct immunofluorescence should be performed to evaluate for the presence of immunoglobulins. If no systemic symptoms are present, laboratory testing, including a complete blood count, measurement of the erythrocyte sedimentation rate, basic metabolic panel, liver function tests, and urinalysis should be done as well. If there is concern for systemic involvement, more extensive workup can be fulfilled. Around 90% of leukocytoclastic vasculitis cases are self-limited, showing spontaneous resolution within weeks to months. The treatment depends on the severity of the disease and can range from an oral corticosteroid course to various steroid-sparing agents [113,114].

There are sporadic reports about the association between CD and cutaneous vasculitis (CV) [115–119]. The coexistence of these two entities might be related to increased intestinal permeability [120], and immune complexes, originating from exogenous or endogenous antigens, might circulate because of the impaired phagocytic function of the reticular endothelium system and be deposited in the skin. As seen in inflammatory bowel disease (IBD), exogenous antigens may permeate the damaged CD mucous in larger quantities than normal. This is reflected by significant serum milk and gluten fraction antibody titers. Moreover, autoimmune sensitization may result because of the release of endogenous antigens from the damaged small bowel mucosa. Meyers et al. [118] described a case of CV associated with CD and the remission of skin lesions after the treatment with a strict GFD. Treatment with a GFD may improve CV lesions in cases associated with CD [9–11].

11. Other Skin Conditions Found in Patients with CD

As reported by Humbert et al. and Caproni et al., in addition to skin diseases with proven association with CD and those improved by a GFD and/or with positivity of celiac serological markers, there are also fortuitous associations with other skin conditions [9–11]. Some of these associations are more common than others.

Juvenile dermatomyositis and dermatomyositis have been reported in association with CD in adult patients. In particular, when patients are newly diagnosed with these conditions, even in the absence of gastrointestinal symptoms, screening for CD should be performed. Clinical manifestations of dermatomyositis may respond to a GFD [121–124].

The possible association between CD and vitiligo is controversial. There are few cases that have reported the improvement of vitiligo in patients that started a GFD. A common basic autoimmune mechanism has been hypothesized [125,126].

Many similarities exist between the pathogeneses of CD and SLE, but it is still unknown whether there is a true association or not [127–129].

Other reported and less frequent associations include lichen planus and lichen sclerosus [130–138], linear IgA bullous dermatosis [139,140], prurigo nodularis [141], pityriasis rubra pilaris and erythroderma [142], erythema elevatum diutinum [143–145], necrolytic migratory erythema [146–148], pityriasis lichenoides [140], erythema nodosum [140,149–151], porphyria [152,153], cutaneous amyloidosis [154], generalized acquired cutis laxa [155,156], acquired hypertrichosis lanuginosa [157], ichthyosis [158], partial lipodystrophy [159], transverse leukonychia [160], atypical mole syndrome, and congenital giant nevus [161]. Finally, we want to mention that earlier studies reported an increased risk of malignant melanoma in patients with CD, but a recent study refuted this relation [162].

12. Other Oral Cavity Disorders

Other oral cavity manifestations among patients with CD have also been described [18,97–99,110,163,164]. Rashid et al. described oral and dental manifestations of CD, consisting of enamel defects, delayed eruption, recurrent aphthous ulcers, cheilitis, and atrophic glossitis [96]. Bramanti et al. found atrophic glossitis, angular cheilitis, and burning tongue to be more frequent in CD patients than in control patients [165].

13. Conclusions

CD is a systemic process of autoimmune nature that affects genetically predisposed people in relation to a permanent intolerance to gluten and related proteins. It has a worldwide distribution, a slight female predominance, and can appear at any age, with a variable clinical course, ranging from subclinical or asymptomatic cases to very severe ones. In the physical examination of these patients, it is very important to recognize the presence of several types of dermatitis which are found in association with CD, such as urticaria (HR: 1.51, CI: 1.36–1.68), chronic urticaria (HR: 1.92, CI: 1.48–2.48), atopic dermatitis (OR: 3.17, CI: 1.02–9.82), psoriasis (HR: 1.72, CI = 1.54–1.92), aphthous stomatitis (OR: 3.79, CI = 2.67–5.39) and rosacea (HR: 1.46, CI = 1.11–1.93), and other skin affectation processes that are not so clearly related to CD. All of these diseases may occur in the form of outbreaks, accompanied generally by pruritus, which negatively affects their quality of life. Their relationship with gluten is through allergic, inflammatory, immunological, and mixed processes. The recognition of their probable relationship facilitates the diagnosis of CD, and the establishment of a GFD improves the evolution of cutaneous lesions and in some cases, full recovery is achieved.

It is very important to emphasize that the classic presentations of CD with associated malabsorption syndrome are currently considered to be exceptional, especially from the age of two years, and the predominant forms are those with mild, fluctuating, or even absent digestive symptoms and a wide range of extra-intestinal manifestations [166–170]. Many undiagnosed celiac patients underestimate their multiple and frequent discomfort from digestive and more general causes because they have grown accustomed to living with a state of chronic poor health as though it is normal. They are only able to recognize that they really did have symptoms related to the consumption of gluten when they start the GFD and the improvement becomes obvious [171,172].

Author Contributions: L.R., V.-B.G., and N.A. designed the study and wrote the abstract, the introduction and the Dermatitis herpetiformis description. C.G.d.C. wrote the Alopecia areata, urticaria and cutaneous vasculitis descriptions, A.d.D. and L.P. contributed to the description of atopic dermatitis and psoriasis. J.S.-J. wrote the sections about the oral mucosal and other CD-associated skin conditions. J.S.-J., V.-B.G. and A.d.D. made all the selected figures in this review. All the authors reviewed and approved the final version of the manuscript.

Funding: This research received no external funding.

Conflicts of Interest: The authors declare no conflict of interest.

References

1. Bai, J.; Fried, M.; Corazza, G.; Schuppan, D.; Farthing, M.; Catassi, C.; Greco, L.; Cohen, H.; Ciacci, C.; Eliakim, R.; et al. World Gastroenterology Organisation Global Guidelines on celiac disease. *J. Clin. Gastroenterol.* **2013**, *47*, 121–126. [CrossRef] [PubMed]
2. Lebwohl, B.; Sanders, D.S.; Green, P.H.R. Coeliac disease. *Lancet* **2018**, *391*, 70–81. [CrossRef]
3. Collin, P.; Vilppula, A.; Luostarinen, L.; Holmes, G.K.T.; Kaukinen, K. Review article: Coeliac disease in later life must not be missed. *Aliment. Pharmacol. Ther.* **2018**, *47*, 563–572. [CrossRef] [PubMed]
4. Rodrigo, L. Celiac disease. *World J. Gastroenterol.* **2006**, *12*, 6585–6593. [CrossRef] [PubMed]
5. Freeman, H.J. Endocrine manifestations in celiac disease. *World J. Gastroenterol.* **2016**, *22*, 8472–8479. [CrossRef] [PubMed]
6. Elli, L.; Bonura, A.; Garavaglia, D.; Rulli, E.; Floriani, I.; Tagliabue, G.; Contiero, P.; Bardella, M. Immunological comorbity in coeliac disease: Associations, risk factors and clinical implications. *J. Clin. Immunol.* **2012**, *32*, 984–990. [CrossRef] [PubMed]
7. Ciccocioppo, R.; Kruzliak, P.; Cangemi, G.; Pohanka, M.; Betti, E.; Lauret, E.; Rodrigo, L. The spectrum of differences between childhood and adulthood celiac disease. *Nutrients* **2015**, *7*, 8733–8751. [CrossRef] [PubMed]
8. Green, P.H.; Cellier, C. Celiac disease. *N. Engl. J. Med.* **2007**, *357*, 1731–1743. [CrossRef] [PubMed]
9. Abenavoli, L.; Proietti, I.; Leggio, L.; Ferrulli, A.; Vonghia, L.; Capizzi, R.; Rotoli, M.; Amerio, P.L.; Gasbarrini, G.; Addolorato, G. Cutaneous manifestations in celiac disease. *World J. Gastroenterol.* **2006**, *12*, 843–852. [CrossRef] [PubMed]
10. Humbert, P.; Pelletier, F.; Dreno, B.; Puzenat, E.; Aubin, F. Gluten intolerance and skin diseases. *Eur. J. Dermatol.* **2006**, *16*, 4–11. [PubMed]
11. Caproni, M.; Bonciolini, V.; D'Errico, A.; Antiga, E.; Fabbri, P. Celiac disease and dermatologic manifestations: Many skin clue to unfold gluten-sensitive enteropathy. *Gastroenterol. Res. Pract.* **2012**, *2012*, 952753. [CrossRef] [PubMed]
12. Ludvigsson, J.F.; Lindelöf, B.; Rashtak, S.; Rubio-Tapia, A.; Murray, J.A. Does urticaria risk increase in patients with celiac disease? A large population-based cohort study. *Eur. J. Dermatol.* **2013**, *23*, 681–687. [CrossRef] [PubMed]
13. Ciacci, C.; Cavallaro, R.; Iovino, P.; Sabbatini, F.; Palumbo, A.; Amoruso, D.; Tortora, R.; Mazzacca, G. Allergy prevalence in adult celiac disease. *J. Allergy Clin. Immunol.* **2004**, *113*, 1199–1203. [CrossRef] [PubMed]
14. Ludvigsson, J.F.; Lindelöf, B.; Zingone, F.; Ciacci, C. Psoriasis in a nationwide cohort study of patients with celiac disease. *J. Investig. Dermatol.* **2011**, *131*, 2010–2016. [CrossRef] [PubMed]
15. Egeberg, A.; Griffiths, C.E.M.; Mallbris, L.; Gislason, G.H.; Skov, L. The association between psoriasis and coeliac disease. *Br. J. Dermatol.* **2017**, *177*, e329–e330. [CrossRef] [PubMed]
16. Ungprasert, P.; Wijarnpreecha, K.; Kittanamongkolchai, W. Psoriasis and risk of celiac disease: A systematic review and meta-analysis. *Indian J. Dermatol.* **2017**, *62*, 41–46. [CrossRef] [PubMed]
17. Bhatia, B.; Millsop, J.; Debbaneh, M.; Koo, J.; Linos, E.; Liao, W. Diet and psoriasis, part II: Celiac disease and role of a gluten-free diet. *Am. Acad. Dermatol.* **2014**, *71*, 350–358. [CrossRef] [PubMed]
18. Nieri, M.; Tofani, E.; Defraia, E.; Giuntini, V.; Franchi, L. Enamel defects and aphthous stomatitis in celiac and healthy subjects: Systematic review and meta-analysis of controlled studies. *J. Dent.* **2017**, *65*, 1–10. [CrossRef] [PubMed]
19. Egeberg, A.; Weinstock, L.B.; Thyssen, E.P.; Gislason, G.H.; Thyssen, J.P. Rosacea and gastrointestinal disorders: A population-based cohort study. *Br. J. Dermatol.* **2017**, *176*, 100–106. [CrossRef] [PubMed]

20. Bonciolini, V.; Bianchi, B.; Del Bianco, E.; Verdelli, A.; Caproni, M. Cutaneous manifestations of non-celiac gluten sensitivity: Clinical histological and immunopathological features. *Nutrients* **2015**, *7*, 7798–7805. [CrossRef] [PubMed]

21. Losurdo, G.; Principi, M.; Iannone, A.; Amoruso, A.; Ierardi, E.; Di Leo, A.; Barone, M. Extra-intestinal manifestations of non-celiac gluten sensitivity: An expanding paradigm. *World J. Gastroenterol.* **2018**, *24*, 1521–1530. [CrossRef] [PubMed]

22. Catassi, C.; Bai, J.C.; Bonaz, B.; Bouma, G.; Calabrò, A.; Carroccio, A.; Castillejo, G.; Ciacci, C.; Cristofori, F.; Dolinsek, J.; et al. Non-Celiac Gluten sensitivity: The new frontier of gluten related disorders. *Nutrients* **2013**, *5*, 3839–3853. [CrossRef] [PubMed]

23. Catassi, C.; Elli, L.; Bonaz, B.; Bouma, G.; Carroccio, A.; Castillejo, G.; Cellier, C.; Cristofori, F.; de Magistris, L.; Dolinsek, J.; et al. Diagnosis of Non-Celiac Gluten Sensitivity (NCGS): The Salerno Experts' Criteria. *Nutrients* **2015**, *7*, 4966–4977. [CrossRef] [PubMed]

24. Leffler, D.A.; Green, P.H.; Fasano, A. Extraintestinal manifestations of coeliac disease. *Nat. Rev. Gastroenterol. Hepatol.* **2015**, *12*, 561–567. [CrossRef] [PubMed]

25. Hadjivassiliou, M.; Grünewald, R.A.; Davies-Jones, G.A. Gluten sensitivity as a neurological illness. *J. Neurol. Neurosurg. Psychiatry* **2002**, *72*, 560–563. [CrossRef] [PubMed]

26. Spencer, J.; Sollid, L.M. The human intestinal B-cell response. *Mucosal Immunol.* **2016**, *9*, 1113–1124. [CrossRef] [PubMed]

27. Jabri, B.; Sollid, L.M. T Cells in Celiac Disease. *J. Immunol.* **2017**, *198*, 3005–3014. [CrossRef] [PubMed]

28. Reunala, T.; Salmi, T.T.; Hervonen, K.; Kaukinen, K.; Collin, P. Dermatitis Herpetiformis: A Common Extraintestinal Manifestation of Coeliac Disease. *Nutrients* **2018**, *10*, E602. [CrossRef] [PubMed]

29. Champion, R.H.; Roberts, S.O.; Carpenter, R.G.; Roger, J. Urticaria and angio-oedema. A review of 554 patients. *Br. J. Dermatol.* **1969**, *81*, 588–597. [CrossRef] [PubMed]

30. Toubi, E.; Kessel, A.; Avshovich, N.; Bamberger, E.; Sabo, E.; Nusem, D.; Panasoff, J. Clinical and laboratory parameters in predicting chronic urticaria duration: A prospective study of 139 patients. *Allergy* **2004**, *59*, 869–873. [CrossRef] [PubMed]

31. O'Donnell, B.; Lawlor, F.; Simpson, J.; Morgan, M.; Greaves, M. The impact of chronic urticaria on the quality of life. *Br. J. Dermatol.* **1997**, *136*, 197–201. [CrossRef] [PubMed]

32. Palikhe, N.; Sin, H.; Kim, S.; Sin, H.; Hwang, E.; Ye, Y.; Park, H. Genetic variability of prostaglandin E2 receptor subtype EP4 gene in aspirin-intolerant chronic urticaria. *J. Hum. Genet.* **2012**, *57*, 494–499. [CrossRef] [PubMed]

33. Dice, J.P. Physical urticaria. *Immunol. Allergy Clin.* **2004**, *24*, 225–246. [CrossRef] [PubMed]

34. Chang, S.; Carr, W. Urticarial vasculitis. *Allergy Asthma Proc.* **2007**, *28*, 97–100. [CrossRef] [PubMed]

35. Fraser, K.; Robertson, L. Chronic urticaria and autoimmunity. *Skin Ther. Lett.* **2013**, *18*, 5–9.

36. Kolkhir, P.; Church, M.; Weller, K.; Metz, M.; Schmetzer, O.; Maurer, M. Autoimmune chronic spontaneous urticaria: What we know and what we do not know. *J. Allergy Clin. Immunol.* **2017**, *139*, 1772–1781.e1. [CrossRef] [PubMed]

37. O'Donnell, B.; O'Neill, C.; Francis, D.; Niimi, N.; Barr, R.; Barlow, R.; Kobza Black, A.; Welsh, K.; Greaves, M. Human leucocyte antigen class II associations in chronic idiopathic urticaria. *Br. J. Dermatol.* **1999**, *140*, 853–858. [CrossRef] [PubMed]

38. Piccini, B.; Vascotto, M.; Serracca, L.; Luddi, A.; Margollicci, M.; Balestri, P.; Vindigni, C.; Bassotti, G.; Villanacci, V. HLA-DQ typing in the diagnostic algorithm of celiac disease. *Rev. Esp. Enferm. Dig.* **2012**, *104*, 248–254. [CrossRef] [PubMed]

39. Hautekeete, M.; De Clerck, L.; Stevens, W. Chronic urticaria associated with coeliac disease. *Lancet* **1987**, *329*, 157. [CrossRef]

40. Kolkhir, P.; Borzova, E.; Grattan, C.; Asero, R.; Pogorelov, D.; Maurer, M. Autoimmune comorbidity in chronic spontaneous urticaria: A systematic review. *Autoimmun. Rev.* **2017**, *16*, 1196–1208. [CrossRef] [PubMed]

41. Caminiti, L.; Passalacqua, G.; Magazzu, G.; Comisi, F.; Vita, D.; Barberio, G.; Sferlazzas, C.; Pajno, G. Chronic urticaria and associated coeliac disease in children: A case-control study. *Pediatr. Allergy Immunol.* **2005**, *16*, 428–432. [CrossRef] [PubMed]

42. Greaves, M.W. Chronic idiophatic urticarial. *Curr. Opin. Allergy Clin. Immunol.* **2003**, *4*, 363–368. [CrossRef]

43. Vakharia, P.; Chopra, R.; Sacotte, R.; Patel, K.; Singam, V.; Patel, N.; Immaneni, S.; White, T.; Kantor, R.; Hsu, D.; et al. Burden of skin pain in atopic dermatitis. *Ann. Allergy Asthma Immunol.* **2017**, *119*, 548–552. [CrossRef] [PubMed]

44. Silverberg, J.; Garg, N.; Paller, A.; Fishbein, A.; Zee, P. Sleep Disturbances in Adults with Eczema Are Associated with Impaired Overall Health: A US Population-Based Study. *J. Investig. Dermatol.* **2015**, *135*, 56–66. [CrossRef] [PubMed]

45. Yu, S.; Attarian, H.; Zee, P.; Silverberg, J. Burden of Sleep and Fatigue in US Adults With Atopic Dermatitis. *Dermatitis* **2016**, *27*, 50–58. [CrossRef] [PubMed]

46. Yu, S.; Silverberg, J. Association between Atopic Dermatitis and Depression in US Adults. *J. Investig. Dermatol.* **2015**, *135*, 3183–3186. [CrossRef] [PubMed]

47. Yaghmaie, P.; Koudelka, C.; Simpson, E. Mental health comorbidity in patients with atopic dermatitis. *J. Allergy Clin. Immunol.* **2013**, *131*, 428–433. [CrossRef] [PubMed]

48. Strom, M.; Fishbein, A.; Paller, A.; Silverberg, J. Association between atopic dermatitis and attention deficit hyperactivity disorder in U.S. children and adults. *Br. J. Dermatol.* **2016**, *175*, 920–929. [CrossRef] [PubMed]

49. Silverberg, J. Associations between atopic dermatitis and other disorders. *F1000Resarch* **2018**, *7*, 303. [CrossRef] [PubMed]

50. Plötz, S.; Wiesender, M.; Todorova, A.; Ring, J. What is new in atopic dermatitis/eczema? *Expert Opin. Emerg. Drugs* **2014**, *19*, 441–458. [CrossRef] [PubMed]

51. Herd, R.M.; Tidman, M.J.; Prescott, R.J.; Hunter, J.A. Prevalence of atopic eczema in the community: The Lothian atopic dermatitis study. *Br. J. Dermatol.* **1996**, *135*, 18–19. [CrossRef] [PubMed]

52. Bieber, T. Atopic Dermatitis. *N. Engl. J. Med.* **2008**, *358*, 1483–1494. [CrossRef] [PubMed]

53. Alduraywish, S.; Lodge, C.; Campbell, B.; Allen, K.; Erbas, B.; Lowe, A.; Dharmage, S. The march from early life food sensitization to allergic disease: A systematic review and meta-analyses of birth cohort studies. *Allergy* **2015**, *71*, 77–89. [CrossRef] [PubMed]

54. Saunders, S.; Moran, T.; Floudas, A.; Wurlod, F.; Kaszlikowska, A.; Salimi, M.; Quinn, E.; Oliphant, C.; Núñez, G.; McManus, R.; et al. Spontaneous atopic dermatitis is mediated by innate immunity, with the secondary lung inflammation of the atopic march requiring adaptive immunity. *J. Allergy Clin. Immunol.* **2016**, *137*, 482–491. [CrossRef] [PubMed]

55. Lee, H.; Lee, N.; Kim, B.; Jung, M.; Kim, D.; Moniaga, C.; Kabashima, K.; Choi, E. Acidification of stratum corneum prevents the progression from atopic dermatitis to respiratory allergy. *Exp. Dermatol.* **2017**, *26*, 66–72. [CrossRef] [PubMed]

56. Kabashima, K.; Otsuka, A.; Nomura, T. Linking air pollution to atopic dermatitis. *Nat. Immunol.* **2016**, *18*, 5–6. [CrossRef] [PubMed]

57. Dainichi, T.; Hanakawa, S.; Kabashima, K. Classification of inflammatory skin diseases: A proposal based on the disorders of the three-layered defense systems, barrier, innate immunity and acquired immunity. *J. Dermatol. Sci.* **2014**, *76*, 81–89. [CrossRef] [PubMed]

58. Kashiwakura, J.; Okayama, Y.; Furue, M.; Kabashima, K.; Shimada, S.; Ra, C.; Siraganian, R.; Kawakami, Y.; Kawakami, T. Most Highly Cytokinergic IgEs Have Polyreactivity to Autoantigens. *Allergy Asthma Immunol. Res.* **2012**, *4*, 332–340. [CrossRef] [PubMed]

59. Rerknimitr, P.; Otsuka, A.; Nakashima, C.; Kabashima, K. The etiopathogenesis of atopic dermatitis: Barrier disruption, immunological derangement, and pruritus. *Inflamm. Regen.* **2017**, *37*, 14. [CrossRef] [PubMed]

60. Ress, K.; Annus, T.; Putnik, U.; Luts, K.; Uibo, R.; Uibo, O. Celiac Disease in Children with Atopic Dermatitis. *Pediatr. Dermatol.* **2014**, *31*, 483–488. [CrossRef] [PubMed]

61. Rachakonda, T.; Schupp, C.; Armstrong, A. Psoriasis prevalence among adults in the United States. *J. Am. Acad. Dermatol.* **2014**, *70*, 512–516. [CrossRef] [PubMed]

62. Christophers, E. Psoriasis—Epidemiology and clinical spectrum. *Clin. Exp. Dermatol.* **2001**, *26*, 314–320. [CrossRef] [PubMed]

63. Takeshita, J.; Grewal, S.; Langan, S.; Mehta, N.; Ogdie, A.; Van Voorhees, A.; Gelfand, J. Psoriasis and comorbid diseases. *J. Am. Acad. Dermatol.* **2017**, *76*, 377–390. [CrossRef] [PubMed]

64. Boehncke, W.; Boehncke, S. More than skin-deep: The many dimensions of the psoriatic disease. *Swiss Med. Wkly.* **2014**, *144*, w13968. [CrossRef] [PubMed]

65. Marks, J.; Shuster, S. Intestinal malabsorption and the skin. *Gut* **1971**, *12*, 938–947. [CrossRef] [PubMed]

66. Ojetti, V.; Aguilar Sánchez, J.; Guerriero, C.; Fossati, B.; Capizzi, R.; De Simmone, C.; Migneco, A.; Amerio, P.; Gasbarrini, G.; Gasbarrini, A. High prevalence of celiac disease in psoriasis. *Am. J. Gastroenterol.* **2003**, *98*, 2574–2575. [CrossRef]

67. Michaelsson, G.; Gerden, B.; Ottosson, M.; Parra, A.; Sjoberg, O.; Hjelmquist, G.; Loof, L. Patients with psoriasis often have increased serum levels of IgA antibodies to gliadin. *Br. J. Dermatol.* **1993**, *129*, 667–673. [CrossRef] [PubMed]

68. Akbulut, S.; Gür, G.; Topal, F.; Senel, E.; Topal, F.; Alli, N.; Saritas, Ü. Coeliac Disease-Associated Antibodies in Psoriasis. *Ann. Dermatol.* **2013**, *25*, 298. [CrossRef] [PubMed]

69. Nagui, N.; El Nabarawy, E.; Mahgoub, D.; Mashaly, H.; Saad, N.; El-Deeb, D. Estimation of (IgA) anti-gliadin, anti-endomysium and tissue transglutaminase in the serum of patients with psoriasis. *Clin. Exp. Dermatol.* **2011**, *36*, 302–304. [CrossRef] [PubMed]

70. Damasiewicz-Bodzek, A.; Wielkoszyński, T. Serologic markers of celiac disease in psoriatic patients. *J. Eur. Acad. Dermatol. Venereol.* **2008**, *22*, 1055–1061. [CrossRef] [PubMed]

71. Singh, S.; Sonkar, G.; Usha; Singh, S. Celiac disease-associated antibodies in patients with psoriasis and correlation with HLA Cw6. *J. Clin. Lab. Anal.* **2010**, *24*, 269–272. [CrossRef] [PubMed]

72. Ojetti, V.; De Simone, C.; Aguilar Sanchez, J.; Capizzi, R.; Migneco, A.; Guerriero, C.; Cazzato, A.; Gasbarrini, G.; Amerio, P.; Gasbarrini, A. Malabsorption in psoriatic patients: Cause or consequence? *Scand. J. Gastroenterol.* **2006**, *41*, 1267–1271. [CrossRef] [PubMed]

73. De Vos, R.; Boer, W.; Haas, F. Is there a relationship between psoriasis and coeliac disease? *J. Intern. Med.* **1995**, *237*, 118. [CrossRef] [PubMed]

74. Sultan, S.; Ahmad, Q.; Sultan, S. Antigliadin antibodies in psoriasis. *Australas. J. Dermatol.* **2010**, *51*, 238–242. [CrossRef] [PubMed]

75. Zamani, F.; Alizadeh, S.; Amiri, A.; Shakeri, R.; Robati, M.; Alimohamadi, S.; Abdi, H.; Malekzadeh, R. Psoriasis and Coeliac Disease; Is There Any Relationship? *Acta Derm.-Venereol.* **2010**, *90*, 295–296. [CrossRef] [PubMed]

76. Kia, K.; Nair, R.; Ike, R.; Hiremagalore, R.; Elder, J.; Ellis, C. Prevalence of Antigliadin Antibodies in Patients with Psoriasis is Not Elevated Compared with Controls. *Am. J. Clin. Dermatol.* **2007**, *8*, 301–305. [CrossRef] [PubMed]

77. Cardinali, C.; Degl'innocenti, D.; Caproni, M.; Fabbri, P. Is the search for serum antibodies to gliadin, endomysium and tissue transglutaminase meaningful in psoriatic patients? Relationship between the pathogenesis of psoriasis and coeliac disease. *Br. J. Dermatol.* **2002**, *147*, 187–188. [CrossRef] [PubMed]

78. Woo, W.; McMillan, S.; Watson, R.; Mccluggage, W.; Sloan, J.; McMillan, J. Coeliac disease-associated antibodies correlate with psoriasis activity. *Br. J. Dermatol.* **2004**, *151*, 891–894. [CrossRef] [PubMed]

79. Lindqvist, U.; Rudsander, Å.; Boström, Å.; Nilsson, B.; Michaëlsson, G. IgA antibodies to gliadin and coeliac disease in psoriatic arthritis. *Rheumatology* **2002**, *41*, 31–37. [CrossRef] [PubMed]

80. Pietrzak, D.; Pietrzak, A.; Krasowska, D.; Borzęcki, A.; Franciszkiewicz-Pietrzak, K.; Polkowska-Pruszyńska, B.; Baranowska, M.; Reich, K. Digestive system in psoriasis: An update. *Arch. Dermatol. Res.* **2017**, *309*, 679–693. [CrossRef] [PubMed]

81. Counsell, C.E.; Taha, A.; Ruddell, W. Coeliac disease and autoimmune thyroid disease. *Gut* **1994**, *35*, 844–846. [CrossRef] [PubMed]

82. Schuppan, D.; Hahn, E. Celiac Disease and its Link to Type 1 Diabetes Mellitus. *J. Pediatr. Endocrinol. Metab.* **2001**, *14* (Suppl. S1), 597–605. [CrossRef] [PubMed]

83. Lu, Y.; Chen, H.; Nikamo, P.; Qi Low, H.; Helms, C.; Seielstad, M.; Liu, J.; Bowcock, A.; Stahle, M.; Liao, W. Association of Cardiovascular and Metabolic Disease Genes with Psoriasis. *J. Investig. Dermatol.* **2013**, *133*, 836–839. [CrossRef] [PubMed]

84. Trynka, G.; Hunt, K.; Bockett, N.; Romanos, J.; Mistry, V.; Szperl, A.; Bakker, S.; Bardella, M.; Bhaw-Rosun, L.; Castillejo, G.; et al. Dense genotyping identifies and localizes multiple common and rare variant association signals in celiac disease. *Nat. Genet.* **2011**, *43*, 1193–1201. [CrossRef] [PubMed]

85. Tsoi, L.; Spain, S.; Knight, J.; Ellinghaus, E.; Stuart, P.; Capon, F.; Ding, J.; Li, Y.; Tejasvi, T.; Gudjonsson, J.; et al. Identification of 15 new psoriasis susceptibility loci highlights the role of innate immunity. *Nat. Genet.* **2012**, *44*, 1341–1348. [CrossRef] [PubMed]

86. Birkenfeld, S.; Dreiher, J.; Weitzman, D.; Cohen, A. Coeliac disease associated with psoriasis. *Br. J. Dermatol.* **2009**, *161*, 1331–1334. [CrossRef] [PubMed]

87. Ventura, A.; Magazzù, G.; Greco, L. Duration of exposure to gluten and risk for autoimmune disorders in patients with celiac disease. *Gastroenterology* **1999**, *117*, 297–303. [CrossRef] [PubMed]
88. Holick, M. Vitamin D: A millenium perspective. *J. Cell. Biochem.* **2003**, *88*, 296–307. [CrossRef] [PubMed]
89. De Bastiani, R.; Gabrielli, M.; Lora, L.; Napoli, L.; Tosetti, C.; Pirrotta, E.; Ubaldi, E.; Bertolusso, L.; Zamparella, M.; De Polo, M.; et al. Association between Coeliac Disease and Psoriasis: Italian Primary Care Multicentre Study. *Dermatology* **2015**, *230*, 156–160. [CrossRef] [PubMed]
90. Kolchak, N.; Tetarnikova, M.; Theodoropoulou, M.; Michalopoulou, A.; Theodoropoulos, D. Prevalence of antigliadin IgA antibodies in psoriasis vulgaris and response of seropositive patients to a gluten-free diet. *J. Multidiscip. Healthc.* **2017**, *11*, 13–19. [CrossRef] [PubMed]
91. Pastore, L.; Carroccio, A.; Compilato, D.; Panzarella, V.; Serpico, R.; Muzio, L. Oral Manifestations of Celiac Disease. *J. Clin. Gastroenterol.* **2008**, *42*, 224–232. [CrossRef] [PubMed]
92. Chavan, M.; Jain, H.; Diwan, N.; Khedkar, S.; Shete, A.; Durkar, S. Recurrent aphthous stomatitis: A review. *J. Oral Pathol. Med.* **2012**, *41*, 577–583. [CrossRef] [PubMed]
93. Lahteenoja, H.; Toivanen, A.; Viander, M.; Maki, M.; Irjala, K.; Raiha, I.; Syrjanen, S. Oral mucosal changes in coeliac patients on a gluten-free diet. *Eur. J. Oral Sci.* **1998**, *106*, 899–906. [CrossRef] [PubMed]
94. Bucci, P.; Carile, F.; Sangianantoni, A.; D'Angiò, F.; Santarelli, A.; Muzio, L. Oral aphthous ulcers and dental enamel defects in children with coeliac disease. *Acta Paediatr.* **2007**, *95*, 203–207. [CrossRef]
95. Macho, V.; Coelho, A.; Veloso e Silva, D.M.; Andrade, D. Oral Manifestations in Pediatric Patients with Coeliac Disease—A Review Article. *Open Dent. J.* **2017**, *11*, 539–545. [CrossRef] [PubMed]
96. Rashid, M.; Zarkadas, M.; Anca, A.; Limeback, H. Oral manifestations of celiac disease: A clinical guide for dentists. *J. Can. Dent. Assoc.* **2011**, *77*, b39. [PubMed]
97. Ferguson, R.; Basu, M.; Asquith, P.; Cooke, W. Jejunal mucosal abnormalities in patients with recurrent aphthous ulceration. *BMJ* **1976**, *1*, 11–13. [CrossRef] [PubMed]
98. Ferguson, M.; Wray, D.; Carmichael, H.; Russell, R.; Lee, F. Coeliac disease associated with recurrent aphthae. *Gut* **1980**, *21*, 223–226. [CrossRef] [PubMed]
99. Wray, D. Gluten-sensitive recurrent aphthous stomatitis. *Dig. Dis. Sci.* **1981**, *26*, 737–740. [CrossRef] [PubMed]
100. Two, A.M.; Wu, W.; Gallo, R.L.; Hata, T.R. Rosacea: Part I. Introduction, categorization, histology, pathogenesis, and risk factors. *J. Am. Acad. Dermatol.* **2015**, *72*, 749–758. [CrossRef] [PubMed]
101. Holmes, A.D.; Steinhoff, M. Integrative concepts of rosacea pathophysiology, clinical presentation and new therapeutics. *Exp. Dermatol.* **2017**, *26*, 659–667. [CrossRef] [PubMed]
102. Chang, A.L.S.; Raber, I.; Xu, J.; Li, R.; Spitale, R.; Chen, J.; Kiefer, A.K.; Tian, C.; Eriksson, N.K.; Hinds, D.A.; et al. Assessment of the genetic basis of rosacea by genome-wide association study. *J. Investig. Dermatol.* **2015**, *135*, 1548–1555. [CrossRef] [PubMed]
103. Egeberg, A.; Hansen, P.; Gislason, G.; Thyssen, J. Clustering of autoimmune diseases in patients with rosacea. *J. Am. Acad. Dermatol.* **2016**, *74*, 667–672. [CrossRef] [PubMed]
104. Darwin, E.; Hirt, P.A.; Fertig, R.; Doliner, B.; Delcanto, G.; Jimenez, J.J. Alopecia Areata: Review of Epidemiology, Clinical Features, Pathogenesis, and New Treatment Options. *Int. J. Trichol.* **2018**, *10*, 51–60. [CrossRef] [PubMed]
105. Strazzulla, L.; Wang, E.H.C.; Avila, L.; Lo Sicco, K.; Brinster, N.; Christiano, A.M.; Shapiro, J. Alopecia areata: Disease characteristics, clinical evaluation, and new perspectives on pathogenesis. *J. Am. Acad. Dermatol.* **2018**, *78*, 1–12. [CrossRef] [PubMed]
106. Ertekin, V.; Tosun, M.; Erdem, T. Screening of celiac disease in children with alopecia areata. *Indian J. Dermatol.* **2014**, *59*, 317. [CrossRef] [PubMed]
107. Corazza, G.R.; Andreani, M.L.; Venturo, N.; Bernardi, M.; Tosti, A.; Gasbarrini, G. Celiac disease and alopecia areata: Report of a new association. *Gastroenterology* **1995**, *109*, 1333–1337. [CrossRef]
108. Volta, U.; Bardazzi, F.; Zauli, D.; Franceschi, L.; Tosti, A.; Mounaro, N.; Ghetti, S.; Tetta, C.; Grassi, A.; Bianchi, F. Serological screening for coeliac disease in vitiligo and alopecia areata. *Br. J. Dermatol.* **1997**, *136*, 801–802. [CrossRef] [PubMed]
109. Hallaji, Z.; Akhyani, M.; Ehsani, A.H.; Noormohammadpour, P.; Gholamali, F.; Bagheri, M.; Jahromi, J. Prevalence of anti-gliadin antibody in patients with alopecia areata: A case-control study. *Tehran Univ. Med. J.* **2011**, *68*, 738–742.

110. Collin, P.; Reunala, T. Recognition and Management of the Cutaneous Manifestations of Celiac Disease. *Am. J. Clin. Dermatol.* **2003**, *4*, 13–20. [CrossRef] [PubMed]
111. Mokhtari, F.; Panjehpour, T.; Naeini, F.; Hosseini, S.; Nilforoushzadeh, M.; Matin, M. The frequency distribution of celiac autoantibodies in alopecia areata. *Int. J. Prev. Med.* **2016**, *7*, 109. [CrossRef] [PubMed]
112. Naveh, Y.; Rosenthal, E.; Ben-Arieh, Y.; Etzioni, A. Celiac disease-associated alopecia in childhood. *J. Pediatr.* **1999**, *134*, 362–364. [CrossRef]
113. Baigrie, D.; Crane, J.S. *Leukocytoclastic Vasculitis (Hypersensitivity Vasculitis)*; StatPearls [Internet]; StatPearls Publishing: Treasure Island, FL, USA, 2018.
114. Pulido-Pérez, A.; Avilés-Izquierdo, J.; Suárez-Fernández, R. Cutaneous vasculitis. *Actas Dermo-Sifiliogr.* **2012**, *103*, 179–191. [CrossRef] [PubMed]
115. Holdstock, D.; Oleesky, S. Vasculitis in coeliac diseases. *BMJ* **1970**, *4*, 369. [CrossRef] [PubMed]
116. Jones, F.A. The skin: A mirror of the gut. *Geriatrics* **1973**, *28*, 75–81. [CrossRef] [PubMed]
117. Similä, S.; Kokkonen, J.; Kallioinen, M. Cutaneous vasculitis as a manifestation of coeliac disease. *Acta Paediatr. Scand.* **1982**, *71*, 1051–1054. [CrossRef] [PubMed]
118. Meyers, S.; Dikman, S.; Spiera, H.; Schultz, N.; Janowitz, H. Cutaneous vasculitis complicating coeliac disease. *Gut* **1981**, *22*, 61–64. [CrossRef] [PubMed]
119. Alegre, V.; Winkelmann, R.; Diez-Martin, J.; Banks, P. Adult celiac disease, small and medium vessel cutaneous necrotizing vasculitis, and T cell lymphoma. *J. Am. Acad. Dermatol.* **1988**, *19*, 973–978. [CrossRef]
120. Menzies, I.; Pounder, R.; Heyer, S.; Laker, M.; Bull, J.; Wheeler, P.; Creamer, B. Abnormal intestinal permeability to sugars in villous atrophy. *Lancet* **1979**, *314*, 1107–1109. [CrossRef]
121. Buderus, S.; Wagner, N.; Lentze, M. Concurrence of Celiac Disease and Juvenile Dermatomyositis: Result of a Specific Immunogenetic Susceptibility? *J. Pediatr. Gastroenterol. Nutr.* **1997**, *25*, 101–103. [CrossRef] [PubMed]
122. Song, M.; Farber, D.; Bitton, A.; Jass, J.; Singer, M.; Karpati, G. Dermatomyositis Associated with Celiac Disease: Response to a Gluten-Free Diet. *Can. J. Gastroenterol.* **2006**, *20*, 433–435. [CrossRef] [PubMed]
123. Evron, E.; Abarbanel, J.M.; Branski, D.; Sthoeger, Z.M. Polymyositis, arthritis, and proteinuria in a patient with adult celiac disease. *J. Rheumatol.* **1996**, *23*, 782–783. [PubMed]
124. Hadjivassiliou, M.; Chattopadhyay, A.; Grünewald, R.; Jarratt, J.; Kandler, R.; Rao, D.; Sanders, D.; Wharton, S.; Davies-Jones, G. Myopathy associated with gluten sensitivity. *Muscle Nerve* **2007**, *35*, 443–450. [CrossRef] [PubMed]
125. Shahmoradi, Z.; Najafian, J.; Naeini, F.F.; Fahimipour, F. Vitiligo and autoantibodies of celiac disease. *Int. J. Prev. Med.* **2013**, *4*, 200–203. [PubMed]
126. Rodríguez-García, C.; González-Hernández, S.; Pérez-Robayna, N.; Guimerá, F.; Fagundo, E.; Sánchez, R. Repigmentation of Vitiligo Lesions in a Child with Celiac Disease after a Gluten-Free Diet. *Pediatr. Dermatol.* **2011**, *28*, 209–210. [CrossRef] [PubMed]
127. Mirza, N.; Bonilla, E.; Phillips, P. Celiac disease in a patient with systemic lupus erythematosus: A case report and review of literature. *Clin. Rheumatol.* **2006**, *26*, 827–828. [CrossRef] [PubMed]
128. Freeman, H.J. Adult celiac disease followed by onset of systemic lupus erythematosus. *J. Clin. Gastroenterol.* **2008**, *42*, 252–255. [CrossRef] [PubMed]
129. Latif, S.; Jamal, A.; Memon, I.; Yasmeen, S.; Tresa, V.; Shaikh, S. Multiple autoimmune syndrome: Hashimoto's thyroiditis, Coeliac disease and systemic lupus erythematosus (SLE). *J. Pak. Med. Assoc.* **2010**, *60*, 863–865. [PubMed]
130. Cigic, L.; Gavic, L.; Simunic, M.; Ardalic, Z.; Biocina-Lukenda, D. Increased prevalence of celiac disease in patients with oral lichen planus. *Clin. Oral Investig.* **2015**, *19*, 627–635. [CrossRef] [PubMed]
131. De, D. Eruptive lichen planus in a child with celiac disease. *Indian J. Dermatol. Venereol. Leprol.* **2008**, *74*, 164–165. [CrossRef] [PubMed]
132. Ruiz Villaverde, R.; Blasco Melguizo, J.; Menéndez García Estrada, A.; Díez García, F. Erosive mucosal lichen associated to hyper IgE syndrome and coeliac disease. *An. Pediatr.* **2004**, *60*, 281–282. [CrossRef]
133. Scully, C.; Porter, S.R.; Eveson, J.W. Oral lichen planus and coeliac disease. *Lancet* **1993**, *341*, 1660. [CrossRef]
134. Fortune, F.; Buchanan, J. Oral lichen planus and coeliac disease. *Lancet* **1993**, *341*, 1154–1155. [CrossRef]
135. Compilato, D.; Carroccio, A.; Campisi, G. Hidden coeliac disease in patients suffering from oral lichen planus. *J. Eur. Acad. Dermatol. Venereol.* **2012**, *26*, 390–391. [CrossRef] [PubMed]

136. Karadag, A.; Kavala, M.; Ozlu, E.; Zindancı, İ.; Ozkanlı, S.; Turkoglu, Z.; Zemheri, E. The co-occurrence of lichen sclerosus et atrophicus and celiac disease. *Indian Dermatol. Online J.* **2014**, *5*, 106. [CrossRef] [PubMed]

137. Jacobs, L.; Gilliam, A.; Khavari, N.; Bass, D. Association between Lichen Sclerosus and Celiac Disease: A Report of Three Pediatric Cases. *Pediatr. Dermatol.* **2014**, *31*, e128–e131. [CrossRef] [PubMed]

138. Essoussi, A.S.; Jomaa, B.; El Fehaiel, A. Association of celiac disease with sclero-atrophic lichen in a child with the HLA-B8 group. *Tunis. Med.* **1981**, *59*, 506–507. [PubMed]

139. Daoud, W.; El Euch, D.; Mokni, M.; Cherif, F.; Ben Tekaya, N.; Azaiz, M.I.; Ben Osman-Dhahri, A. Linear IgA bullous dermatosis associated with celiac disease. *Ann. Dermatol. Venereol.* **2006**, *133*, 588–589. [CrossRef]

140. Vaz, S.; Franco, C.; Santos, P.; Amaral, R. Skin and coeliac disease, a lot to think about: A case series. *BMJ Case Rep.* **2018**. [CrossRef] [PubMed]

141. Bonciolini, V.; Antiga, E.; Fabbri, P.; Caproni, M. Skin manifestations of celiac disease: Not always dermatitis herpetiformis. *Int. J. Dermatol.* **2014**, *53*, e352–e353. [CrossRef] [PubMed]

142. Randle, H.W.; Winkelmann, R.K. Pityriasis rubra pilaris and celiac sprue with malabsorption. *Cutis* **1980**, *25*, 626–627. [PubMed]

143. Tasanen, K.; Raudasoja, R.; Kallioinen, M.; Ranki, A. Erythema elevatum diutinum in association with coeliac disease. *Br. J. Dermatol.* **1997**, *136*, 624–627. [CrossRef] [PubMed]

144. Collin, P.; Korpela, M.; Hällström, O.; Viander, M.; Keyriläinen, O.; Mäki, M. Rheumatic Complaints as a Presenting Symptom in Patients with Coeliac Disease. *Scand. J. Rheumatol.* **1992**, *21*, 20–23. [CrossRef] [PubMed]

145. Rodriguez-Serna, M.; Fortea, J.; Perez, A.; Febrer, I.; Ribes, C.; Aliaga, A. Erythema elevatum diutinum associated with celiac disease: Response to a gluten-free diet. *Pediatr. Dermatol.* **1993**, *10*, 125–128. [CrossRef] [PubMed]

146. Goodenberger, D.M.; Lawley, T.J.; Strober, W.; Wyatt, L.; Sangree, M.H., Jr.; Sherwin, R.; Rosenbaum, H.; Braverman, I.; Katz, S.I. Necrolytic Migratory Erythema Without Glucagonoma. *Arch. Dermatol.* **1979**, *115*, 1429–1432. [CrossRef] [PubMed]

147. Kelly, C.; Johnston, C.; Nolan, N.; Keeling, P.; Weir, D. Necrolytic Migratory Erythema with Elevated Plasma Enteroglucagon in Celiac Disease. *Gastroenterology* **1989**, *96*, 1350–1353. [CrossRef]

148. Thorisdottir, K.; Camisa, C.; Tomecki, K.; Bergfeld, W. Necrolytic migratory erythema: A report of three cases. *J. Am. Acad. Dermatol.* **1994**, *30*, 324–329. [CrossRef]

149. Cribier, B.; Caille, A.; Heid, E.; Grosshans, E. Erythema nodosum and associated diseases. A study of 129 cases. *Int. J. Dermatol.* **1998**, *37*, 667–672. [CrossRef] [PubMed]

150. Durand, J.; Lefevre, P.; Weiller, C. Erythema nodosum and coeliac disease. *Br. J. Dermatol.* **1991**, *125*, 291–292. [CrossRef] [PubMed]

151. Bartyik, K.; Varkonyi, A.; Kirschner, A.; Endreffy, E.; Turi, S.; Karg, E. Erythema Nodosum in Association with Celiac Disease. *Pediatr. Dermatol.* **2004**, *21*, 227–230. [CrossRef] [PubMed]

152. Twaddle, S.; Wassif, W.S.; Deacon, A.C.; Peters, T.J. Celiac disease in patients with variegate porphyria. *Dig. Dis. Sci.* **2001**, *46*, 1506–1508. [CrossRef] [PubMed]

153. Moore, M.; Disler, P. Drug sensitive diseases-I-acute porphyrias. *Advers. Drug React. Bull.* **1988**, *129*, 484–487. [CrossRef]

154. Katsikas, G.; Maragou, M.; Rontogianni, D.; Gouma, P.; Koutsouvelis, I.; Kappou-Rigatou, I. Secondary cutaneous nodular AA amyloidosis in a patient with primary Sjögren syndrome and celiac disease. *J. Clin. Rheumatol.* **2008**, *14*, 27–29. [CrossRef] [PubMed]

155. Lewis, F.; Lewis-Jones, S.; Gipson, M. Acquired cutis laxa with dermatitis herpetiformis and sarcoidosis. *J. Am. Acad. Dermatol.* **1993**, *29*, 846–848. [CrossRef]

156. García-Patos, V.; Pujol, R.; Barnadas, M.; Pérez, M.; Moreno, A.; Condomines, J.; Gelpi, C.; Rodríguez, J.; De Moragas, J. Generalized acquired cutis laxa associated with coeliac disease: Evidence of immunoglobulin A deposits on the dermal elastic fibres. *Br. J. Dermatol.* **1996**, *135*, 130–134. [CrossRef] [PubMed]

157. Russell, P.; Floridis, J. Hypertrichosis Lanuginosa acquisita: A rare dermatological disorder. *Lancet* **2016**, *387*, 2035. [CrossRef]

158. Menni, S.; Boccardi, D.; Brusasco, A. Ichthyosis revealing coeliac disease. *Eur. J. Dermatol.* **2000**, *10*, 398–399. [PubMed]

159. O'Mahony, D.; O'Mahony, S.; Whelton, M.; McKiernan, J. Partial lipodystrophy in coeliac disease. *Gut* **1990**, *31*, 717–718. [CrossRef] [PubMed]

160. Foti, C.; Cassano, N.; Palmieri, V.O.; Portincasa, P.; Conserva, A.; Lamuraglia, M.; Palasciano, G.; Vena, G.A. Transverse leukonychia in severe hypocalcemia. *Eur. J. Dermatol.* **2004**, *14*, 67–68. [PubMed]

161. Montalto, M.; Diociaiuti, A.; Alvaro, G.; Manna, R.; Amerio, P.L.; Gasbarrini, G. Atypical mole syndrome and congenital giant naevus in a patient with celiac disease. *Panminerva Med.* **2003**, *45*, 219–221. [PubMed]

162. Lebwohl, B.; Eriksson, H.; Hansson, J.; Green, P.; Ludvigsson, J. Risk of cutaneous malignant melanoma in patients with celiac disease: A population-based study. *J. Am. Acad. Dermatol.* **2014**, *71*, 245–248. [CrossRef] [PubMed]

163. Pastore, L.; De Benedittis, M.; Petruzzi, M.; Tatò, D.; Napoli, C.; Montagna, M.T.; Catassi, C.; Serpico, R. Importance of oral signs in the diagnosis of atypical forms of celiac disease. *Recenti Prog. Med.* **2004**, *95*, 482–490. [PubMed]

164. Lahteenoja, H. Oral Mucosa Is Frequently Affected in Patients with Dermatitis Herpetiformis. *Arch. Dermatol.* **1998**, *134*, 756–758. [CrossRef] [PubMed]

165. Bramanti, E.; Cicciù, M.; Matacena, G.; Costa, S.; Magazzù, G. Clinical Evaluation of Specific Oral Manifestations in Pediatric Patients with Ascertained versus Potential Coeliac Disease: A Cross-Sectional Study. *Gastroenterol. Res. Pract.* **2014**, *2014*, 1–9. [CrossRef] [PubMed]

166. Fasano, A. Clinical presentation of celiac disease in the pediatric population. *Gastroenterology* **2005**, *128*, S68–S73. [CrossRef] [PubMed]

167. Husby, S.; Koletzko, S.; Korponay-Szabó, I.R.; Mearin, M.L.; Phillips, A.; Shamir, R.; Troncone, R.; Giersiepen, K.; Branski, D.; Catassi, C.; et al. European Society for Pediatric Gastroenterology, Hepatology, and Nutrition guidelines for the diagnosis of coeliac disease. *J. Pediatr. Gastroenterol. Nutr.* **2012**, *54*, 136–160. [CrossRef] [PubMed]

168. Newnham, E.D. Coeliac disease in the 21st century: Paradigm shifts in the modern age. *J. Gastroenterol. Hepatol.* **2017**, *32*, 82–85. [CrossRef] [PubMed]

169. Rostami Nejad, M.; Hogg-Kollars, S.; Ishaq, S.; Rostami, K. Subclinical celiac disease and gluten sensitivity. *Gastroenterol. Hepatol. Bed Bench* **2011**, *4*, 102–108. [PubMed]

170. Tonutti, E.; Bizzaro, N. Diagnosis and classification of celiac disease and gluten sensitivity. *Autoimmun. Rev.* **2014**, *13*, 472–476. [CrossRef] [PubMed]

171. Lionetti, E.; Gatti, S.; Pulvirenti, A.; Catassi, C. Celiac disease from a global perspective. *Best Pract. Res. Clin. Gastroenterol.* **2015**, *29*, 365–379. [CrossRef] [PubMed]

172. Ludvigsson, J.F.; Card, T.R.; Kaukinen, K.; Bai, J.; Zingone, F.; Sanders, D.S.; Murray, J.A. Screening for celiac disease in the general population and in high-risk groups. *United Eur. Gastroenterol. J.* **2015**, *3*, 106–120. [CrossRef] [PubMed]

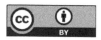

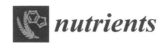

Review

Celiac Disease and Glandular Autoimmunity

George J. Kahaly [1,*], Lara Frommer [1] and Detlef Schuppan [2,3]

[1] Department of Medicine I, Johannes Gutenberg University (JGU) Medical Center, 55101 Mainz, Germany;
     Lara.Frommer@unimedizin-mainz.de
[2] Institute for Translational Immunology and Research Center for Immunotherapy (FZI), Johannes Gutenberg
     University (JGU) Medical Center, 55101 Mainz, Germany; Detlef.Schuppan@unimedizin-mainz.de
[3] Division of Gastroenterology, Beth Israel Deaconess Medical Center, Harvard Medical School,
     Boston, MA 02215, USA
* Correspondence: george.kahaly@unimedizin-mainz.de; Tel.: +49-6131-17-2290

Received: 6 June 2018; Accepted: 21 June 2018; Published: 25 June 2018

Abstract: Celiac disease is a small intestinal inflammatory disease with autoimmune features that is triggered and maintained by the ingestion of the storage proteins (gluten) of wheat, barley, and rye. Prevalence of celiac disease is increased in patients with mono- and/or polyglandular autoimmunity and their relatives. We have reviewed the current and pertinent literature that addresses the close association between celiac disease and endocrine autoimmunity. The close relationship between celiac disease and glandular autoimmunity can be largely explained by sharing of a common genetic background. Further, between 10 and 30% of patients with celiac disease are thyroid and/or type 1 diabetes antibody positive, while around 5–7% of patients with autoimmune thyroid disease, type 1 diabetes, and/or polyglandular autoimmunity are IgA anti-tissue transglutaminase antibody positive. While a gluten free diet does not reverse glandular autoimmunity, its early institution may delay or even prevent its first manifestation. In conclusion, this brief review highlighting the close association between celiac disease and both monoglandular and polyglandular autoimmunity, aims to underline the need for prospective studies to establish whether an early diagnosis of celiac disease and a prompt gluten-free diet may positively impact the evolution and manifestation of glandular autoimmunity.

Keywords: celiac disease; glandular autoimmunity; autoimmune thyroid disease; type 1 diabetes; polyglandular autoimmune syndrome

---

1. Celiac Disease

Celiac disease (CeD) is defined as a life-long intolerance to dietary gluten that results in small intestinal inflammation, villous atrophy, crypt hyperplasia, and often malabsorption. The ingestion of gluten containing cereal grains, mainly wheat, rye, and barley, drives this T cell driven auto-destructive process within the small intestinal mucosa which usually recovers when these cereals and gluten are rigorously withdrawn from the diet [1–4].

At least 50% of CeD is diagnosed in adulthood, and in the majority of adolescents and adults clinical features at diagnosis are subtle, with mild abdominal discomfort, fatigue, low bone mineralisation and hypocalcaemia, and only rarely manifest anemia, weight loss, infertility, or recurrent aphtous stomatitis. However, up to one third of adults suffer from one or more CeD-associated autoimmune diseases, prominently with autoimmune thyroid disease (AITD) and type 1 diabetes mellitus (T1D), but also rheumatoid diseases including systemic lupus erythematodes, Sjoegren's syndrome, autoimmune liver diseases, and others [5]. Severe complications, like refractory CeD type 2, a premalignant condition, and overt enteropathy-associated T-cell lymphoma, occur in patients with longstanding undetected and untreated CeD, but remain rare [6,7]. Iron, zinc, vitamin D, vitamin B12, or folic acid deficiency, iron deficiency or overt anemia are the most common laboratory finding.

Frequent episodes of hypoglycemia, a reduction of insulin requirements and brittle diabetes may indicate the presence of CeD in patients with T1D [8]. CeD is considered sufficiently prevalent and the benefits of diagnosis and treatment by gluten withdrawal are such that it is advocated to screen all patients with T1D (and autoimmune thyroid disease) for this disorder.

Both endoscopic-histological diagnosis and the presence of circulating IgA antibodies (Ab) to tissue transglutaminase (TG2) confirm the diagnosis. As shown in Table 1, anti-transglutaminase antibodies may be of IgG isotype in the presence, but also in the absence of a selective IgA deficiency. This suggests that the gluten-triggered autoantibody response shows mucosal IgA as its main component, while systemic IgG may represent a long-term reaction probably related to the occurrence of extra-intestinal manifestations. Consistently, it has been reported previously that the prevalence of CeD in T1D increases dramatically when the detection of both IgA and IgG autoantibodies is used in the screening. After a gluten-free diet the IgA-TG2-Ab disappear in most patients with CeD, usually with a half-life between 30 and 60 days.

Table 1. Autoimmune disease specific antibodies.

Disease	Autoantibodies
Celiac disease	Tissue transglutaminase IgA (IgG)
Type 1 diabetes	Glutamate decarboxylase (GAD) Tyrosine phosphatase (IA2) Islet cell (IC) Insulin Zinc transporter (ZnT8)
Autoimmune thyroid disease	Thyro-peroxidase (TPO) Thyroglobulin (Tg) TSH receptor

Genetic factors greatly determine susceptibility to CeD. All CeD patients carry HLA DR3/DQ2 (mainly DQA1*0501-DQB1*0201; 85–95%), or HLA DR4/DQ8 (DQA1*0301-DQB1*0302; 5–15%), or both haplotypes [1–3]. Exceptions are certain Native American populations that mainly carry DQ8 [9]. Since, e.g., the prevalence of HLA DQ2 in most populations is between 25 and 50%, only a minority with this necessary but insufficient genetic predisposition will ever develop CeD. This implies the involvement of additional, non-HLA linked genes, as well as environmental factors in CeD manifestation, as discussed below.

The ubiquitous enzyme TG2, the CeD autoantigen, is central to the pathogenesis of CeD, since it can deamidate specific glutamine residues in certain gluten peptides that remain undigested and reach the subepithelial small intestinal lamina propria. This deamidation of the gluten peptides and their haptenization by binding to TG2 itself (autocatalysis) thereby increases their affinity to DQ2 or DQ8 on professional antigen presenting cells like macrophages, dendritic, and B cells, favoring the subsequent gluten specific destructive T cell response [1,10–12].

2. Monoglandular and Polyglandular Autoimmunity

Patients with CeD show a high prevalence of glandular autoimmune disorders [13–16]. CeD is associated with T1D, AITD i.e., Hashimoto's thyroiditis (HT), Graves' disease (GD), and the polyglandular autoimmune syndrome (PAS) [17].

2.1. Type 1 Diabetes

T1D is a T-cell mediated glandular autoimmune disease that develops in genetically susceptible individuals and results in destruction of the insulin-producing β cells. Of T1D patients, 15–30% have AITD and 3–12% present with CeD [18]. The close relationship between CeD and glandular autoimmunity can be widely explained by sharing of a common genetic background. However, some common pathogenic mechanisms have been further implicated, such as increased intestinal permeability resulting from zonulin upregulation and dysfunction of tight junctions in both CeD and T1D [19]. T1D is characterized by the infiltration of the pancreatic islets by lymphocytes and macrophages, the presence of autoantibodies to *islet cell antigens (ICA), tyrosine phosphatase (IA2), glutamic acid decarboxylase-65 (GAD), insulin (IAA)*, and *zinc transporter ZnT8 (Slc30A8)*, an increased prevalence of organ-specific autoimmune disorders in T1D, a preferential occurrence of T1D in persons carrying specific allelic combinations at immune response loci within the *HLA* gene complex. The disease can be transferred by spleen or bone marrow cells and animal models of T1D show a defect in immunoregulation contributing to the onset of disease [20].

2.2. Hashimoto's Thyroiditis

HT is currently the most common autoimmune disease and frequently clusters with other autoimmune endocrinopathies. It is defined by the presence of thyro-peroxidase (TPO) or thyroglobulin (Tg) Ab and either normal or elevated serum thyroid stimulating hormone (TSH) concentrations. The majority of patients with HT are hypothyroid; however there is a subgroup of thyroid Ab-positive cases who are euthyroid. HT frequently occurs with T1D, with a prevalence of 13–20% of subclinical hypothyroidism in T1D patients compared with 3–6% in a non-diabetic population. Overt hypothyroidism is present in 4–18% of subjects with T1D. TPO-Ab are present in 15–30% of adults and in 5–22% of children with T1D, compared with 2–10% and 1–4%, respectively, in healthy controls. Up to 50% of TPO-Ab positive T1D patients progress to overt AITD. As many as 30% of patients with T1D develop AITD. Age, duration of T1D, and female preponderance impact the link between T1D and AITD [21,22]. In a prospective controlled study, celiac patients had an increased risk of thyroid autoimmune disorders when compared to non-celiac controls on normal gluten-containing diet [23]. However, in this Scandinavian trial, a gluten-free diet seemed not to prevent the progression of autoimmune process during a follow-up of one year.

2.3. Graves' Disease

GD is meanwhile less prevalent than HT; it affects approximately 1–1.5% of the general population worldwide and is the underlying cause of 50–80% of cases of thyrotoxicosis. GD and HT share many immunological features, including high serum concentrations of Ab against Tg and TPO. GD is caused by TSH receptor stimulating Ab [24–26] that bind to and activate the TSH receptor on thyroid cells. These Ab not only cause hypersecretion of thyroid hormone, but also promote hypertrophy and hyperplasia of thyroid follicles, resulting in an enhanced vascularization of the gland and in a diffuse goiter. Women are five to ten times more at risk of developing GD than men, due to the relevant involvement of sex hormones. Also, stress and negative life events are regarded as risk factors for GD and may trigger the disease. Subclinical endogenous hyperthyroidism can be diagnosed in 6–10% of T1D patients, compared with 0.1–2% in the non-diabetic population. The incidence of overt autoimmune hyperthyroidism in persons with a suppressed serum TSH is calculated at 2–4% per year [27].

2.4. Polyglandular Autoimmune Syndrome

The association of two or more glandular autoimmune diseases is designated as PAS. Especially in adults, the presence of one autoimmune endocrine disorder increases the risk of developing other autoimmune diseases. CeD is a strong predictor not only of glandular but also polyglandular autoimmunity. PAS shows a great heterogeneity of syndromes and usually manifests sequentially, with a variable time interval between the occurrence of the first and second glandular autoimmune disease component. It also clusters with several non-endocrine autoimmune diseases [28]. PAS is divided into two major subtypes, which are distinguished according to age of presentation, characteristic patterns of disease combinations and different modes of inheritance. Juvenile PAS I, also known as autoimmune polyendocrinopathy-candidiasis-ectodermal dystrophy, usually manifests in infancy or childhood at age three to five years, or in early adolescence, It is characterized by a persistent fungal infection (chronic mucocutaneous candidiasis), the presence of acquired hypoparathyroidism and adrenal failure. In most patients mucocutaneous candidiasis precedes the other immune disorders, usually followed by hypoparathyroidism. The female-to-male ratio varies from 0.8:1 to 2.4:1. The highest prevalence of PAS I has been found in populations characterized by a high degree of consanguinity or descendants of small founder populations, particularly in Iranian Jews and Fins. PAS I is a monogenic disease with autosomal recessive inheritance caused by mutations in the autoimmune regulatory gene (AIRE) on chromosome 21. Adult PAS occurs mainly in the third or fourth decade. Adult PAS subtype II encompasses adrenal failure or Addison's disease (AD) with other autoimmune endocrine disorders, i.e., AITD and/or T1D. AD may precede other endocrinopathies. In contrast to the juvenile type, family members of adult PAS II patients are often affected. PAS II is believed to be polygenic, characterized by autosomal dominant inheritance [29–34].

The adult PAS type III is the most frequent PAS type and is characterized by AITD and T1D and the absence of AD. In contrast, the poorly defined PAS type IV is very heterogeneous involving a large variety of glandular autoimmune diseases that are not considered within adult PAS types 2 and 3. Being less well defined, it is often incorrectly described as a combination of monoglandular autoimmune disease with one non-glandular autoimmune disease. In fact, PAS type IV includes various combinations of autoimmune hypopituitarism, hypergonadotropic hypogonadism, or hypoparathyroidism with T1D or an AITD. The adult form of PAS has a prevalence of 1:20,000, and is far more prevalent than the juvenile type, with an annual incidence of 1–2:100,000. The gender ratio of adult PAS types II–IV shows a female predominance of 75% [35,36]. The manifestation peaks in the fourth and fifth decade depending on the combination of the various autoimmune endocrinopathies [37].

Even if the time between the manifestations of CeD and other autoimmune endocrinopathies, as well as the time until a PAS can be diagnosed, is highly variable, many patients with one autoimmune disease already have Ab against other, often endocrine, tissues (Table 2). The reason is the tendency of autoimmune diseases to associate with one another, especially when they share a genetic basis, of the metachronous manifestations of the component diseases, and of the often subclinical initial course. Mainly first but also second degree family members of patients are often at risk for developing related autoimmunities and are already Ab positive.

Table 2. Prevalence of autoimmune thyroid disease auto antibodies in patients with celiac disease.

CeD Patients Studied (N)	Prevalence of Thyroid Autoantibodies, N	Prevalence of Thyroid Autoantibodies in %	Reference
107	Tg Ab, N = 12	11.2	[38]
	TMA, N = 16	15	
70	TMA, N = 15	21	[39]
47	TPO, N = 14	29.7	[40]
	TMA, N = 5	14.7	
34	Tg Ab, N = 11	32.4	[41]
	TPO, N = 4	11.8	
90	TPO, N = 13	14.4	[42]
36	TPO, N = 11	30.5	[43]

Modified according to reference [44]. CeD: celiac disease, Tg-Ab: thyroglobulin antibodies; TMA: thyroid microsomal antibodies; TPO-Ab: thyro-peroxidase antibodies.

3. The Role of a Gluten Free Diet in Preventing Celiac Disease and Glandular Autoimmunity

A large prospective study demonstrated that in infants at genetic risk for CeD and T1D (i.e., from families with at least one affected parent and the *DR3/DQ2* and/or *DR4/DQ8* risk genes) a careful early introduction of 100 mg gluten per day in the diet from month 5–6 did not prevent celiac autoimmunity compared to placebo [45]. Moreover, the introduction of gluten at 12 instead of 6 months of age only delayed the onset of CeD, with similar prevalences at age 5 years [46]. However, a retrospective study indicated that patients on a long-term gluten free diet developed 50% fewer autoimmune diseases in up to 15 years of follow up [47]. The (retrospective) studies that examined the effect of a gluten free versus gluten containing diet on the development and severity of T1D and AITD remain controversial (Tables 3 and 4). Interestingly, T1D appears to precede the development of CeD, as determined by IgA-TG2 Ab positivity, which would assign a less important role to the gluten free diet in the prevention of glandular autoimmunity [19].

Table 3. Gluten exposure and occurrence of type 1 diabetes.

Patients (*N*)	Duration of Follow-up (Years)	Early CeD Dx Protective?	GFD Protective?	Reference
90	2	NE	Yes	[42]
44	1.6	No	Yes	[48]
383	7.6	No	NE	[49]
1183	0.9	NE	Yes	[50]
19796	NE	No	NE	[51]
4322	NE	No	NE	[52]
150	3	NE	Yes	[53]

Table 4. Gluten exposure and occurrence of autoimmune thyroid disease (AITD).

Patients (*N*)	Duration of Follow-up (Years)	Early CeD Dx Protective?	GFD Protective?	Reference
909	>0.5	Yes	NE	[42]
44	1.6	No	Yes	[48]
66	1–5	Yes	Yes	[54]
343	0.25–16	NE	No	[55]
324	8	Yes	No	[56]
135	8.9	No	No	[57]
545	2	No	No	[58]
335	9	No	No	[59]

Dx: diagnosis; GFD: gluten free diet; NE: not evaluated.

Several mainly retrospective and correlative studies, often based on registries, have tried to address the question, how far an early diagnosis of CeD and/or a gluten free diet may protect from AITD or T1D. As shown in tables 3 and 4, in these studies early diagnosis of CeD did not appear to protect from the development of T1D [42,48–53]; whereas some studies suggested such protection in AITD [42,48,54–59]. In comparison, a gluten free diet (GFD) may positively impact the occurrence of T1D rather than of AITD. These somewhat conflicting data need validation in large, prospective studies with well-defined diagnosis and markers of CeD, T1D, and AITD. Such studies are currently performed in children with an increased risk for the three diseases (being offspring of affected parents and carrying the *DQ2* and/or *DQ8* genes. However, a beneficial effect of a gluten free diet may be expected, since in general, in children as well as in adults, intestinal inflammation and the associated dysbiosis, with or without underlying CeD, are known to promote extra intestinal autoimmune diseases [60–62]. Therefore, any measure that would dampen gut inflammation in CeD patients will likely positively impact the evolution and perhaps the manifestation of glandular autoimmunity.

Author Contributions: G.J.K., L.F., and D.S. jointly drafted and edited the article.

Funding: D.S. receives CeD related funding form the German Research Foundation (DFG 646/17-1).

Acknowledgments: The authors are grateful to Tanja Diana, Elisa Schulze, and Marie Kuschnereit, JGU Thyroid Research Lab, Mainz, Germany for data collection.

Conflicts of Interest: The authors declare no conflict of interest.

References

1. Schuppan, D.; Junker, Y.; Barisani, D. Celiac disease: From pathogenesis to novel therapies. *Gastroenterology* **2009**, *137*, 1912–1933. [CrossRef] [PubMed]

2. Fasano, A.; Catassi, C. Clinical practice. Celiac disease. *N. Engl. J. Med.* **2012**, *367*, 2419–2426. [CrossRef] [PubMed]

3. Sollid, L.M.; Jabri, B. Triggers and drivers of autoimmunity: Lessons from coeliac disease. *Nat. Rev. Immunol.* **2013**, *13*, 294–302. [CrossRef] [PubMed]

4. Lundin, K.E.; Sollid, L.M. Advances in coeliac disease. *Curr. Opin. Gastroenterol.* **2014**, *30*, 154–162. [CrossRef] [PubMed]

5. Ventura, A.; Magazzu, G.; Greco, L. Duration of exposure to gluten and risk for autoimmune disorders in patients with celiac disease. Sigep study group for autoimmune disorders in celiac disease. *Gastroenterology* **1999**, *117*, 297–303. [CrossRef] [PubMed]

6. Malamut, G.; Meresse, B.; Cellier, C.; Cerf-Bensussan, N. Refractory celiac disease: From bench to bedside. *Semin. Immunopathol.* **2012**, *34*, 601–613. [CrossRef] [PubMed]

7. Van Gils, T.; Nijeboer, P.; van Wanrooij, R.L.; Bouma, G.; Mulder, C.J. Mechanisms and management of refractory coeliac disease. *Nat. Rev. Gastroenterol. Hepatol.* **2015**, *12*, 572–579. [CrossRef] [PubMed]

8. Pham-Short, A.; Donaghue, K.C.; Ambler, G.; Garnett, S.; Craig, M.E. Greater postprandial glucose excursions and inadequate nutrient intake in youth with type 1 diabetes and celiac disease. *Sci. Rep.* **2017**, *7*, 45286. [CrossRef] [PubMed]

9. Vazquez, H.; de la Paz Temprano, M.; Sugai, E.; Scacchi, S.M.; Souza, C.; Cisterna, D.; Smecuol, E.; Moreno, M.L.; Longarini, G.; Mazure, R.; et al. Prevalence of celiac disease and celiac autoimmunity in the toba native amerindian community of Argentina. *Can. J. Gastroenterol. Hepatol.* **2015**, *29*, 431–434. [CrossRef] [PubMed]

10. Dieterich, W.; Ehnis, T.; Bauer, M.; Donner, P.; Volta, U.; Riecken, E.O.; Schuppan, D. Identification of tissue transglutaminase as the autoantigen of celiac disease. *Nat. Med.* **1997**, *3*, 797–801. [CrossRef] [PubMed]

11. Molberg, O.; McAdam, S.N.; Korner, R.; Quarsten, H.; Kristiansen, C.; Madsen, L.; Fugger, L.; Scott, H.; Noren, O.; Roepstorff, P.; et al. Tissue transglutaminase selectively modifies gliadin peptides that are recognized by gut-derived t cells in celiac disease. *Nat. Med.* **1998**, *4*, 713–717. [CrossRef] [PubMed]

12. Van de Wal, Y.; Kooy, Y.M.; van Veelen, P.A.; Pena, S.A.; Mearin, L.M.; Molberg, O.; Lundin, K.E.; Sollid, L.M.; Mutis, T.; Benckhuijsen, W.E.; et al. Small intestinal T cells of celiac disease patients recognize a natural pepsin fragment of gliadin. *Proc. Natl. Acad. Sci. USA* **1998**, *95*, 10050–10054. [CrossRef] [PubMed]

13. Frohlich-Reiterer, E.E.; Hofer, S.; Kaspers, S.; Herbst, A.; Kordonouri, O.; Schwarz, H.P.; Schober, E.; Grabert, M.; Holl, R.W.; Group, D.P.-W.S. Screening frequency for celiac disease and autoimmune thyroiditis in children and adolescents with type 1 diabetes mellitus—Data from a German/Austrian multicentre survey. *Pediatr. Diabetes* **2008**, *9*, 546–553. [CrossRef] [PubMed]

14. Boelaert, K.; Newby, P.R.; Simmonds, M.J.; Holder, R.L.; Carr-Smith, J.D.; Heward, J.M.; Manji, N.; Allahabadia, A.; Armitage, M.; Chatterjee, K.V.; et al. Prevalence and relative risk of other autoimmune diseases in subjects with autoimmune thyroid disease. *Am. J. Med.* **2010**, *123*, e181–e189. [CrossRef] [PubMed]

15. Dittmar, M.; Libich, C.; Brenzel, T.; Kahaly, G.J. Increased familial clustering of autoimmune thyroid diseases. *Horm. Metab. Res.* **2011**, *43*, 200–204. [CrossRef] [PubMed]

16. Villano, M.J.; Huber, A.K.; Greenberg, D.A.; Golden, B.K.; Concepcion, E.; Tomer, Y. Autoimmune thyroiditis and diabetes: Dissecting the joint genetic susceptibility in a large cohort of multiplex families. *J Clin. Endocrinol. Metab.* **2009**, *94*, 1458–1466. [CrossRef] [PubMed]

17. Kahaly, G.J.; Schuppan, D. Celiac disease and endocrine autoimmunity. *Dig. Dis.* **2015**, *33*, 155–161. [CrossRef] [PubMed]

18. Kordonouri, O.; Dieterich, W.; Schuppan, D.; Webert, G.; Muller, C.; Sarioglu, N.; Becker, M.; Danne, T. Autoantibodies to tissue transglutaminase are sensitive serological parameters for detecting silent coeliac disease in patients with type 1 diabetes mellitus. *Diabet. Med.* **2000**, *17*, 441–444. [CrossRef] [PubMed]

19. Hagopian, W.; Lee, H.S.; Liu, E.; Rewers, M.; She, J.X.; Ziegler, A.G.; Lernmark, A.; Toppari, J.; Rich, S.S.; Krischer, J.P.; et al. Co-occurrence of type 1 diabetes and celiac disease autoimmunity. *Pediatrics* **2017**, *140*. [CrossRef] [PubMed]

20. Kahaly, G.J.; Hansen, M.P. Type 1 diabetes associated autoimmunity. *Autoimmun. Rev.* **2016**, *15*, 644–648. [CrossRef] [PubMed]
21. Ponto, K.A.; Schuppan, D.; Zwiener, I.; Binder, H.; Mirshahi, A.; Diana, T.; Pitz, S.; Pfeiffer, N.; Kahaly, G.J. Thyroid-associated orbitopathy is linked to gastrointestinal autoimmunity. *Clin. Exp. Immunol.* **2014**, *178*, 57–64. [CrossRef] [PubMed]
22. Schuppan, D.; Ciccocioppo, R. Coeliac disease and secondary autoimmunity. *Dig. Liver. Dis.* **2002**, *34*, 13–15. [CrossRef]
23. Metso, S.; Hyytia-Ilmonen, H.; Kaukinen, K.; Huhtala, H.; Jaatinen, P.; Salmi, J.; Taurio, J.; Collin, P. Gluten-free diet and autoimmune thyroiditis in patients with celiac disease. A prospective controlled study. *Scand. J. Gastroenterol.* **2012**, *47*, 43–48. [CrossRef] [PubMed]
24. Diana, T.; Wuster, C.; Olivo, P.D.; Unterrainer, A.; Konig, J.; Kanitz, M.; Bossowski, A.; Decallonne, B.; Kahaly, G.J. Performance and specificity of 6 immunoassays for TSH receptor antibodies: A multicenter study. *Eur. Thyroid. J.* **2017**, *6*, 243–249. [CrossRef] [PubMed]
25. Diana, T.; Wuster, C.; Kanitz, M.; Kahaly, G.J. Highly variable sensitivity of five binding and two bio-assays for TSH-receptor antibodies. *J. Endocrinol. Invest.* **2016**, *39*, 1159–1165. [CrossRef] [PubMed]
26. Diana, T.; Brown, R.S.; Bossowski, A.; Segni, M.; Niedziela, M.; Konig, J.; Bossowska, A.; Ziora, K.; Hale, A.; Smith, J.; et al. Clinical relevance of thyroid-stimulating autoantibodies in pediatric graves' disease—A multicenter study. *J. Clin. Endocrinol. Metab.* **2014**, *99*, 1648–1655. [CrossRef] [PubMed]
27. Ross, D.S.; Burch, H.B.; Cooper, D.S.; Greenlee, M.C.; Laurberg, P.; Maia, A.L.; Rivkees, S.A.; Samuels, M.; Sosa, J.A.; Stan, M.N.; et al. 2016 American thyroid association guidelines for diagnosis and management of hyperthyroidism and other causes of thyrotoxicosis. *Thyroid* **2016**, *26*, 1343–1421. [CrossRef] [PubMed]
28. Kahaly, G.J.; Frommer, L. Polyglandular autoimmune syndromes. *J. Endocrinol. Invest.* **2018**, *41*, 91–98. [CrossRef] [PubMed]
29. Kahaly, G.J. Polyglandular autoimmune syndromes. *Eur. J. Endocrinol.* **2009**, *161*, 11–20. [CrossRef] [PubMed]
30. Dittmar, M.; Kahaly, G.J. Polyglandular autoimmune syndromes: Immunogenetics and long-term follow-up. *J. Clin. Endocrinol. Metab.* **2003**, *88*, 2983–2992. [CrossRef] [PubMed]
31. Weinstock, C.; Matheis, N.; Barkia, S.; Haager, M.C.; Janson, A.; Markovic, A.; Bux, J.; Kahaly, G.J. Autoimmune polyglandular syndrome type 2 shows the same HLA class ii pattern as type 1 diabetes. *Tissue Antigens* **2011**, *77*, 317–324. [CrossRef] [PubMed]
32. Selmi, C. Autoimmunity in 2011. *Clin. Rev. Allergy Immunol.* **2012**, *43*, 194–206. [CrossRef] [PubMed]
33. Anaya, J.M. The diagnosis and clinical significance of polyautoimmunity. *Autoimmun. Rev.* **2014**, *13*, 423–426. [CrossRef] [PubMed]
34. Cutolo, M. Autoimmune polyendocrine syndromes. *Autoimmun. Rev.* **2014**, *13*, 85–89. [CrossRef] [PubMed]
35. Betterle, C.; Zanchetta, R. Update on autoimmune polyendocrine syndromes (aps). *Acta. Biomed.* **2003**, *74*, 9–33. [PubMed]
36. Betterle, C.; Lazzarotto, F.; Presotto, F. Autoimmune polyglandular syndrome type 2: The tip of an iceberg? *Clin. Exp. Immunol.* **2004**, *137*, 225–233. [CrossRef] [PubMed]
37. Houcken, J.; Degenhart, C.; Bender, K.; Konig, J.; Frommer, L.; Kahaly, G.J. PTPN22 and CTLA-4 polymorphisms are associated with polyglandular autoimmunity. *J. Clin. Endocrinol. Metab.* **2018**. [CrossRef] [PubMed]
38. Counsell, C.E.; Taha, A.; Ruddell, W.S. Coeliac disease and autoimmune thyroid disease. *Gut* **1994**, *35*, 844–846. [CrossRef] [PubMed]
39. Volta, U.; de Franceschi, L.; Molinaro, N.; Tetta, C.; Bianchi, F.B. Organ-specific autoantibodies in coeliac disease: Do they represent an epiphenomenon or the expression of associated autoimmune disorders? *Ital. J. Gastroenterol. Hepatol.* **1997**, *29*, 18–21. [PubMed]
40. Velluzzi, F.; Caradonna, A.; Boy, M.F.; Pinna, M.A.; Cabula, R.; Lai, M.A.; Piras, E.; Corda, G.; Mossa, P.; Atzeni, F.; et al. Thyroid and celiac disease: Clinical, serological, and echographic study. *Am. J. Gastroenterol.* **1998**, *93*, 976–979. [CrossRef] [PubMed]
41. Kowalska, E.; Wasowska-Krolikowska, K.; Toporowska-Kowalska, E. Estimation of antithyroid antibodies occurrence in children with coeliac disease. *Med. Sci. Monit.* **2000**, *6*, 719–721. [PubMed]
42. Ventura, A.; Neri, E.; Ughi, C.; Leopaldi, A.; Citta, A.; Not, T. Gluten-dependent diabetes-related and thyroid-related autoantibodies in patients with celiac disease. *J. Pediatr.* **2000**, *137*, 263–265. [CrossRef] [PubMed]

43. Carta, M.G.; Hardoy, M.C.; Boi, M.F.; Mariotti, S.; Carpiniello, B.; Usai, P. Association between panic disorder, major depressive disorder and celiac disease: A possible role of thyroid autoimmunity. *J. Psychosom. Res.* **2002**, *53*, 789–793. [CrossRef]

44. Ch'ng, C.L.; Jones, M.K.; Kingham, J.G. Celiac disease and autoimmune thyroid disease. *Clin. Med. Res.* **2007**, *5*, 184–192. [CrossRef] [PubMed]

45. Vriezinga, S.L.; Auricchio, R.; Bravi, E.; Castillejo, G.; Chmielewska, A.; Crespo Escobar, P.; Kolacek, S.; Koletzko, S.; Korponay-Szabo, I.R.; Mummert, E.; et al. Randomized feeding intervention in infants at high risk for celiac disease. *N. Engl. J. Med.* **2014**, *371*, 1304–1315. [CrossRef] [PubMed]

46. Lionetti, E.; Castellaneta, S.; Francavilla, R.; Pulvirenti, A.; Tonutti, E.; Amarri, S.; Barbato, M.; Barbera, C.; Barera, G.; Bellantoni, A.; et al. Introduction of gluten, HLA status, and the risk of celiac disease in children. *N. Engl. J. Med.* **2014**, *371*, 1295–1303. [CrossRef] [PubMed]

47. Cosnes, J.; Cellier, C.; Viola, S.; Colombel, J.F.; Michaud, L.; Sarles, J.; Hugot, J.P.; Ginies, J.L.; Dabadie, A.; Mouterde, O.; et al. Incidence of autoimmune diseases in celiac disease: Protective effect of the gluten-free diet. *Clin. Gastroenterol. Hepatol.* **2008**, *6*, 753–758. [CrossRef] [PubMed]

48. Toscano, V.; Conti, F.G.; Anastasi, E.; Mariani, P.; Tiberti, C.; Poggi, M.; Montuori, M.; Monti, S.; Laureti, S.; Cipolletta, E.; et al. Importance of gluten in the induction of endocrine autoantibodies and organ dysfunction in adolescent celiac patients. *Am. J. Gastroenterol.* **2000**, *95*, 1742–1748. [CrossRef] [PubMed]

49. Valerio, G.; Maiuri, L.; Troncone, R.; Buono, P.; Lombardi, F.; Palmieri, R.; Franzese, A. Severe clinical onset of diabetes and increased prevalence of other autoimmune diseases in children with coeliac disease diagnosed before diabetes mellitus. *Diabetologia* **2002**, *45*, 1719–1722. [PubMed]

50. Norris, J.M.; Barriga, K.; Hoffenberg, E.J.; Taki, I.; Miao, D.; Haas, J.E.; Emery, L.M.; Sokol, R.J.; Erlich, H.A.; Eisenbarth, G.S.; et al. Risk of celiac disease autoimmunity and timing of gluten introduction in the diet of infants at increased risk of disease. *JAMA* **2005**, *293*, 2343–2351. [CrossRef] [PubMed]

51. Kaspers, S.; Kordonouri, O.; Schober, E.; Grabert, M.; Hauffa, B.P.; Holl, R.W. Anthropometry, metabolic control, and thyroid autoimmunity in type 1 diabetes with celiac disease: A multicenter survey. *J. Pediatr.* **2004**, *145*, 790–795. [CrossRef] [PubMed]

52. Cerutti, F.; Bruno, G.; Chiarelli, F.; Lorini, R.; Meschi, F.; Sacchetti, C.; the Diabetes Study Group of Italian Society of Pediatric Endocrinology and Diabetology. Younger age at onset and sex predict celiac disease in children and adolescents with type 1 diabetes: An Italian multicenter study. *Diabetes Care* **2004**, *27*, 1294–1298. [CrossRef] [PubMed]

53. Hummel, S.; Pfluger, M.; Hummel, M.; Bonifacio, E.; Ziegler, A.G. Primary dietary intervention study to reduce the risk of islet autoimmunity in children at increased risk for type 1 diabetes: The babydiet study. *Diabetes Care* **2011**, *34*, 1301–1305. [CrossRef] [PubMed]

54. Oderda, G.; Rapa, A.; Zavallone, A.; Strigini, L.; Bona, G. Thyroid autoimmunity in childhood celiac disease. *J. Pediatr. Gastroenterol. Nutr.* **2002**, *35*, 704–705. [CrossRef] [PubMed]

55. Ansaldi, N.; Palmas, T.; Corrias, A.; Barbato, M.; D'Altiglia, M.R.; Campanozzi, A.; Baldassarre, M.; Rea, F.; Pluvio, R.; Bonamico, M.; et al. Autoimmune thyroid disease and celiac disease in children. *J. Pediatr. Gastroenterol. Nutr.* **2003**, *37*, 63–66. [CrossRef] [PubMed]

56. Meloni, A.; Mandas, C.; Jores, R.D.; Congia, M. Prevalence of autoimmune thyroiditis in children with celiac disease and effect of gluten withdrawal. *J. Pediatr.* **2009**, *155*, 51–55. [CrossRef] [PubMed]

57. Cassio, A.; Ricci, G.; Baronio, F.; Miniaci, A.; Bal, M.; Bigucci, B.; Conti, V.; Cicognani, A. Long-term clinical significance of thyroid autoimmunity in children with celiac disease. *J. Pediatr.* **2010**, *156*, 292–295. [CrossRef] [PubMed]

58. Diamanti, A.; Ferretti, F.; Guglielmi, R.; Panetta, F.; Colistro, F.; Cappa, M.; Daniele, A.; Sole Basso, M.; Noto, C.; Crisogianni, M.; et al. Thyroid autoimmunity in children with coeliac disease: A prospective survey. *Arch. Dis. Child.* **2011**, *96*, 1038–1041. [CrossRef] [PubMed]

59. Van der Pals, M.; Ivarsson, A.; Norstrom, F.; Hogberg, L.; Svensson, J.; Carlsson, A. Prevalence of thyroid autoimmunity in children with celiac disease compared to healthy 12-year olds. *Autoimmune Dis.* **2014**, *2014*, 417356. [CrossRef] [PubMed]

60. Li, C.; Xu, M.M.; Wang, K.; Adler, A.J.; Vella, A.T.; Zhou, B. Macrophage polarization and meta-inflammation. *Transl. Res.* **2018**, *191*, 29–44. [CrossRef] [PubMed]

61. De Oliveira, G.L.V.; Leite, A.Z.; Higuchi, B.S.; Gonzaga, M.I.; Mariano, V.S. Intestinal dysbiosis and probiotic applications in autoimmune diseases. *Immunology* **2017**, *152*, 1–12. [CrossRef] [PubMed]

62. Thaiss, C.A.; Zmora, N.; Levy, M.; Elinav, E. The microbiome and innate immunity. *Nature* **2016**, *535*, 65–74. [CrossRef] [PubMed]

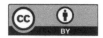

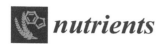

Article

A Serological Diagnosis of Coeliac Disease Is Associated with Osteoporosis in Older Australian Adults

Michael D. E. Potter [1,2,3,*], Marjorie M. Walker [1,2], Stephen Hancock [1], Elizabeth Holliday [1], Gregory Brogan [1,2], Michael Jones [4], Mark McEvoy [1], Michael Boyle [1,3], Nicholas J. Talley [1,2,3] and John Attia [1,3]

[1] Faculty of Health and Medicine, University of Newcastle, Level 3 East, HMRI Building, Lookout Road, New Lambton Heights 2305, Australia; marjorie.walker@newcastle.edu.au (M.M.W.); Stephen.hancock@newcastle.edu.au (S.H.); liz.holliday@newcastle.edu.au (E.H.); gregory.brogan@hnehealth.nsw.gov.au (G.B.); Mark.McEvoy@newcastle.edu.au (M.M.); Michael.boyle@hnehealth.nsw.gov.au (M.B.); nicholas.talley@newcastle.edu.au (N.J.T.); john.attia@newcastle.edu.au (J.A.)
[2] Australian Gastrointestinal Research Alliance (AGIRA), Newcastle 2305, Australia
[3] Department of Medicine, John Hunter Hospital, Newcastle 2305, Australia
[4] Department of Psychology, Macquarie University, Sydney 2109, Australia; mike.jones@mq.edu.au
* Correspondence: michael.potter@newcastle.edu.au

Received: 30 May 2018; Accepted: 26 June 2018; Published: 29 June 2018

Abstract: Previously thought to be mainly a disorder of childhood and early adult life, coeliac disease (CeD) is increasingly diagnosed in older adults. This may be important given the association between CeD and osteoporosis. The primary aim of this study was to determine the seroprevalence of undiagnosed CeD ('at-risk serology') in an older Australian community and relate this to a diagnosis of osteoporosis and fractures during a follow-up period of 12 years. We included participants from the Hunter Community Study (2004–2007) aged 55–85, who had anti-tissue transglutaminase (tTG) titres, human leukocyte antigen (HLA) genotypes, and bone mineral density measurements at baseline. Follow-up data included subsequent diagnosis of CeD and fractures using hospital information. 'At-risk' serology was defined as both tTG and HLA positivity. Complete results were obtained from 2122 patients. The prevalence of 'at-risk' serology was 5%. At baseline, 3.4% fulfilled criteria for a diagnosis of osteoporosis. During a mean of 9.7 years of follow-up, 7.4% of the cohort suffered at least one fracture and 0.7% were subsequently diagnosed with CeD. At-risk serology was significantly associated with osteoporosis in a multivariate model (odds ratio 2.83, 95% confidence interval 1.29–6.22); there was insufficient power to look at the outcome of fractures. The results of this study demonstrate that at-risk CeD serology was significantly associated with concurrent osteoporosis but not future fractures. Most individuals with a serological diagnosis of CeD were not diagnosed with CeD during the follow-up period according to medical records. Coeliac disease likely remains under-diagnosed.

Keywords: coeliac disease; osteoporosis; fractures

1. Introduction

Coeliac disease (CeD), once considered rare, is now estimated to affect 1–2% of the population in Western countries [1,2]. It is an immune-mediated systemic condition, manifested by small intestinal enteropathy triggered by exposure to gluten (a complex of water insoluble proteins in wheat, rye, and barley) in the diet [1]. CeD occurs almost exclusively in those who are genetically predisposed with the haplotypes human leukocyte antigen (HLA)-DQA1*05-DQB1*02 (DQ2) and/or

DQA1*03-DQB1*03:02 (DQ8) [1]. Previously thought to be a childhood disorder, CeD is increasingly diagnosed in older patients with longstanding atypical symptoms in whom the diagnosis has not previously been pursued [3,4]. The reported biopsy proven prevalence in older populations (over 55 years) has been reported to be 0.1–2.3% [5]. This may be important given the known association between CeD and diseases such as cancer and osteoporosis [6]. A recent study on case finding in the general community for individuals with undiagnosed CeD showed that these subjects were more likely to develop osteoporosis [7].

Osteoporosis is characterized by low bone mineral density (BMD) and architectural distortion of bone tissue that leads to bone fragility and an increased risk of fractures [8]. Age and gender are the major risk factors for the condition, which predominantly affect post-menopausal females [9]. Osteoporosis is a major public health problem, and over 4.7 million Australians over the age of 50 have low BMD [10]. This results in fractures, with over 140,000 fractures occurring in 2012 attributed to osteoporosis [10]. This is estimated to cost the Australian health care system over AU$3 billion per year [10].

Osteoporosis is common in CeD, and approximately 40% of patients with newly diagnosed CeD demonstrate a low BMD [11]. Patients with CeD are at higher risk of osteoporotic fractures [12], a risk which persists after diagnosis [13,14] for up to 20 years [15], although the absolute increase in fracture risk is low [12,16]. Importantly, BMD improves with a gluten free diet [17–19], although recovery is slow, taking up to 5 years to obtain complete recovery [20], in line with the slow rate of mucosal recovery in CeD [21]. The degree of adherence to the gluten free diet [18], and degree of mucosal damage at follow-up [22], has been shown to correlate with the degree of BMD recovery.

The aim of this study was to determine the seroprevalence of undiagnosed CeD in an older Australian community and relate this to a diagnosis of osteoporosis and fractures during long-term follow-up. Secondary aims included evaluation of the association between at-risk serology at baseline, and the presence of other autoimmune antibodies, and the rate of CeD diagnoses and death during the follow-up period.

2. Methods

2.1. Ethics

The research was approved by the Human Research Ethics Committees of the Hunter New England Local Health District and the University of Newcastle, Australia.

2.2. Participants

Data for this study is from the Hunter Community Study, a prospective cohort of community-dwelling older men and women (aged 55–96 years) from Newcastle, New South Wales, Australia. The sample characteristics and recruitment strategy has been described previously in detail [23]. Participants were randomly selected from the electoral roll between 2004 and 2007 and recruited using a modified Dillman strategy which included two letters of invitation followed by a phone call to non-responders. Invitation letters were sent to 9784 individuals, of whom 7575 responded and 3877 agreed to participate. A total of 3253 eventually participated in the study (a response rate of 44.5%). The sample has been shown previously to be comparable to the general Australian population in terms of gender and marital status, but is slightly younger in age [23].

2.3. Baseline Measures

Several self-report questionnaires were sent to participants at baseline, covering demographics, self-reported diseases, and prescribed and over the counter medication use. Anthropometric measurements including standing height (measured from the floor to the vertex of the head) and weight (measured using Tanita digital scales, Tanita, IL, USA) were taken at an initial face-to-face clinic visit. Bone mineral density was measured by heel ultrasound using the Sahara clinical bone sonometer (Hologic, Bedford, MA, USA) [24]. Osteoporosis was defined as a T score of less than or equal to −2.5 [25]. A measurement of functional capacity was performed by a 'timed up and go test' [26]. Physical activity was measured using a pedometer worn for seven consecutive days during waking hours to record step count [23]. Samples of serum and plasma were taken for serological measures (including anti-tissue transglutaminase (anti-tTG) antibodies, anti-nuclear antibodies (ANA), and anti-thyroid peroxidase antibodies (TPO)). Samples of serum and plasma were cryopreserved in 1 mL aliquots at −80 degrees Celsius and subsequently thawed for serological measures (including anti-tTG antibodies, anti-nuclear antibodies (ANA), and anti-thyroid peroxidase antibodies (TPO)), as well as DNA isolation and genotyping. Hazardous alcohol intake was defined for males and females, respectively, as greater than five or seven standard drinks per day or more than seven or eleven drinks on any occasion based on national guidelines [27]. Current smoking status was self-reported.

2.4. Follow-Up Measures

Non-traumatic fractures during follow-up were determined using linkage with hospital inpatient codes arising from contact with both public and private hospitals in the state of NSW from enrolment until 2017; data were obtained from the Centre for Health Record Linkage (CHeReL). Fractures were excluded if they were associated with a hospital code for trauma. A subsequent diagnosis of CeD was determined by self-report at follow-up contact made at 5 and 10 years and using hospital inpatient codes (ICD_10). Details regarding medications targeting low bone density (including hormone replacement therapy, selective estrogen receptor modulators, bisphosphonates, denosumab, or teriparatide) were available via linkages with the national Pharmaceutical Benefits Scheme (PBS) as well as through self-reporting at baseline and follow-up. Date of death was obtained through the National Death Index.

2.5. Coeliac Serology and Genotype

Anti-tissue transglutaminase antibody levels (anti-tTG) were measured by the hospital reference laboratory on enrolment to the study, using the AESKULISA human recombinant combined Immunoglobulin A (IgA) and IgG anti-tTG assay (Aesku.Diagnostics, Wendelsheim, Germany). A cut-off of ≥25 IU/mL was considered positive in line with the local reference laboratory. HLA genotyping was performed on thawed samples using an Affymetrix Kaiser Axiom array (ThermoFisher scientific, Waltham, MA, USA). Single nucleotide polymorphisms (SNPs) on chromosome 6 were used to locate HLA-DQ-2.5 and 8. Three SNPs were selected for tagging the HLA-DQ2.2 haplotype, and haplotype phasing for the three DQ2.2 tag SNPs was performed using SHAPEIT software [28]. Those HLA-DQ2- or DQ8-positive were considered to have a permissive genotype for CeD. "At-risk serology" for CeD was defined as a combination of anti-tTG antibodies greater than or equal to 25 IU/mL, and a permissive genotype for CeD (positive HLA-DQ2.2, 2.5 or DQ8).

2.6. Autoimmune Serology

ANA was assessed using HEp-2 ANA slides (Bio-Rad Laboratories, Hercules, CA, USA); ANA titre of >1/160 was defined as positive. TPO-Abs were analysed by ELISA testing (Aesku.Diagnostics, Wendelsheim, Germany).

2.7. Statistical Analysis

Statistical analysis was performed using STATA software (StataCorp, Texas, USA). Confidence intervals were calculated using the binomial exact method. Two models examining the association between "at-risk serology" and osteoporosis and fractures, respectively, were constructed; adjustment for several other potential risk factors was based on pre-designed directed acyclic graphs [29] (see Appendixs A and B). Given that there was no difference in the mean follow-up times or mortality between at-risk serology groups, simple and multiple unconditional logistic regression was used.

No multivariate analysis was conducted for the outcome of fractures according to the direct acyclic graph in order to avoid over adjustment bias for the exposure of at-risk serology (see Appendix B).

3. Results

3.1. Sample Characteristics

Of the original sample, 2121 had serum available for serology and genotype analysis and were included in the study. The included sample was slightly older (mean age 75.9 vs. 75.3 years, $p < 0.0001$) and more likely to be female than the original cohort (58.2% vs. 50.0%, $p < 0.0001$). The mean follow-up time was 9.7 years (range 0.2–12.4 years).

3.2. Prevalence of 'At-Risk' Serology, Osteoporosis, and Fracture during Follow-Up

Of the 2121 participants included in the analysis, 59.1% (95% confidence interval (CI) 56.7–61.2) had a permissive genotype and 7.3% (95%% CI 6.2–8.4) were determined to have a positive anti-tTG, with 0.8% having a high titre anti-tTG (>10 time the upper limit of normal) [21]. The mean anti-tTG was 11.4 IU/mL (range 1–313). In the entire cohort, 22.3% (95% CI 20.5–24.1) possessed at least one allele of HLA-DQ2.2, 27.2% (95% CI 25.3–29.1) possessed at least one HLA-DQ2.5 allele, and 18.9% (95% CI 17.3–20.6) possessed at least one HLA-DQ8 allele. 'At-risk serology' was present in 5.0% (95% CI 4.1–6.0), and 2.3% of participants who had positive anti-tTG but a non-permissive genotype for CeD (see Figure 1). Of those with a high titre anti-tTG, 88% (15/17) had a permissive HLA. There was no difference between those with and without at-risk serology in terms of mean follow-up time ($p = 0.50$).

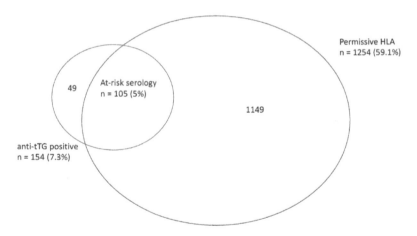

Figure 1. Overlap between participants with positive anti-tissue transglutaminase (anti-tTG) serology and permissive human leukocyte antigen (HLA) genotype from the overall sample of 2121 subjects.

A diagnosis of osteoporosis was present in 3.4% (95% CI 2.6–4.2) of participants at baseline (2.2% in males, 3.6% in females). At least one fracture (limb or other) occurred in 7.4% (95% CI 6.3–8.7) of participants ($n = 1883$) during follow-up (see Figure 2). Of those with a baseline diagnosis of osteoporosis, 10.2% received medication targeting bone density during the study period. Diagnosis of CeD during follow-up was reported in only 0.7% (95% CI 0.4–1.1) of participants ($n = 2081$), representing only 5.8% of the at-risk serology group. By the end of the follow-up period, 14.1% of the cohort had died, with no significant difference between those with and without at-risk serology (15.2% vs. 14.1%, $p = 0.74$).

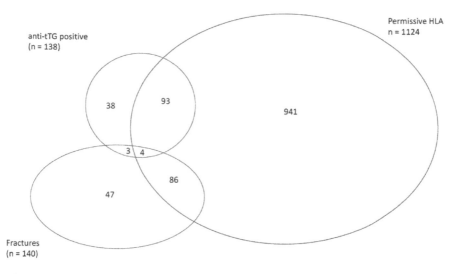

Figure 2. Overlap between participants with positive anti-tissue transglutaminase (tTG) serology, permissive HLA genotype, and fractures during the follow-up period from the overall sample of 1883 subjects.

3.3. Association between Coeliac Serology and Other Autoimmune Markers

Positive anti-tTG antibodies were associated with positive TPO antibodies but not ANA. In those with positive anti-tTG antibodies, 9.5% had a positive ANA compared with 6.8% of those without ($p = 0.07$), and 17.5% had a positive TPO antibodies compared with 10.0% without ($p = 0.003$).

3.4. Osteoporosis

In a univariate analysis, at-risk serology was associated with a diagnosis of osteoporosis at baseline (Odds Ratio [OR] 2.56, 95% CI 1.19–5.49) (see Table 1). Other factors significantly influencing the presence of osteoporosis at baseline included positive anti-tTG, age, gender, body mass index (BMI), and alcohol intake (see Table 1); no significant association was found for smoking or physical activity. In the multivariate model, at-risk serology, BMI, gender, smoking status, and age, but not alcohol intake, were all significantly associated with osteoporosis (see Table 2).

Table 1. Univariate analysis of risk factors associated with osteoporosis (OP). Risk factors are expressed as percentages in the osteoporotic and non-osteoporotic groups unless otherwise specified. CI—confidence interval. SD—standard deviation. BMI—body mass index.

	OP—%(95% CI)	No OP—%(95% CI)	Odds Ratio (95% CI)
At-risk serology	11.3 (3.7–18.8)	4.7 (3.8–5.7)	2.56 (1.19–5.49)
Anti-tTG (IU/mL); mean (SD)	20.3 (50.4)	11.1 (31.0)	1.01 (1.00–1.01)
Positive anti-tTG	15.5 (6.9–24.1)	7.0 (5.9–8.1)	2.44 (1.26–4.75)
Positive HLA	63.4 (51.9–74.9)	59.0 (56.8–61.1)	1.20 (0.74–1.97)
Age (years); mean (SD)	80.2 (7.4)	75.8 (7.2)	1.08 (1.05–1.11)
BMI (kg/m^2); mean (SD)	27.3 (5.3)	28.8 (4.9)	0.93 (0.88–0.98)
Gender (male)	36.6 (25.1–48.1)	50.4 (48.3–52.6)	0.57 (0.35–0.93)
Current smoker	6.1 (5.1–7.2)	9.9 (2.8–17.0)	1.67 (0.75–3.72)
Hazardous alcohol intake	1.4 (0.0–4.2)	9.7 (8.4–10.9)	0.13 (0.02–0.97)
Physical activity (step count per day); mean (SD)	6160 (5106–7216)	6700 (6530–6871)	1.00 (1.00–1.00)

Table 2. Odds ratios from the multivariate analysis of factors associated with osteoporosis.

	Odds Ratio	95% CI	*p* Value
At-risk serology	3.09	1.32–7.23	0.009
BMI	0.94	0.89–1.00	0.04
Gender (male)	0.51	0.29–0.89	0.02
Current smoking	3.22	1.36–7.61	0.008
Hazardous alcohol intake	0.22	0.30–1.66	0.14
Age	1.08	1.04–1.12	<0.001

3.5. Fracture Risk

In those with osteoporosis, 21.2% sustained a fracture during the follow-up period, compared with only 6.9% of the non-osteoporotic group (*p* < 0.001). There was no significant difference in the rate of fractures in those with at-risk serology compared to those without (4.1% vs. 7.6%, *p* = 0.2) (see Figure 2). None of the subjects with a high titre anti-tTG sustained a fracture during the follow-up period. In the univariate analysis, fracture during follow-up was also significantly associated with age and gender, but not BMI, smoking status, alcohol intake, physical activity, or the timed up and go test (see Table 3). A multivariate analysis was not performed in order to avoid over adjustment bias in accordance with the pre-constructed directed acyclic graph.

Table 3. Univariate analysis of factors associated with fractures during the follow-up period (*n* = 1, 883). Risk factors are expressed as percentages in the fracture and no-fracture groups unless otherwise specified.

	Fracture—% (95% CI)	No Fracture—% (95% CI)	Odds Ratio (95% CI)
Osteoporosis (baseline)	10.0 (5.0–15.0)	3.0 (2.2–3.8)	3.6 (1.9–6.7)
At-risk serology	2.9 (0.1–5.7)	5.3 (4.3–6.4)	0.52 (0.19–1.44)
Anti-tTG (IU/mL); mean (SD)	8.0 (5.1–10.8)	11.6 (10.1–13.2)	0.99 (0.98–1.00)
Positive anti-tTG	5.0 (1.3–8.7)	7.5 (6.3–8.8)	0.64 (0.30–1.41)
Positive HLA	6.4 (5.6–7.2)	5.9 (5.7–6.2)	1.2 (0.9–1.8)
Positive tTG with non-permissive HLA	2.3 (−0.3–4.6)	2.2 (1.5–2.9)	0.98 (0.30–3.22)
Age (years); mean (SD)	80.4 (79.0–81.7)	76.0 (75.6–76.3)	1.08 (1.06–1.11)
BMI (kg/m^2); mean (SD)	28.9 (27.9–29.9)	28.9 (28.6–29.1)	1.00 (0.97–1.04)
Gender (male)	33.6 (25.7–41.5)	51.7 (49.3–54.0)	0.47 (0.33–0.68)
Current smoker	5.0 (1.3–8.7)	6.0 (4.9–7.1)	0.83 (0.38–1.82)
Hazardous alcohol intake	7.1 (2.8–11.5)	9.8 (8.4–11.2)	0.71 (0.36–1.37)
Physical activity (step count per day); mean	6282 (5554–7101)	6615 (6433–6797)	1.00 (1.00–1.00)
Timed up and go test (seconds)	10.7 (10.0–11.4)	9.9 (8.8–11.1)	1.00 (1.00–1.01)

4. Discussion

We report a high prevalence of at-risk serology, with 5% of the sample having an elevated anti-tTG and a permissive genotype for CeD. However, 2.3% of the cohort returned a positive anti-tTG in the absence of permissive genotype, likely representing false positives. It follows that a proportion of the 'at-risk' group would not have CeD if gastroscopy and duodenal biopsy were undertaken. This is consistent with a previous seroprevalence study from Australia by Anderson et al. [30], which reported anti-tTG IgA antibody positivity in 5.7% of a general population cohort (median age 54–56 years in two combined cohorts), in whom approximately one-third had a non-permissive genotype for CeD. The eventual prevalence of CeD in this cohort, estimated based on biopsy or extended serological screening, was 1.2–1.9%. They suggested that in those who screen positive on anti-tTG, testing for HLA-DQ status would reduce unnecessary gastroscopies due to false positive serology by 40% [30]. Our findings of similarly high rates of positive anti-tTG in the presence of non-permissive genotype support these observations.

Second generation anti-tTG assays, employing human purified or human recombinant anti-tTG antigen (as used in our assay) have been shown to be highly sensitive and specific, with a positive predictive value of 85–100% [31,32]. These studies, however, are generally performed in cohorts with a high prevalence of disease and therefore high pre-test probabilities for an eventual diagnosis, and their performance in general population screening cohorts is likely to be lower [33]. Furthermore, there are no studies, to our knowledge, examining the performance of these assays specifically in older adults. Reports regarding false positive anti-tTG results are not uncommon, and high rates of false positivity have been demonstrated in cohorts with other autoimmune diseases [34], inflammatory bowel disease [35,36], congestive heart failure [37], and liver disease [38,39]. The link between osteoporosis and chronic diseases such as these is well established [40], and may partially explain the link between positive serology and osteoporosis, although we did not evaluate these conditions in this study. High rates of autoimmune markers have been previously reported in our own cohort, with 8% of the overall cohort testing positive for anti-TPO antibodies, and 27% testing positive for ANA antibodies [41]. We observed higher rates of both ANA and TPO antibodies in those testing positive for anti-tTG antibodies, although this result was only statistically significant for TPO antibodies and approached significance ($p = 0.07$) for ANA. There are two potential explanations for this. The first is that autoantibody findings are common in an ageing population, explaining the association between these autoantibodies and a positive anti-tTG. The second, specifically in regard to thyroid specific antibodies, is that CeD and autoimmune thyroid disease are associated [21,42], and the association between these antibodies in our cohort represents an underlying association between undiagnosed CeD and thyroid disease. Although some have called for serological diagnosis of CeD in adults (without biopsy) [43], the observations reported here do not support this diagnostic approach in older adults.

Whilst the worldwide prevalence of CeD is thought to be 1–2% [42], this may be higher in older cohorts. A study by Vilppula et al. [6] of 2815 subjects over 55 years of age in Finland screened participants for CeD using serology, with positive cases going on to have duodenal biopsy to confirm the presence of CeD. They reported positive serology in 2.5% of the group, but only 2.1% were subsequently biopsy proven. A subset of this group was rescreened again 3 years later, of whom six had undergone seroconversion and five had developed biopsy proven CeD, representing an increase in seroprevalence to 2.7% and a biopsy proven prevalence to 2.3%, and suggesting an incidence rate of 0.08% per year [6].

The link between biopsy proven CeD and osteoporosis is well established, with a prevalence of around 40% [11]. We report an association between positive serology (in the absence of biopsy confirmation) and osteoporosis. This is consistent with previous literature which has also associated anti-tTG seropositivity with low bone mineral density. Duerksen et al. [44] retrospectively evaluated 376 women who had both coeliac serology (anti-endomysial /tTG Ab) and bone mineral density tested (with bone mineral density preceding coeliac serology by at least 6 months). They reported higher rates of osteoporosis (68% vs. 45%, $p < 0.05$) in seropositive compared with seronegative women, respectively. This has also been confirmed in a study from the USA in which undiagnosed CeD patients were more likely to develop osteoporosis and autoimmune conditions, heralding CeD in older life rather than classic malabsorption [7].

A gluten free diet improves bone mineral density in CeD patients, with complete resolution of low BMD in younger patients after two years treatment with a gluten free diet [45]. The addition of bisphosphonates, traditionally the first line pharmacologic therapy for osteoporosis, has been shown to be no more effective than a gluten free diet alone [46]. Other traditional adjunctive therapies, such as exercise, have also been shown to contribute little to BMD recovery in the context of gluten withdrawal [19]. This suggests that the pathogenesis of osteoporosis is different in CeD, and related to malabsorption of nutrients involved in bone mineralisation such as vitamin D [47], rather than hormonal regulation of bone architecture.

If indeed a relationship exists between CeD serology and osteoporosis, this may be mediated by a combination of factors, including a subset with undiagnosed CeD who develop osteoporosis secondary to enteropathy, malabsorption, and low-grade inflammation, as well as a relationship between chronic diseases that increase the likelihood of having both osteoporosis and false positive CeD serology.

There was no significant association between at-risk serology and fractures sustained during the follow-up period (20,181 person years). However, with only four participants with at-risk serology sustaining a fracture during follow-up, it is likely that the analysis was underpowered to evaluate this outcome. A systematic review by Olmos et al. [12] of case-control and cross sectional studies examining fracture risk in CeD, which included eight studies of 20,995 CeD patients and 96,777 controls, reported a fracture risk of 8.7% in CeD and 6.15% in controls (OR 1.43, 95% CI 1.15–1.78). A more recent meta-analysis by Heikkila et al. [48] limited to six prospective studies reported a slightly increased risk of bone fractures (random effects estimate: 1.30, 95% CI 1.14–1.50). Few prospective studies have examined the association between undiagnosed CeD and osteoporosis or fracture risk [48]. Agardh et al. [49] reported a study of 6480 women aged 50–64 years old (mean age 56 years) in whom both BMD (by wrist dual X-ray absorptiometry) and anti-tTG measurements were taken; they found that those with elevated tTG ($\geq$17 IU/mL), representing approximately 0.9% of the sample, were significantly more likely to have osteoporosis (13.4% vs. 6.5%, $p = 0.008$) and fracture risk (32% vs. 19%, $p = 0.009$).

This study has a number of strengths, including the relatively unique demographic profile of the cohort, the availability of both serological measures and bone mineral density measurements at baseline, as well as long-term follow-up allowing us to estimate fractures over a 12-year period. One significant limitation of this study is the lack of confirmatory biopsy for the diagnosis of CeD. We defined a subsequent diagnosis of CeD based on hospital coding information and self-report at follow-up as available tools of diagnosis. As mentioned, the high rate of false positivity of the anti-tTG assay means that a significant proportion of the 'at-risk' group are likely not to have CeD on confirmatory biopsy. Another limitation of this study is the measurement of bone mineral density, which was performed by heel ultrasound as opposed to dual X-ray absorptiometry (DXA) which is considered the gold standard [50]. Although quantitative heel ultrasound performs well against DXA in predicting fracture risk [51,52], it generally underestimates bone mineral density when compared with DXA, with lower sensitivity (21–45%) but high specificity (87–96%) at a cut-off of −2.5 for an equivalent DXA score [52]. This reflects our relatively low prevalence figures when compared to other local prevalence studies that have reported osteoporosis in 3–12% of males and 8–43% of females over age 50 [10,53].

5. Conclusions

At-risk coeliac serology, defined by the presence of an elevated anti-tTG antibody and a permissive genotype, is highly prevalent in older Australian adults and is significantly associated with low bone mineral density as measured by quantitative heel ultrasound. Few with at-risk serology were diagnosed with CeD during long-term follow-up. The issue of false positive serology should be addressed in studies where biopsy is used to confirm disease, as high anti-tTG levels are documented in autoimmune and liver disease. We did not find a significant relationship between at-risk serology and fractures during the follow-up period, as our analysis was underpowered for this outcome. The findings in this study would support considering the diagnosis of osteoporosis in older patients with newly diagnosed CeD.

Author Contributions: Conceptualization of the project, J.A., S.H., M.M., M.M.W., M.B., and N.J.T.; Methodology, J.A., S.H., M.M, and E.H. Formal Analysis, M.D.E.P., G.B., and J.A.; Resources, S.H.; Data Curation, J.A., M.M., and S.H.; Original Draft Preparation, M.D.E.P., M.M.W., and J.A.; Review and Editing, M.D.E.P., M.M.W., J.A., N.J.T., S.H., M.J., M.M., E.H., and G.B.; Supervision, J.A., M.M.W., and N.J.T.; Funding Acquisition, J.A., M.M., and S.H.

Funding: The study was funded by the University of Newcastle, the Hunter Medical Research Institute, and the Vincent Fairfax Family Foundation.

Conflicts of Interest: The authors declare no conflicts of interest.

Disclosures: M.M.W.: Grant/Research Support: Prometheus Laboratories Inc. (Irritable bowel syndrome (IBS Diagnostic), Commonwealth Diagnostics International (Biomarkers for FGIDs)). N.J.T.: Grant/Research Support: Rome Foundation; Abbott Pharmaceuticals; Datapharm; Pfizer; Salix (Irritable bowel syndrome); Prometheus

Laboratories Inc. (Irritable bowel syndrome (IBS Diagnostic)); Janssen (Constipation). Consultant/Advisory Boards: Adelphi Values (Functional dyspepsia (patient-reported outcome measures)); (Budesonide); GI therapies (Chronic constipation (Rhythm IC)); Allergens PLC; Napo Pharmaceutical; Outpost Medicine; Samsung Bioepis; Yuhan (IBS); Synergy (IBS); Theravance (Gastroparesis). Patent Holder: Biomarkers of irritable bowel syndrome (Irritable bowel syndrome) Licensing Questionnaires (Mayo Clinic Talley Bowel Disease Questionnaire—Mayo Dysphagia Questionnaire); Nestec European Patent (Application No. 12735358.9); Singapore 'Provisional' Patent (NTU Ref: TD/129/17 "Microbiota Modulation of BDNF Tissue Repair Pathway).

Appendix A

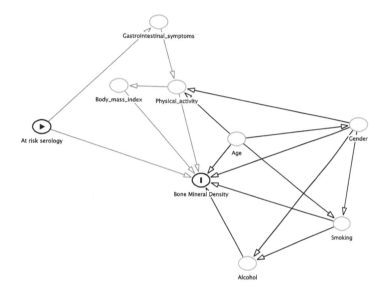

Figure A1. Directed acyclic graph to determine relationship between at-risk serology and osteoporosis.

Appendix B

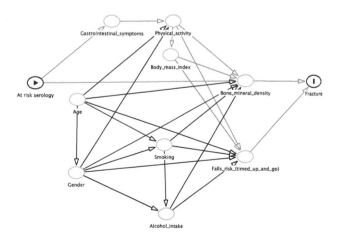

Figure A2. Directed acyclic graph to determine relationship between at-risk serology and fracture.

References

1. Fasano, A.; Catassi, C. Clinical practice. Celiac disease. *N. Engl. J. Med.* **2012**, *367*, 2419–2426. [CrossRef] [PubMed]
2. Walker, M.M.; Ludvigsson, J.F.; Sanders, D.S. Coeliac disease—Review of practice issues, diagnosis and management—Guidance to the guidelines. *Med. J. Aust.* **2017**, in press. [CrossRef] [PubMed]
3. Robson, K.; Alizart, M.; Martin, J.; Nagel, R. Coeliac patients are undiagnosed at routine upper endoscopy. *PLoS ONE* **2014**, *9*, e90552. [CrossRef] [PubMed]
4. Hankey, G.L.; Holmes, G.K. Coeliac disease in the elderly. *Gut* **1994**, *35*, 65–67. [CrossRef] [PubMed]
5. Collin, P.; Vilppula, A.; Luostarinen, L.; Holmes, G.K.T.; Kaukinen, K. Review article: Coeliac disease in later life must not be missed. *Aliment. Pharmacol. Ther.* **2018**, *47*, 563–572. [CrossRef] [PubMed]
6. Vilppula, A.; Kaukinen, K.; Luostarinen, L.; Krekela, I.; Patrikainen, H.; Valve, R.; Maki, M.; Collin, P. Increasing prevalence and high incidence of celiac disease in elderly people: A population-based study. *BMC Gastroenterol.* **2009**, *9*, 49. [CrossRef] [PubMed]
7. Hujoel, I.A.; Van Dyke, C.T.; Brantner, T.; Larson, J.; King, K.S.; Sharma, A.; Murray, J.A.; Rubio-Tapia, A. Natural history and clinical detection of undiagnosed coeliac disease in a north american community. *Aliment. Pharmacol. Ther.* **2018**, *47*, 1358–1366. [CrossRef] [PubMed]
8. Di Stefano, M.; Mengoli, C.; Bergonzi, M.; Corazza, G.R. Bone mass and mineral metabolism alterations in adult celiac disease: Pathophysiology and clinical approach. *Nutrients* **2013**, *5*, 4786–4799. [CrossRef] [PubMed]
9. Lane, N.E. Epidemiology, etiology, and diagnosis of osteoporosis. *Am. J. Obstet. Gynecol.* **2006**, *194*, S3–S11. [CrossRef] [PubMed]
10. Watts, J.J.; Abimanyi-Ochom, J.; Sanders, K.M. Osteoporosis Costing All Australians a New Burden of Disease Analysis—2012 to 2022. Osteoporosis Australia. 2013. Available online: https://www.osteoporosis.org.au/sites/default/files/files/Burden%20of%20Disease%20Analysis%202012-2022.pdf (accessed on 29 June 2018).
11. Lucendo, A.J.; Garcia-Manzanares, A. Bone mineral density in adult coeliac disease: An updated review. *Rev. Esp. Enferm. Dig.* **2013**, *105*, 154–162. [CrossRef] [PubMed]
12. Olmos, M.; Antelo, M.; Vazquez, H.; Smecuol, E.; Maurino, E.; Bai, J.C. Systematic review and meta-analysis of observational studies on the prevalence of fractures in coeliac disease. *Dig. Liver Dis.* **2008**, *40*, 46–53. [CrossRef] [PubMed]
13. Jafri, M.R.; Nordstrom, C.W.; Murray, J.A.; Van Dyke, C.T.; Dierkhising, R.A.; Zinsmeister, A.R.; Melton, L.J., 3rd. Long-term fracture risk in patients with celiac disease: A population-based study in olmsted county, minnesota. *Dig. Dis. Sci.* **2008**, *53*, 964–971. [CrossRef] [PubMed]
14. McFarlane, X.A.; Bhalla, A.K.; Reeves, D.E.; Morgan, L.M.; Robertson, D.A. Osteoporosis in treated adult coeliac disease. *Gut* **1995**, *36*, 710–714. [CrossRef] [PubMed]
15. Ludvigsson, J.F.; Michaelsson, K.; Ekbom, A.; Montgomery, S.M. Coeliac disease and the risk of fractures—A general population-based cohort study. *Aliment. Pharmacol. Ther.* **2007**, *25*, 273–285. [CrossRef] [PubMed]
16. West, J.; Logan, R.F.; Card, T.R.; Smith, C.; Hubbard, R. Fracture risk in people with celiac disease: A population-based cohort study. *Gastroenterology* **2003**, *125*, 429–436. [CrossRef]
17. Sategna-Guidetti, C.; Grosso, S.B.; Grosso, S.; Mengozzi, G.; Aimo, G.; Zaccaria, T.; Di Stefano, M.; Isaia, G.C. The effects of 1-year gluten withdrawal on bone mass, bone metabolism and nutritional status in newly-diagnosed adult coeliac disease patients. *Aliment. Pharmacol. Ther.* **2000**, *14*, 35–43. [CrossRef] [PubMed]
18. Bai, J.C.; Gonzalez, D.; Mautalen, C.; Mazure, R.; Pedreira, S.; Vazquez, H.; Smecuol, E.; Siccardi, A.; Cataldi, M.; Niveloni, S.; et al. Long-term effect of gluten restriction on bone mineral density of patients with coeliac disease. *Aliment. Pharmacol. Ther.* **1997**, *11*, 157–164. [CrossRef] [PubMed]
19. Passananti, V.; Santonicola, A.; Bucci, C.; Andreozzi, P.; Ranaudo, A.; Di Giacomo, D.V.; Ciacci, C. Bone mass in women with celiac disease: Role of exercise and gluten-free diet. *Dig. Liver Dis.* **2012**, *44*, 379–383. [CrossRef] [PubMed]
20. Grace-Farfaglia, P. Bones of contention: Bone mineral density recovery in celiac disease—A systematic review. *Nutrients* **2015**, *7*, 3347–3369. [CrossRef] [PubMed]

21. Ludvigsson, J.F.; Bai, J.C.; Biagi, F.; Card, T.R.; Ciacci, C.; Ciclitira, P.J.; Green, P.H.; Hadjivassiliou, M.; Holdoway, A.; van Heel, D.A.; et al. Diagnosis and management of adult coeliac disease: Guidelines from the british society of gastroenterology. *Gut* **2014**, *63*, 1210–1228. [CrossRef] [PubMed]

22. Lebwohl, B.; Michaelsson, K.; Green, P.H.; Ludvigsson, J.F. Persistent mucosal damage and risk of fracture in celiac disease. *J. Clin. Endocrinol. Metab.* **2014**, *99*, 609–616. [CrossRef] [PubMed]

23. McEvoy, M.; Smith, W.; D'Este, C.; Duke, J.; Peel, R.; Schofield, P.; Scott, R.; Byles, J.; Henry, D.; Ewald, B.; et al. Cohort profile: The hunter community study. *Int. J. Epidemiol.* **2010**, *39*, 1452–1463. [CrossRef] [PubMed]

24. Hololologic. Sahara Clinical Bone Sonometer. 2000. Available online: http://www.alpha-imaging.com/files/document%20library/hologic/hologic%20brochures/hologic%20sahara%20brochure.pdf (accessed on 29 June 2018).

25. WHO. *Who Scientific Group on the Assessment of Osteoporosis at Primary Health Care Level*; WHO: Geneva, Switzerland, 2007.

26. Podsiadlo, D.; Richardson, S. The timed "up & go": A test of basic functional mobility for frail elderly persons. *J. Am. Geriatr. Soc.* **1991**, *39*, 142–148. [PubMed]

27. National Health and Medical Research Council. *Australian Alcohol Guidelines, Health Risks and Benefits*; National Health and Medical Research Council: Canberra, Australia, 2001.

28. Delaneau, O.; Zagury, J.F.; Marchini, J. Improved whole-chromosome phasing for disease and population genetic studies. *Nat. Methods* **2013**, *10*, 5–6. [CrossRef] [PubMed]

29. Attia, J.R.; Oldmeadow, C.; Holliday, E.G.; Jones, M.P. Deconfounding confounding part 2: Using directed acyclic graphs (dags). *Med. J. Aust.* **2017**, *206*, 480–483. [CrossRef] [PubMed]

30. Anderson, R.P.; Henry, M.J.; Taylor, R.; Duncan, E.L.; Danoy, P.; Costa, M.J.; Addison, K.; Tye-Din, J.A.; Kotowicz, M.A.; Knight, R.E.; et al. A novel serogenetic approach determines the community prevalence of celiac disease and informs improved diagnostic pathways. *BMC Med.* **2013**, *11*, 188. [CrossRef] [PubMed]

31. Hill, I.D. What are the sensitivity and specificity of serologic tests for celiac disease? Do sensitivity and specificity vary in different populations? *Gastroenterology* **2005**, *128*, S25–S32. [CrossRef] [PubMed]

32. Hill, P.G.; Holmes, G.K. Coeliac disease: A biopsy is not always necessary for diagnosis. *Aliment. Pharmacol. Ther.* **2008**, *27*, 572–577. [CrossRef] [PubMed]

33. Rostom, A.; Dube, C.; Cranney, A.; Saloojee, N.; Sy, R.; Garritty, C.; Sampson, M.; Zhang, L.; Yazdi, F.; Mamaladze, V.; et al. The diagnostic accuracy of serologic tests for celiac disease: A systematic review. *Gastroenterology* **2005**, *128*, S38–S46. [CrossRef] [PubMed]

34. Sardy, M.; Csikos, M.; Geisen, C.; Preisz, K.; Kornsee, Z.; Tomsits, E.; Tox, U.; Hunzelmann, N.; Wieslander, J.; Karpati, S.; et al. Tissue transglutaminase elisa positivity in autoimmune disease independent of gluten-sensitive disease. *Clin. Chim. Acta* **2007**, *376*, 126–135. [CrossRef] [PubMed]

35. Alper, A.; Rojas-Velasquez, D.; Pashankar, D.S. Prevalence of anti-tissue transglutaminase (tTG) antibodies and celiac disease in children with IBD. *J. Pediatr. Gastroenterol. Nutr.* **2017**, *66*, 934–936. [CrossRef] [PubMed]

36. Watanabe, C.; Komoto, S.; Hokari, R.; Kurihara, C.; Okada, Y.; Hozumi, H.; Higashiyama, M.; Sakuraba, A.; Tomita, K.; Tsuzuki, Y.; et al. Prevalence of serum celiac antibody in patients with IBD in japan. *J. Gastroenterol.* **2014**, *49*, 825–834. [CrossRef] [PubMed]

37. Castillo, N.E.; Theethira, T.G.; Leffler, D.A. The present and the future in the diagnosis and management of celiac disease. *Gastroenterol. Rep.* **2015**, *3*, 3–11. [CrossRef] [PubMed]

38. Sood, A.; Khurana, M.S.; Mahajan, R.; Midha, V.; Puri, S.; Kaur, A.; Gupta, N.; Sharma, S. Prevalence and clinical significance of IgA anti-tissue transglutaminase antibodies in patients with chronic liver disease. *J. Gastroenterol. Hepatol.* **2017**, *32*, 446–450. [CrossRef] [PubMed]

39. Bizzaro, N.; Villalta, D.; Tonutti, E.; Doria, A.; Tampoia, M.; Bassetti, D.; Tozzoli, R. Iga and igg tissue transglutaminase antibody prevalence and clinical significance in connective tissue diseases, inflammatory bowel disease, and primary biliary cirrhosis. *Dig. Dis. Sci.* **2003**, *48*, 2360–2365. [CrossRef] [PubMed]

40. Kanis, J.A. Diagnosis of osteoporosis and assessment of fracture risk. *Lancet* **2002**, *359*, 1929–1936. [CrossRef]

41. Napthali, K.; Boyle, M.; Tran, H.; Schofield, P.W.; Peel, R.; McEvoy, M.; Oldmeadow, C.; Attia, J. Thyroid antibodies, autoimmunity and cognitive decline: Is there a population-based link? *Dement. Geriatr. Cogn. Dis. Extra* **2014**, *4*, 140–146. [CrossRef] [PubMed]

42. Walker, M.M.; Ludvigsson, J.F.; Sanders, D.S. Coeliac disease: Review of diagnosis and management. *Med. J. Aust.* **2017**, *207*, 173–178. [CrossRef] [PubMed]

43. Holmes, G.K.T.; Hill, P.G. Coeliac disease: Further evidence that biopsy is not always necessary for diagnosis. *Eur. J. Gastroenterol. Hepatol.* **2017**, *29*, 1189–1190. [CrossRef] [PubMed]

44. Duerksen, D.R.; Leslie, W.D. Positive celiac disease serology and reduced bone mineral density in adult women. *Can. J. Gastroenterol.* **2010**, *24*, 103–107. [CrossRef] [PubMed]

45. Mora, S.; Barera, G.; Ricotti, A.; Weber, G.; Bianchi, C.; Chiumello, G. Reversal of low bone density with a gluten-free diet in children and adolescents with celiac disease. *Am. J. Clin. Nutr.* **1998**, *67*, 477–481. [CrossRef] [PubMed]

46. Kumar, M.; Rastogi, A.; Bhadada, S.K.; Bhansali, A.; Vaiphei, K.; Kochhar, R. Effect of zoledronic acid on bone mineral density in patients of celiac disease: A prospective, randomized, pilot study. *Indian J. Med. Res.* **2013**, *138*, 882–887. [PubMed]

47. Nuti, R.; Martini, G.; Valenti, R.; Giovani, S.; Salvadori, S.; Avanzati, A. Prevalence of undiagnosed coeliac syndrome in osteoporotic women. *J. Intern. Med.* **2001**, *250*, 361–366. [CrossRef] [PubMed]

48. Heikkila, K.; Pearce, J.; Maki, M.; Kaukinen, K. Celiac disease and bone fractures: A systematic review and meta-analysis. *J. Clin. Endocrinol. Metab.* **2015**, *100*, 25–34. [CrossRef] [PubMed]

49. Agardh, D.; Bjorck, S.; Agardh, C.D.; Lidfeldt, J. Coeliac disease-specific tissue transglutaminase autoantibodies are associated with osteoporosis and related fractures in middle-aged women. *Scand. J. Gastroenterol.* **2009**, *44*, 571–578. [CrossRef] [PubMed]

50. Cosman, F.; de Beur, S.J.; LeBoff, M.S.; Lewiecki, E.M.; Tanner, B.; Randall, S.; Lindsay, R.; National Osteoporosis, F. Clinician's guide to prevention and treatment of osteoporosis. *Osteoporos. Int.* **2014**, *25*, 2359–2381. [CrossRef] [PubMed]

51. Moayyeri, A.; Adams, J.E.; Adler, R.A.; Krieg, M.A.; Hans, D.; Compston, J.; Lewiecki, E.M. Quantitative ultrasound of the heel and fracture risk assessment: An updated meta-analysis. *Osteoporos. Int.* **2012**, *23*, 143–153. [CrossRef] [PubMed]

52. Nayak, S.; Olkin, I.; Liu, H.; Grabe, M.; Gould, M.K.; Allen, I.E.; Owens, D.K.; Bravata, D.M. Meta-analysis: Accuracy of quantitative ultrasound for identifying patients with osteoporosis. *Ann. Intern. Med.* **2006**, *144*, 832–841. [CrossRef] [PubMed]

53. Henry, M.J.; Pasco, J.A.; Nicholson, G.C.; Kotowicz, M.A. Prevalence of osteoporosis in Australian men and women: Geelong osteoporosis study. *Med. J. Aust.* **2011**, *195*, 321–322. [CrossRef] [PubMed]

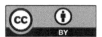

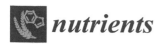

Review

Psychiatric Comorbidity in Children and Adults with Gluten-Related Disorders: A Narrative Review

Mahmoud Slim [1], Fernando Rico-Villademoros [2] and Elena P. Calandre [2,*]

[1] Division of Neurology, The Hospital for Sick Children, The Peter Gilgan Centre for Research and Learning, 686 Bay St., Toronto, ON M5G 0A4, Canada; mahmoud.slim@gmail.com

[2] Instituto de Neurociencias, Universidad de Granada, Avenida del Conocimiento s/n, 18100 Armilla, Granada, Spain; fernando.ricovillademoros@gmail.com

* Correspondence: calandre@gmail.com; Tel.: +34-958-244-033

Received: 7 June 2018; Accepted: 4 July 2018; Published: 6 July 2018

Abstract: Gluten-related disorders are characterized by both intestinal and extraintestinal manifestations. Previous studies have suggested an association between gluten-related disorder and psychiatric comorbidities. The objective of our current review is to provide a comprehensive review of this association in children and adults. A systematic literature search using MEDLINE, Embase and PsycINFO from inception to 2018 using terms of 'celiac disease' or 'gluten-sensitivity-related disorders' combined with terms of 'mental disorders' was conducted. A total of 47 articles were included in our review, of which 28 studies were conducted in adults, 11 studies in children and eight studies included both children and adults. The majority of studies were conducted in celiac disease, two studies in non-celiac gluten sensitivity and none in wheat allergy. Enough evidence is currently available supporting the association of celiac disease with depression and, to a lesser extent, with eating disorders. Further investigation is warranted to evaluate the association suggested with other psychiatric disorders. In conclusion, routine surveillance of potential psychiatric manifestations in children and adults with gluten-related disorders should be carried out by the attending physician.

Keywords: celiac disease; non-celiac gluten sensitivity; psychiatric disorders; depression; anxiety disorders; eating disorders; ADHD; autism; psychosis

1. Introduction

Gluten-related disorders include three pathologies caused by the ingestion of gluten-containing cereals grains, namely celiac disease (CD), non-celiac gluten sensitivity (NCGS) and wheat allergy (WA) [1]. Although all of them are due to the toxicity of gluten proteins in the sensitive subject, their respective pathogenetic mechanisms differ.

Celiac disease is a systemic autoimmune disease due to a permanent intolerance to gluten which causes villous atrophy of the intestinal mucosa. It involves both innate and adaptive immune responses that appear in genetically predisposed subjects exposed to gluten and, unlike food allergies, it is not mediated by an immediate hypersensitivity reaction. It is a polygenic multifactorial disorder whose development depends on the genetic constitution of the subject, on his/her exposure to gluten intake, and on different environmental factors [2,3]. To date, the only effective treatment for the disease is to observe a life-long strict gluten-free diet although other therapeutic approaches are being explored [4].

In relation to the genetic background of the disease, two HLA class II genes, the HLA-DQ2 and the HLA-DQ8 heterodimers are present in almost all CD patients and their simultaneous absence in a subject usually rules out a diagnosis of CD. However, these genes are also common in the general population and the implication of other non-HLA genes is being investigated by genome wide association studies [5]. Environmental factors that facilitate or, conversely, protect against the development of CD are defectively known although they are considered important given that the genetic background is not enough to explain the increasing incidence and prevalence of CD [2]. Infant feeding practices such as the timing of the first gluten introduction in the diet and the presumed protective role of maternal breastfeeding that were once considered important, have been recently shown to be irrelevant in relation to the development of CD [6]. In contrast, gastrointestinal infections and antibiotics use during the first year of life seem to be associated with a higher risk of developing CD [7]; these latter factors could be related with the composition of gut microbiota that seems to be different between children with and without CD [8].

As both the two most relevant genes associated with the development of CD as well as the consumption gluten-containing foods are fairly prevalent in most of the world, it is not surprising that there is high worldwide prevalence of CD [9]. The global worldwide prevalence of CD has been shown to be higher when diagnosed only by serological tests, i.e., anti-tissue transglutaminase and/or antiendomysial antibodies (1.4%, 95% confidence interval [CI] 1.1–1.7%) than when diagnosed with intestinal biopsy (0.7%, 95% CI 0.5–0.9%) [10]. Some striking differences have been found among different geographic areas; differences that are probably due to different genetic haplotypes, different patterns of gluten-containing foods intake, and environmental differences. CD has been found to be more frequent in females than in males and in children than in adults [10]. A fact worthy of mention is that the CD prevalence has been increasing during the last decades [2,10]. This increase must be partially attributed to an augmented awareness about the disease and more accurate diagnosis, but environmental factors are also responsible for being the most relevant the increase to gluten exposure in countries where nutrition traditionally relied on the intake of gluten-free grains such as rice or corn [3].

The clinical manifestations of CD can be both gastrointestinal and extraintestinal. Gastrointestinal symptoms include diarrhea, steatorrhea, abdominal pain, abdominal bloating, vomiting and failure to thrive due to the malabsorption process. This kind of symptomatology is more frequent in children and was formerly called "typical CD", a term that has currently been replaced by "classic" CD [3]. Among the extraintestinal manifestations, some of them such as ferropenic anemia, osteopenia and osteoporosis, short stature or dental enamel hypoplasia, are a consequence of the intestinal malabsorption process. Others, however, seem to be due to the noxious effect of gluten in the affected organs; dermatitis herpetiformis, gluten ataxia, gluten encephalopathy, epileptic seizures or elevation of liver enzymes are examples of the latter. Extraintestinal symptoms, which are more frequently found among adolescents and adults, were initially known as "atypical" CD, a term that has now been replaced by "symptomatic" CD [3].

CD is frequently comorbid with mainly other autoimmune disorders, although non-exclusively, type1 diabetes, Graves' disease and inflammatory bowel diseases [11,12]. It has also been found to be associated with a higher risk of non-Hodgkin lymphoma [13,14] and with Down [15,16] and Turner syndromes [15,17].

Unlike CD, NCGS has not been shown to be associated with underlying autoimmune mechanisms. Similar to patients with CD, subjects that experience NCGS may, after gluten intake, suffer a wide variety of intestinal and/or extraintestinal symptoms that improve after following a gluten-free diet. Contrarily to CD, the presence of anti-tissue transglutaminase and/or antiendomysial antibodies is always negative, the HLA-DQ2/HLA-DQ8 combination in these patients is only slightly more frequent than in the general population, and there is no atrophy of the small intestine mucosa although a rise in intraepithelial intestinal lymphocytes has been observed [18]. Its prevalence is not yet well-known although it does not seem to be an uncommon disease [19]. The pathogenetic mechanisms of NCGS are, at present, poorly understood. Patients with NCGS benefit from a gluten-free diet but they have been also shown to improve following a low FODMAPs (fermentable, oligo-, di-, monosaccharides and polyols) diet, a fact that suggests that other constituents of grains may be responsible for the symptoms of the disease [20].

Wheat allergy is an IgE-mediated reaction to the proteins contained in wheat and in particular, although not exclusively, the omega-5-gliadin. WA can be developed by inhalation of wheat flour, the so-called baker's asthma and baker's rhinitis which are considered occupational diseases, or by wheat ingestion [21]. The latter case, which is the most frequent, may cause urticaria, angioedema and/or gastrointestinal symptoms such as nausea, vomiting, abdominal bloating, abdominal pain and diarrhea; in the most severe cases it can induce systemic anaphylaxis [18]. WA is especially frequent in children, being less commonly seen in adolescents and adults. The treatment is based on the avoidance of wheat-containing foods, being less restrictive compared to gluten-free diet in CD, as it does not require the restriction of rye and barley-containing foods [22].

Psychiatric disturbances have frequently been reported in patients with CD. Several narrative reviews of the literature undertaken in the last five years indicate that CD could be associated with a wide spectrum of psychiatric disorders, including anxiety disorders, dysthymia, major depression, bipolar disorders, schizophrenia, eating disorders, autism spectrum disorders, and attention-deficit hyperactive disorders [23–27]. However, these otherwise important reviews have several limitations. Several of them were focused on specific psychiatric disorders such as anxiety and depression [24], mood disorders and schizophrenia [25], or severe psychiatric disorders [27]. Some others, according to their objectives comprised the whole spectrum of psychiatric disorders, but they do not specify their search strategies and/or the biomedical literature database used for the review [23,26]. Finally, when specified, literature searches were almost restricted to PubMed, thus providing a limited review of the literature on this topic. Moreover, none of the previous have evaluated the association of psychiatric disorders in children and adults with gluten-related disorders separately. The aim of this manuscript is presenting a comprehensive review of the literature on the potential association of gluten-related disorders with the whole spectrum of psychiatric disorders using the most common literature databases for this kind of evaluation (namely, Medline, EMBASE and PyscINFO).

2. Methodology

2.1. Search Strategy

We searched the medical literature for published studies indexed in the Medline (1966 to January 2018), EMBASE (1947 to January 2018), and PsycINFO (1967 to January 2018). The search strategy included terms of 'celiac disease' or 'gluten-sensitivity related disorders' combined with terms of 'mental disorders' as described in Supplementary Table S1. No limits or restrictions were applied. Retrieved references were pooled and managed using EndNote X8 (Clarivate Analytics, Philadelphia, PA, USA).

2.2. Inclusion Criteria

We included studies that investigated the prevalence, incidence or the likelihood of presenting mental or psychiatric disorders in patients with CD or gluten-sensitivity related disorders. For that purpose, comparative observational or interventional studies, including meta-analysis, assessing the aforementioned objectives as part of their primary or secondary objectives were included. Only studies published in English, Spanish, French, Portuguese, or Italian were included. Case-reports, case-series, abstracts and editorials were excluded. The relationship between CD and psychiatric disorders may be bidirectional. Our purpose was to assess the comorbidity between gluten-related disorders and psychiatric manifestations; thus, those studies assessing the prevalence, incidence or likelihood of presenting CD or gluten-related disorders in patients with diagnosed psychiatric disorders were excluded.

Study eligibility was independently evaluated by the three investigators (MS, EPC, FRV). Discrepancies in the evaluation were resolved by consensus among study investigators.

2.3. Data Extraction

Standardized data collection forms were used to extract data that included: (1) name of the first author; (2) year of publication; (3) country where the study was conducted; (4) study objective(s);

(5) study design; (6) assessment tools used in psychiatric comorbidities evaluation; (7) Disease diagnostic criteria; (8) sample size and demographic characteristics; and (9) summary of outcomes. Data extraction was independently completed by two investigators (MS and FRV). Discrepancies in data extraction were solved by consensus.

3. Results

3.1. Study Selection

Our systematic search strategy identified 1375 potentially relevant articles (730 articles from EMBASE, 453 articles from MEDLINE and 192 articles from PsycINFO). After removing 461 duplicate articles, 914 articles underwent title and abstract screening. Seven hundred and eighty-eight articles were excluded as they were case-reports, editorials, animal studies, basic science studies, did not include comparator group, or were published in a language other than those specified in the inclusion criteria, leaving 126 articles for a full-text screening. Two studies were excluded because we were unable to obtain their full text [28,29]. A total of 77 were excluded following full-text review because they were either published in abstract form, did not meet the specific objectives set for our current review or did not report outcomes of interest, leaving a total of 47 articles that were included in our review, of which 28 studies were conducted in the adult population, 11 studies were conducted in the pediatric population and eight studies included both adults and children. Mixed studies (including children and adults, $n = 8$) were classified under the corresponding population group with a larger sample size (pediatrics ($n = 4$), adults ($n = 4$)) (Figure 1).

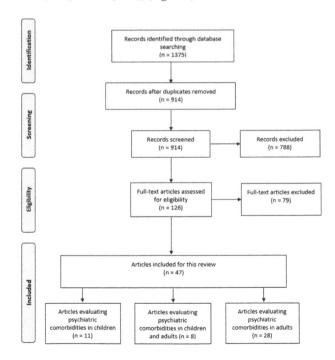

Figure 1. PRISMA flow chart.

3.2. Studies Conducted in Children with CD

We found 15 studies that evaluated psychiatric disorders in children or young adults with CD, 11 of which were conducted in clinical-based settings and four were conducted in community-based settings (Table 1). Studies were published between 1997 and 2018 [30–44]. Most studies (*n* = 12) were cross-sectional, although one of them included a subsequent longitudinal phase [41]. Three studies used a population-based cohort design and were conducted in Sweden using the same data source for patients with CD [31,34,44]. Finally, one study used a cohort design [38]. With the exception of this later study which was conducted in several countries [38], the remaining studies were conducted in European countries or Turkey.

According to a population-based cohort study, children with CD have a 70% increased likelihood of presenting a psychiatric disorder with intellectual disability being the most likely disorder (HR 1.7, 95% CI 1.4 to 2.1) [44]. A summary of results of studies evaluating the association between CD and the occurrence or presence of psychiatric disorders is presented in Table 2. Regarding specific conditions, cohort studies have shown that CD is associated with an increased likelihood of occurrence of depression (HR = 1.8, 95% CI 1.6 to 2.2) [34] or mood disorders (HR 1.2, 95% CI 1.0–1.4) [44], although this latter result did not reach statistical significance. In contrast, most cross-sectional studies have found that the point prevalence of depression or the severity of depressive symptoms did not differ in children with CD as compared with controls [33,35–37]. Pynnonen et al. [32], using a cross sectional study, found no differences between patients with CD and controls in the point prevalence of major depressive disorder, but the lifetime prevalence of major depressive disorder was significantly increased in patients with CD (31% vs. 7%; OR = 6.06, 95% CI 1.18–31.23). Although a population-based study found an increased likelihood of occurrence of anxiety disorder in patients with CD as compared with controls (HR 1.2, 95% CI 1.0 to 1.4, *p* <0.05) [44], cross-sectional studies have not shown differences between patients with CD and controls in the prevalence or severity of symptom of anxiety [32,35,36]. In children, no association has been found between CD and the occurrence of bipolar disorder [34].

The association of CD with psychotic disorders in children has been scarcely investigated, showing no association with the occurrence of schizophrenia [31] or psychotic disorder [44]; an association has been reported between CD and non-schizophrenic non-affective psychosis (HR 1.61, 95% CI 1.19–2.20) [31].

A population-based study found a significant association between CD and the occurrence of an eating disorder (HR 1.4, 95% CI 1.1 to 1.8) [44], and the presence of the disorder seems to have a negative impact on some dimensions of quality of life (namely, ill-being and joy-in-life) [39]. A population-based cohort found an excess likelihood of occurrence of an autism spectrum disorder in patients with CD as compared to controls [44]; however, a cross-sectional study did not find an association between both disorders [30]. A slight, but significant, increase in the likelihood of occurrence of attention deficit and hyperactive disorder (ADHD) in patients with CD has been reported [44].

Several factors have been suggested to contribute to depressive symptomatology in the pediatric population including the presence of parental depressive disorders, low parental educational level, divorce of the parents, presence of functional comorbid conditions and female gender [32,33,43]. Older age, higher body mass index and history of dietary restrictions were linked to higher risk of eating disorders [39,40].

3.3. Studies Conducted in Adults with CD

We found 32 studies that evaluated psychiatric comorbidities in adult patients with CD or NCGS, 18 of which were conducted in clinical-based settings and nine were conducted in community-based settings (Table 3). Studies were published between 1982 and 2018 [45–76]. More than half of these studies were of cross-sectional design [45,48,51,53–57,59,60,63,67,68,71,72,74–76] and four of them were representative of the general population [47,70,73,76].

Table 1. Objectives and design of studies evaluating the association between gluten-related disorders and psychiatric disorders in children and young adults.

Author (Year)	Country	Primary Objective	Design [‡]	Study Setting	Psychiatric Comorbidity Assessment	Celiac Disease Diagnostic Criteria
Autism spectrum disorders						
Pavone (1997) [30]	Italy	To evaluate behavioral problems and autistic features in children with CD	Cross-sectional	Clinical	DSM-III-R	Biopsy
Schizophrenia Spectrum						
Ludvigsson (2007) * [31]	Sweden	To determine the risk of non-affective psychosis in patients with CD in a national general population cohort	Population-based cohort	Community	ICD	ICD
Bipolar, depressive and anxiety disorders						
Pynnonen (2004) [32]	Finland	To compare the prevalence of current and lifetime mental disorders in adolescents with CD and controls	Cross-sectional	Clinical	K-SADS-PL Youth Self-Report BDI and BAI HDRS and HARS	Biopsy
Accomando (2005) * [33]	Italy	To investigate the relationship between CD and depression	Cross-sectional	Clinical	CDQ (adults) CDS (children)	NR
Ludvigsson (2007) * [34]	Sweden	To investigate the risk of subsequent depression and bipolar in patients with CD	Population-based cohort	Community	ICD	NR
Fidan (2013) [35]	Turkey	To investigate the depression and anxiety levels of children and adolescents with celiac disease and the impact of these on quality of life	Cross-sectional	Clinical	CDI STAIC	NR
Esenyel (2014) [36]	Turkey	To explore the diet compliance and depression and anxiety levels of pediatric celiac children and their families after a GFD	Cross-sectional	Clinical	CDI SCARED	ESPGHAN criteria
Simsek (2015) [37]	Turkey	To evaluate depressive symptoms at time of CD diagnosis and 6 months following GFD initiation	Phase 1: Cross-sectional Phase 2: Case-series	Clinical	CDI HRQOL (Kid-KINDL)	Biopsy
Smith (2017) [38]	USA, Finland, Germany, and Sweden	To assess mother's report of psychological functioning in children with CDA	Cohort	Community	CBCL	Serology and optional biopsy
Feeding and eating disorders						
Wagner (2015) [39]	Austria	To assess the determinants of eating disorders in female adolescents with CD	Cross-sectional	Clinical	EDI-2 EDE DSM-IV for subclinical eating disorders CDI (total score ≥ 18)	Both
Babio (2018) * [40]	Spain	To assess the risk of eating disorders in individuals between 10 and 23 years old diagnosed with CD	Cross-sectional	Clinical	CEAT EAT-26 SCFF BITE BSQ	Both

Table 1. *Cont.*

Author (Year)	Country	Primary Objective	Design ‡	Study Setting	Psychiatric Comorbidity Assessment	Celiac Disease Diagnostic Criteria
Overall psychological status						
Terrone (2013) [41]	Italy	To screen for neurological and behavioral disorders in children with CD	Phase 1: cross-sectional Phase 2: cohort	Clinical	PSC (total score ≥ 28)	ESPGHAN criteria
Various psychiatric conditions						
Ruggieri (2008) [42]	Italy	To determine the prevalence of neurologic symptoms in children with gluten sensitivity enteropathy	Cross-sectional	Clinical	NR	Both
Mazzone (2011) [43]	Italy	To identify psychological features in children with CD following strict GFD	Cross-sectional	Clinical	MASC CBCL CDI DSM-IV-TR criteria to assess autistic disorders	ESPGHAN criteria
Butwicka (2017) [44]	Sweden	To examine the risk of psychiatric disorders in children with a biopsy-verified diagnosis of CD and to examine the prevalence of psychiatric disorders before CD is diagnosed in children	Population-based cohort	Community	ICD	Biopsy

* Included patients of all age groups (pediatrics and adults); ‡ The design was determined by the authors of the current review which might not coincide with the design described in the original studies; for studies including multiple methodologies, the design that achieved the objectives of interest was selected; BAI: Beck Anxiety Inventory; BDI: Beck Depression Inventory; BITE: Bulimia Investigatory Test Edinburgh; 3SQ: Body Shape Questionnaire; CBCL: Achenbach Child Behavior Checklist; CD: celiac disease; CDA: celiac disease autoimmunity; CDI: Child Depression Inventory; CDQ: Clinical Depression Questionnaire; CDS: Children Depression Scale; CEAT: Children Eating Attitudes Test; DSM: Diagnostic and Statistical Manual of Mental Disorders; EAT: Eating Attitudes Test; EDE: Eating Disorder Examination; EDI: Eating Disorder Inventory; ESPGHAN: The European Society for Pediatric Gastroenterology, Hepatology, and Nutrition; GFD: gluten-free diet; HARS: Hamilton Anxiety Rating Scale; HDRS: Hamilton Depression Rating Scale; HRQOL: Health-Related Quality of Life; ICD: International Classification of Disease; KINDL: German questionnaire for measuring quality of life in children and adolescents; K-SADS-PL: Schedule for Affective Disorders and Schizophrenia for school-Age Children-Present and Lifetime version; MASC: Multidimensional Anxiety Scale for Children; NR: not reported; PSC: Pediatric Symptom Checklist; SCARED: Childhood Anxiety Disorders Screening Measure; SCFF: Sick Control Fat Food; STAIC: State-Trait Anxiety Inventory for Children.

Table 2. Summary of outcomes evaluating the association between gluten-related disorders and psychiatric disorders in children and young adults.

Author (Year)	Design	Sample Size and Demographic Characteristics	Summary of Outcomes	Associated Factors with Psychiatric Comorbidities and Other Relevant Information
Autism spectrum disorders				
Pavone (1997) [30]	Cross-sectional	CD, *n* = 120 (mean age 9.6 years, 48% females) Recently-diagnosed CD, *n* = 27 CD on strict GFD, *n* = 70 GFD non-adherent CD, *n* = 23 Controls, *n* = 20 (mean age 9.6 years, 48% females)	- Autism diagnosis: none of the recently-diagnosed CD - Language delay: Two subjects in GFD-compliant, one subject in the non-adherent group - Differences were not statistically significant compared to controls	NR
Schizophrenia Spectrum				
Ludvigsson (2007) [31]	Population-based cohort study	CD, *n* = 14,003 (age at diagnosis, 0–15 years 66% & ≥16 years 34%; 59% females) Controls, *n* = 68,125 (matched age and gender)	- Likelihood of psychosis in CD vs. controls using a Cox regression model stratified for gender, age, year of study entry and county: Any non-affective psychosis (schizophrenia and other psychoses) HR = 1.55 (95% CI: 1.16–2.06) Non-schizophrenic non-affective psychosis HR = 1.61 (95% CI: 1.19–2.20) Schizophrenia HR = 1.43 (95% CI: 0.77–2.67)	NR
Bipolar, depressive and anxiety disorders				
Pynnonen (2004) [32]	Cross-sectional	CD, *n* = 29 (mean age 14.2 years, 55% females) Controls, *n* = 29 (mean age 14.4 years, 55% females)	- Lifetime prevalence of major depression disorder (CD vs. controls): 31% vs. 7%, *p* <0.05. OR = 6.06 (95% CI: 1.18–31.23). - Disruptive behavior disorders (CD vs. controls): 28% vs. 3%, *p* <0.05. OR = 10.67 (95% CI: 1.24–92). - Lifetime prevalence of anxiety disorders (CD vs. controls): 21% vs. 24%, *p* = NS - Differences in the prevalence of current depressive, anxiety, or disruptive behavior disorders between the two groups were non-significant	- History of parental depressive disorder was more common in CD patients with depressive symptomatology compared to CD without depressive symptomatology - Parental educational level, divorce of parents, poor weight or height gain, and somatic symptoms were not associated with mental disorders
Accomando (2005) [33]	Cross-sectional	CD, *n* = 42 (17 adults and 25 children) HC, *n* = 42	Prevalence of depression (CD vs. HC): 26.2% vs. 30.9%, *p* = NS	- Females predominated in CD patients with depression (not reaching statistical significance) - Depression was more common in CD with functional comorbid conditions (specific conditions not specified)
Ludvigsson (2007) [34]	Population-based cohort study	CD, *n* = 13,776 (median age at diagnosis 2 years, 58.6% females) Controls, *n* = 66,815 (median age at diagnosis 2 years, 58.7% females)	- CD was associated with an increased risk of subsequent depression (HR = 1.8, 95% CI: 1.6–2.2) - No significant association between CD and bipolar disorder was reported (HR = 1.1, 95% CI: 0.7–1.7)	- Socioeconomic index didn't have any confounding effect on the later schizophrenia diagnosis in CD
Fidan (2013) [35]	Cross-sectional	CD, *n* =30 (mean age 12.4 ± 3.1 years, 57% females). HC, *n* = 30 (mean age NR, 57% females)	- CD vs. HC: CDI: 10.8 ± 7.4 vs. 8.8 ± 6.8, *p*=0.28 STAIC-State Anxiety: 34.6 ± 6.1 vs. 32.8 ± 7.2, *p* = 0.30 STAIC-Trait Anxiety: 33.7 ± 6.5 vs. 33 ± 6.3, *p* =0.64	- Data on the impact of depression and anxiety on HRQOL NR

Table 2. *Cont.*

Author (Year)	Design	Sample Size and Demographic Characteristics	Summary of Outcomes	Associated Factors with Psychiatric Comorbidities and Other Relevant Information
Esenyel (2014) [36]	Cross-sectional	CD, n = 30 (mean age 11.9 ± 2 years, 70% females) HC, n =20 (mean age 12 ± 2 years, 55% females)	- CD vs. HC: CDI points: 8.73 ± 5.51 vs. 8.3 ± 4.02, p = 0.921 SCARED points: 24.5 ± 14.41 vs. 17.85 ± 9.12, p = 0.120 - There were no differences in depression and anxiety scores between patients with CD compliant or non-compliant with a GFD	NR
Simsek (2015) [37]	Phase 1: Cross-sectional Phase 2: Case-series	CD, n = 25 (mean age 11.8 years, 72% females) Controls, n = 25 (mean age 12.2 years, 64%)	- At the time of diagnosis (CD vs. controls): CDI scores: 9 vs. 6, p = NS - 6 months following GFD initiation: CDI scores in CD: 9 before diet vs. 9.5 after diet, p = NS	- Total scores of HRQOL were significantly lower in CD patients (p <0.05)
Smith (2017) [38]	Cohort	Aware-CDA, n = 440 (58% females) Unware-CDA, n = 66 (50% females) No CDA, n = 3651 (NR)	- At 3.5 years of age, unaware-CDA mothers reported more anxious/depressed symptoms, aggressive behavior, and externalizing composite score compared to aware-CDA group (p <0.05) or without CDA (p <0.05) - At 3.5 years of age, Aware-CDA mothers reported significantly fewer problems on the anxious/depressed subscale compared to No CDA group (p = 0.03) - At 4.5 years, there were no significant differences	NR

Feeding and eating disorders

Author (Year)	Design	Sample Size and Demographic Characteristics	Summary of Outcomes	Associated Factors with Psychiatric Comorbidities and Other Relevant Information
Wagner (2015) [39]	Cross-sectional	CD, n = 206 (mean age NR) CD with ED, n = 32 (mean age 16.4 yeas) CD without ED, n = 174 (mean age 14.5 years) Controls, n = 53 (mean age 14.7 years)	- Lifetime prevalence of EDs: 5.3% of girls with CD: anorexia nervosa (n = 1), bulimia nervosa (n = 4), and EDs not otherwise specified (n = 6); 3.9% suffered from current ED - Criteria for lifetime subclinical EDs: 21 girls (10.2%) with CD - Higher BMI and self-directedness were predictors of greater risk of ED - Higher ill-being and lower joy in life were reported by patients with CD with ED compared with patients without EDs, even when controlling for age and depression levels	- No differences between patients (with CD) with and without EDs in coping strategies were found - Higher BMI and lower self-directedness were linked to higher risk of ED in CD
Babio (2018) [40]	Cross-sectional	CD, n = 98 (mean age 15 years, 60% females) Controls, n = 98 (mean age 15 years, 60% females)	- No significant differences in the median scores of the screening tools for EDs between CD and HC - CD vs. HC: β coefficient = 2.15 (1.04); p = 0.04 in a multiple linear regression model for EAT after adjusting for several factors	- Only significant results for one out of the 4 models (one for each screening test) - Age > 13 years old was positively associated with an increase in the score on the EAT

Overall psychological status

Author (Year)	Design	Sample Size and Demographic Characteristics	Summary of Outcomes	Associated Factors with Psychiatric Comorbidities and Other Relevant Information
Terrone (2013) [41]	Phase 1: cross-sectional Phase 2: cohort	CD, n = 139 (mean age 10 years, 64.7% females): Group A (n =40): newly diagnosed CD Group B (n = 54): CD in remission on GFD > 1 year Group C (n = 45): potential CD	- Comparison of mean PSC scores using ANOVA: Group A, 14.8 ± 4.2 (one pathological score) vs. Group B, 12.3 ± 6.4 (one pathological score) vs. Group C, 7.6 ± 6 (p <0.0001)	NR

Table 2. Cont.

Author (Year)	Design	Sample Size and Demographic Characteristics	Summary of Outcomes	Associated Factors with Psychiatric Comorbidities and Other Relevant Information
Various psychiatric conditions				
Ruggieri (2008) [42]	Cross-sectional	GS, n = 835 (demographic characteristics NR) Controls, n = 300 (demographic characteristics NR)	- 3 out of 835 children had bipolar disorders - None of the controls had psychiatric disorders	NR
Mazzone (2011) [43]	Cross-sectional	CD, n = 100 (mean age 10.4 years, 65% females) HC, n = 100 (mean age 11.5 years, 58% females)	- MASC scores: CD children showed significantly higher scores (50 ± 8.3 vs. 42.9 ± 6.6, p <0.01) - CDI scores: CD children showed significantly higher scores (8.1 ± 5.7 vs. 5.6 ± 3.4, p <0.01) - No significant differences were found in CBCL analysis - Two children in the CD group were classified within the spectrum of autistic disorders	- CD males showed significantly higher scores for total CBCL. - CD females showed an increased rate of anxiety and depression symptoms, as indicated by significantly higher MASC and CDI scores
Butwicka (2017) [44]	Population-based cohort study	CD, n = 10,903 (median age 3 years, 62% females) Controls, n = 1,042,072 (age NR but matched, 61% females)	- HRs from a Multivariate Cox regression adjusted for maternal/paternal age at child's birth, maternal/paternal country of birth, level of education of higher-educated parent, gestational age, birth weight, birth cohort, Apgar score, and history of psychiatric disorders before recruitment: Any psychiatric disorder 1.4 (95% CI: 1.3–1.4) Psychotic disorders 1.9 (95% CI: 1.0–3.5) Mood disorders 1.2 (95% CI: 1.0–1.4) Anxiety disorders 1.2 (95% CI: 1.0–1.4) EDs 1.4 (95% CI: 1.1–1.8) Substance misuse 1.0 (95% CI: 0.9–1.3) Behavioral disorders 1.4 (95% CI: 1.2–1.6) ADHD 1.2 (95% CI: 1.0–1.4) Autism spectrum disorder 1.3 (95% CI: 1.1–1.7) Intellectual disability 1.7 (95% CI: 1.4–2.1)	NR

ADHD: Attention-Deficit Hyperactivity Disorder; ANOVA: analysis of variance; BMI: body mass index; CBCL: Achenbach Child Behavior Checklist; CD: celiac disease; CDA: celiac disease autoimmunity; CDI: Child Depression Inventory; CI: confidence interval; EAT: Eating Attitudes Test; ED: eating disorder; GFD: gluten free diet; GS: gluten sensitivity; HC: healthy controls; HR: hazard ratio; HRQOL: Health-Related Quality of Life; MASC: Multidimensional Anxiety Scale for Children; NR: not reported; NS: not significant; OR: odd ratio; PSC: Pediatric Symptom Checklist; SCARED: Childhood Anxiety Disorders Screening Measure; STAIC: State-Trait Anxiety Inventory for Children; vs: versus.

Table 3. Objectives and design of studies evaluating the association between gluten-related disorders and psychiatric disorders in adults.

Author (Year)	Country	Primary Objective	Design [‡]	Study Setting	Psychiatric Comorbidity Assessment	Celiac Disease Diagnostic Criteria
Attention-Deficit/Hyperactivity Disorder						
Zelnik (2004) * [45]	Israel	To evaluate neurologic disorders including ADHD in CD	Cross-sectional	Clinical	DSM criteria for ADHD	Both
Autism spectrum disorders						
Ludvigsson (2013) * [46]	Sweden	To examine the association between autistic spectrum disorder and CD	Cohort study	Community	ICD	Group 1: villous atrophy, Marsh stage 3 Group 2: villous atrophy, Marsh stages 1–2 Group 3: normal mucosa and positive serologic findings
Schizophrenia Spectrum						
West (2006) [47]	UK	To compare the risk of schizophrenia in patients with CD, ulcerative colitis, Crohn's disease with the general population	Population-based cross-sectional	Community	NR	NR
Eaton (2006) [48]	Denmark	To estimate the association of schizophrenia with autoimmune disorders	Cross-sectional	Community	ICD	ICD
Benros (2011) [49]	Denmark	To investigate whether autoimmune diseases are associated with increased risk of schizophrenia	Population-based retrospective cohort	Community	ICD	NR
Wijarnpreecha (2018) [50]	USA	To evaluate the risk of developing schizophrenia among patients with CD	Meta-analysis	NA	NR	NR
Bipolar, depressive or anxiety disorders						
Hallert (1982) [51] Hallert (1983) [52]	Sweden	To compare the prevalence of psychiatric illness among patients with CD vs. controls and to assess the effects of gluten withdrawal and vitamin B6 supplement on depressive symptoms	Phase 1: cross-sectional Phase 2: case-series	Clinical	MMPI	Both (serological and biopsy) combined with morphological improvement with GFD
Addolorato (1996) [53]	Italy	To conduct psychometric evaluation in patients with CD or IBD compared to healthy controls	Cross-sectional	Clinical	STAI IDSQ	Both
Ciacci (1998) [54]	Italy	To explore the relevance of depressive symptoms in a large series of adult celiacs	Cross-sectional	Clinical	SRDS	Both
Addolorato (2001) [55]	Italy	To evaluate state and trait anxiety and depression in adult CD patients before and after 1 year of GFD	Phase 1: Cross-sectional Phase 2: Case-series	Clinical	STAI SRDS	Both
Cicarelli (2003) [56]	Italy	To evaluate the prevalence of headache, mood disorders, epilepsy, ataxia and peripheral neuropathy in adult celiac patients	Cross-sectional	Clinical	DSM-IV	Both
Carta (2002) [57] Carta (2003) [58]	Italy	To evaluate the association between celiac disease and specific anxiety and depressive disorders	Cross-sectional	Clinical	CIDI-DSM-IV	Both
Addolorato (2008) [59]	Italy	To evaluate social phobia in CD patients	Cross-sectional	Clinical	LSAS total > 30 SRDS > 49	Both

115

Table 3. *Cont.*

Author (Year)	Country	Primary Objective	Design ‡	Study Setting	Psychiatric Comorbidity Assessment	Celiac Disease Diagnostic Criteria
Garud (2009) [60]	US	To determine the prevalence of psychiatric and autoimmune disorders in patients with CD in the US compared with control groups	Cross-sectional	Community	Clinical charts	Biopsy
Smith (2012) [61]	Denmark	To investigate whether CD is reliably linked with anxiety and/or depression	Meta-analysis	NA	NA	NA
Peters (2014) [62]	Australia	To investigate the effect of gluten on mental state among patients with NCGS	Randomized, double-blind, cross-over trial	Clinical	STPI	Challenging with varying amounts of gluten
Carta (2015) [63]	Italy	To measure the association between CD and affective disorders	Cross-sectional	Clinical	DSM-IV	NR
Di Sabatino (2015) [64]	Italy	To assess the effects of gluten administration on intestinal and extraintestinal symptoms in subjects with NCGS	Randomized, double-blind, placebo-controlled cross-over trial	Clinical	Extraintestinal symptoms, including depression, were self-reported by patients as absent or present	Self-reported persistence of relevant intestinal and extraintestinal symptoms at low gluten doses
Tortora (2013) [65]	Italy	To evaluate the prevalence of post-partum depression in CD	Cross-sectional	Clinical	EPDS (Total score > 10 possible PPD)	Both
Sainsbury (2018) [66]	UK	To synthesize the evidence on the relationship between depression and degree of adherence to GFD in patients with CD	Meta-analysis	NA	NA	NA
Feeding and eating disorders						
Passananti (2013) [67]	Italy	To investigate the prevalence of eating disorders in patients with celiac disease	Cross-sectional	Clinical	Structured psychological assessment using: BES (Total score ≥ 17) EAT-26 (Total score ≥ 20) EDI-2 M-SDS (Total score > 44) SCL-90	Both
Satherley (2016) [68]	United Kingdom	To examine the prevalence of eating disorders in women with CD	Cross-sectional	Clinical	EAT-26 (Total score > 20) BES (Moderate bingeing, score > 17; severe bingeing, score > 27) DASS-21	Self-reported a biopsy-confirmed diagnosis
Mårild (2017) * [69]	Sweden	To determine whether women with CD are at increased risk of diagnosis of anorexia nervosa	Register-based cohort study	Community	ICD	Group 1: villous atrophy, Marsh stage 3 Group 2: villous atrophy, Marsh stages 1–2 Group 3: normal mucosa and positive serologic findings
Sleep-Wake disorders						
Mårild (2015) * [70]	Sweden	To estimate the risk of repeated use of hypnotics among individuals with CD as a proxy measure for poor sleep	Population-based cohort study	Community	Prescribed Drug Register in Sweden—Use of hypnotics	Biopsy

Table 3. *Cont.*

Author (Year)	Country	Primary Objective	Design [‡]	Study Setting	Psychiatric Comorbidity Assessment	Celiac Disease Diagnostic Criteria
Substance-related and addictive disorders						
Roos (2006) [71]	Sweden	To assess psychological well-being in adults with CD with proven remission (treated for 10 years)	Cross-sectional	Clinical	PGWB	Remission was ascertained with a return of villous structure at repeat biopsy (82%) or negative serology (18%)
Gili (2013) [72]	Spain	To study the impact of alcohol disorders on length of hospital stays, over-expenditures during hospital stays, and excess mortality in CD patients	Cross-sectional	Clinical	ICD	ICD
Neurocognitive Disorders						
Lebwohl (2016) [73]	Sweden	To determine whether patients with CD have an increased risk of dementia	Population-based cohort	Community	ICD	Biopsy
Various psychiatric conditions						
Fera (2003) [74]	Italy	To estimate the incidence of psychiatric disorders in celiac disease patients on gluten withdrawal	Cross-sectional	Clinical	DSM-IV criteria	Biopsy & Clinical history
Sainsbury (2013) [75]	Australia	To compare the relevant impact of psychological symptoms to known negative impacts of gastrointestinal symptoms and adherence to the GFD on quality of life	Study 1: Cross-sectional Study 2: Cross-sectional	Clinical	DASS EDI-3 CISS	Biopsy
Zylberberg (2017) [76]	US	To assess the prevalence of depression and insomnia among patients with CD, both diagnosed and undiagnosed, and people without CD who avoid gluten	Population-based cross-sectional	Community	PHQ-9 (Total score on questions 1–9 ≥ 10) SDQ	Diagnosed CD: self-reported diagnosis Undiagnosed CD: serology

* Included patients of all age groups (pediatrics and adults); [‡] The design was determined by the authors of the current review which might not coincide with the design described in the original studies; for studies including multiple methodologies, the design that achieved the objectives of interest was selected; ADHD: Attention-deficit/hyperactivity disorder; BES: Binge Eating Scale; CD: celiac disease; CDS: Children Depression Scale; DSM: Diagnostic and Statistical Manual of Mental Disorders; CIDI-DSM-IV: Composite International Diagnostic Interview for DSM-IV; CISS: Coping Inventory for Stressful Situations; DASS: Depression Anxiety Stress Scale; DSM: Diagnostic and Statistical Manual of Mental Disorders; EAT: Eating Attitudes Test; EDI: Eating Disorder Inventory; EDRS: Eating Disorder Risk Scale; EPDS: Edinburgh Postnatal Depression Scale; GFD: gluten-free diet; HADS: Hospital Anxiety and Depression Scale; IBD: inflammatory bowel disease; ICD: International Classification of Disease; IDSQ: Ipat Depression Scale Questionnaire; LSAS: Liebowitz Social Anxiety Scale; MMPI: Minnesota Multiphasic Personality Inventory; M-SDS: Modified Zung Self-Rating Depression Scale; NA: not applicable; NCGS: non-celiac gluten sensitivity; NR: not reported; PGWB: Psychological General Well-being; PHQ: Patient Health Questionnaire; PPD: post-partum depression; PSS: Perceived Stress Scale; SCL: Symptom Check List; SDQ: Sleep Disorder Questionnaire; SRDS: Zung Self-Rating Depression Scale; STAI: State and Trait Anxiety Inventory; STAI: State and Trait Anxiety; STPI: Spielberger State Trait Personality Inventory.

117

A summary of results of studies evaluating the association between CD and the occurrence or presence of psychiatric disorders is presented in Table 4.

The prevalence rates of depression or depressive symptomatology were significantly higher in patients with CD compared to controls in the majority of the published studies except for two [56,60]. Nevertheless, significant variability in the point-prevalence of depression or depressive symptomatology exists, ranging from 14% to 68.7% [53,56,57,59,60,63]. In a meta-analysis conducted by Smith et al. [61], depression was shown to be more common and severe in CD than in healthy adults, but not compared to patients with other medical conditions. Comorbid illnesses, including type I diabetes mellitus or subclinical thyroid disease, and stress were associated with the presence of depressive symptomatology in CD [57,60]. Increased severity of gastrointestinal symptoms in CD was linked to worsened depressive symptoms [75] which, in turn, led to poorer QOL compared to controls [63]. Although gluten-free diet (GFD) did not lead to any improvement in depressive symptoms in two longitudinal studies [52,55], a meta-analysis conducted by Sainsbury et al. [66] found a moderate association between poor adherence to GFD and greater depressive symptoms. With respect to post-partum depression, it was assessed in a single study in which it turned out to be significantly more prevalent in women with CD compared to controls (41% vs. 11%, $p < 0.01$) [65].

Nutrients **2018**, *10*, 875

Table 4. Summary of outcomes evaluating the association between gluten-related disorders and psychiatric disorders in adults.

Author (Year)	Design	Sample Size and Demographic Characteristics	Summary of Outcomes	Associated Factors with Psychiatric Comorbidities and other Relevant Information
Attention-Deficit/Hyperactivity Disorder				
Zelnik (2004) [45]	Cross-sectional	CD, *n* = 111 (mean age 20.1 years, 57.7% females) Controls, *n* = 211 (mean age 20.1 years, 56.7% females)	- ADHD diagnosis: 20.7% in CD vs. 10.5% in controls (*p* <0.01) CD, 20.3% of female patients and 21.2% of male patients Controls, 8.7% of females and 12.9% males	-No gender differences were found in the prevalence of ADHD in patients with CD -Differences in ADHD were not different among CD patients presenting with infantile form of CD or late-onset symptoms
Autism spectrum disorders				
Ludvigsson (2013) [46]	Cohort study	Group 1, *n* = 26,995 (age at diagnosis, 0–19 years 40.4%, >20 years 59.6%; 62.1% females); Controls, *n* = 134,076 (matched age and gender) Group 2, *n* = 12,304 (age at diagnosis, 0–19 years 8.9%, >20 years 91.1%; 56.9% females); Controls, *n* = 60,654 (matched age and gender) Group 3, *n* = 3719 (age at diagnosis, 0–19 years 25.3%, >20 years 74.7%; 62.1% females); Controls, *n* = 18,478 (matched age and gender)	- Risk of later ASD diagnosis: Group 1: HR = 1.39 (95% CI: 1.13–1.71) Group 2: HR =2.01 (95% CI: 1.29–3.13) Group 3: HR = 3.09 (95% CI: 1.99–4.8)	NR
Schizophrenia Spectrum				
West (2006) [47]	Population-based case-control	CD, *n* = 4732; matched controls, *n* = 23,620 Crohn's disease, *n* = 5961; matched controls, *n* = 29,843 Ulcerative colitis, *n* = 8301; matched controls, *n* = 41,589 Demographics NR	- Prevalence of schizophrenia 0.25% in CD, 0.27% in Crohn's disease and 0.24% in ulcerative colitis, 0.37% in general population - ORs for schizophrenia compared to controls adjusted for smoking status: 0.76 (95% CI: 0.4–1.4) in CD, 0.74 (95% CI: 0.4–1.3) in Crohn's disease, 0.71 (95% CI 0.4–1.1) in ulcerative colitis	NR
Eaton (2006) [48]	Cross-sectional	Schizophrenia, *n* = 7704, 25 controls for each case. Demographics NR	- Prior CD diagnosis in subjects with schizophrenia: Crude incidence rate: 3.8 (95% CI: 1.3–11) Adjusted incidence rate: 3.6 (95% CI: 1.2–10.6)	NR
Benros (2011) [49]	Population-based cohort	Schizophrenia, *n* = 39,076: Prior diagnosis of autoimmune disease, *n* = 927, autoimmune disease and infections, *n* = 444, without autoimmune disease, *n* = 37,705 Demographics NR	- The risk of schizophrenia among individuals with CD was increased: CD without infection: Incidence rate ratio = 2.11 (95% CI: 1.09–3.61) CD with infections: Incidence rate ratio = 2.47 (95% CI: 1.13–4.61)	NR
Wijarnpreecha (2018) [50]	Meta-analysis	Four studies were included	- Higher risk of schizophrenia among patients with CD was found: pooled OR = 2.03 (95% CI: 1.45–2.86)	NR

Table 4. *Cont.*

Author (Year)	Design	Sample Size and Demographic Characteristics	Summary of Outcomes	Associated Factors with Psychiatric Comorbidities and other Relevant Information
Bipolar, depressive and anxiety disorders				
Hallert (1982) [51] Hallert (1983) [52]	Phase 1: cross-sectional Phase 2: case-series	CD, n = 12 (mean age 47 years, 67% females) Controls undergoing cholecystectomy, n = 12 (mean age 47 years, 67% females)	- MMPI depression subscale: Significantly higher scores in CD vs. controls (70.3 ± 12.5 vs. 59.2 ± 9.3, p <0.01) - MMPI scores: Post-remission in small intestinal mucosa following GFD in CD: no improvement in mood (70 ± 12.5 at point 0 vs. 68 ± 14 at year 1, p = NS) - Post-cholecystectomy in controls: No change in MMPI scores - Supplementation with Vitamin B6 80 mg/day for 6 months: Significant decrease in depressive symptoms (68 ± 14.0 to 56 ± 8.5, p <0.01)	-In patients with CD, significant correlation was found between depression scores and degree of steatorrhea -No correlation was found between abdominal complaints (diarrhea and pain) and depression scores
Addolorato (1996) [53]	Case-control	CD, n = 20 (mean age 37 years, 56% females) IBD, n = 16 (mean age 32 years, 56% females) Controls, n = 16 (mean age 35 years, 56% females)	- Prevalence of State anxiety: 62.5% in CD, 50% in IBD, and 31.3% in controls (p = NS). - Prevalence of depression: 68.7% in CD, 37.5% in IBD, and 18.8% in controls (p <0.01 for CD vs. controls only)	NR
Ciacci (1998) [54]	Cross-sectional	CD, n = 92 (mean age 29.4 years, 70% females) CPH, n = 48 (mean age 31.8 years, 34% females) Controls, n = 100 (mean age 30 years, 71% females)	- Mean scores of the M-SDS: CD: 31.81 ± 7.84 CPH: 28.73 ± 7.09 (p = 0.038 vs. CD) Controls: 27.14 ± 5.26 (p <0.0001 vs. CD)	- Demographic characteristics did not influence M-SDS scores -Depressive symptoms are present to a similar extent in patients with childhood- and adulthood-diagnosed CD
Addolorato (2001) [55]	Phase 1: Cross-sectional Phase 2: Case-series	CD, n = 35 (mean age 29.8 years, 60% females) Controls, n = 59 (mean age 31.7 years, 54% females)	*Before diet:* - Prevalence of high levels of state anxiety: CD vs. control: 71.4% versus 23.7% (p <0.0001) - Prevalence of high levels of trait anxiety: CD vs. controls: 25.7% versus 15.2% (p = NS) - Prevalence of depression CD vs. controls: 57.1% versus 9.6% (p <0.0001) *After 1 year of GFD (T0 vs. T1)* - Prevalence of high levels of state anxiety: T0 71.4% versus T1: 25.7% (p <0.001) - Prevalence of high levels of trait anxiety: T0: 25.7% versus T1: 17.1% (p = NS) - Prevalence of depression T0: 57.1% versus T1:45.7 (p = NS)	NR
Cicarelli (2003) [56]	Cross-sectional	CD, n = 176 (mean age 30.9 years, 75% females) Controls, n = 52 (mean age 31.7 years, 65% females)	- Prevalence of mood disorders (CD vs. controls): Mood disorders 50 (29%) vs. 9 (17%), p = NS Depression episodes 24 (14%) vs. 7 (13%), p = NS Dysthymia 26 (15%) vs. 2 (4%), p <0.05	- Adherence to a strict gluten-free diet was associated with a significant reduction of dysthymia

Table 4. Cont.

Author (Year)	Design	Sample Size and Demographic Characteristics	Summary of Outcomes	Associated Factors with Psychiatric Comorbidities and other Relevant Information
Bipolar, depressive and anxiety disorders				
Carta (2002) [57] Carta (2003) [58]	Cross-sectional	CD, n = 36 (mean age 41.1 years, 75% females) Controls, n = 144 (mean age 41.3 years, 75% females)	- Lifetime prevalence of psychiatric disorders (cases vs. controls): Major depressive disorder 15 (41.7%) vs. 30 (20.8%), p = 0.01 Dysthymic disorder 3 (8.3%) vs. 2 (1.4%), p = 0.05 Adjustment disorders 11 (30.5%) vs. 11 (7.6%), p = 0.001 Generalized anxiety disorder 10 (27.7%) vs. 23 (16%), p = NS Panic disorder 5 (13.9%) vs. 3 (2.1%), p = 0.001 Specific phobia 1 (2.7%) vs. 6 (4.2%), p = NS Social phobia 3 (8.3%) vs. 10 (6.9%), p = NS Recurrent brief depression 36.1% versus 6.9% (OR = 7.6; 95% CI: 3.2–17.8)	- Earlier onset of CD was linked to higher prevalence of major depressive disorder - Subclinical thyroid disease appears to represent a significant risk factor for these psychiatric disorders
Addolorato (2008) [59]	Cross-sectional	CD, n = 40 (mean age 38 years, 86% females) HC, n = 50 (mean age 36 years, 80% females)	- Prevalence of social phobia: 70% in CD vs. 16% in HC (p <0.0001) - Prevalence of depression: 53% in CD vs. 8% in HC (p <0.0001)	- The prevalence of social phobia or depression in patients with CD did not differ among subjects newly diagnosed with CD and those already on GFD
Garud (2009) [60]	Cross-sectional	CD, n = 600 (mean age 54 males & 45 females, 75% females) IBS, n = 200 (mean age 48 males & 45 females, 75% females) Controls, n = 200 (mean age 52 males & 47 females, 75% females)	Prevalence of depression: 17.2% in CD vs. 18.5% in IBS (p = 0.74 vs. CD) and 16% in controls (p = 0.79 vs. CD)	- Among CD patients, type I diabetes mellitus was identified as a significant risk factor for depression (p <0.01) with 37% of patients with both CD and type I DM having clinical depression
Smith (2012) [61]	Meta-analysis	Eleven studies on depression and eight studies on anxiety were included	- Depression is more common and severe in CD than in healthy adults with an overall effect size of 0.97 - Anxiety did not differ significantly between CD and healthy adults - No differences in depression or anxiety in CD vs. other medical disorders	- Other medical conditions included: Crohn's disease, DM, IBD, lactose intolerance, surgery patients, CPH
Peters (2014) [62]	Randomized, double-blind, cross-over trial	NCGS, n = 22 (median age 48 years, 77% females)	- Gluten ingestion effect on STPI depression scores: Significantly higher scores in CD vs. controls (mean difference = 2.03, 95% CI: 0.55–3.51, p = 0.01) - No differences in other STPI state indices or for any STPI trait measures	NR
Carta (2015) [63]	Cross-sectional	CD, n = 46 (mean age 41 years, 83% females) Controls, n = 240 (mean age 41 years, 83% females)	- Prevalence of depression: 30.0% in CD vs. 8.3% in controls, p <0.0001 - Prevalence of panic disorder: 18.3% in CD vs. 5.4% in controls, p <0.001 - Prevalence of bipolar disorder: 4.3% in CD vs. 0.4% in controls, p <0.005	- Patients with CD but without comorbidity with major depression, panic disorder, or bipolar disorder do not show worse QOL than controls
Di Sabatino (2015) [64]	Randomized, double-blind, placebo-controlled cross-over trial	NCGS, n = 61 (mean age 39 years, 87% females) randomly assigned to: Gluten 4.375 mg/day for 1 week Placebo 4.375 g/day rice starch for 1 week Wash-out period: 1 week	- Depression was significantly worsened by gluten ingestion (p = 0.02)	NR

Table 4. *Cont.*

Author (Year)	Design	Sample Size and Demographic Characteristics	Summary of Outcomes	Associated Factors with Psychiatric Comorbidities and other Relevant Information
Bipolar, depressive and anxiety disorders				
Tortora (2013) [65]	Cross-sectional	CD, $n = 70$ (mean age 33 years) Controls, $n = 70$ (mean age 32 years)	- EPDS scores in CD women vs. controls: 9.9 ± 5.9 vs. 6.7 ± 3.7, $p < 0.01$ - EPDS > 10: 47% in CD vs. 14% in controls (OR = 3.3, $p < 0.01$) - PPD diagnosis: 41% of CD women with vs. 11% in controls ($p < 0.01$)	- A significant association was observed between the onset of PPD and a previous menstrual disorder in women suffering from CD - QOL scores were significantly higher in women with CD
Sainsbury (2018) [66]	Meta-analysis	Eight studies were included in quantitative analysis (total $n = 1644$, mean age ranged from 39 to 57 years, % of females ranged from 76.6% to 100%)	- Moderate association between poor adherence to GFD and greater depressive symptoms ($r = 0.398$, 95% CI: 0.32–0.47) with marked heterogeneity in effects ($I^2 = 66.8\%$) - Exclusion of studies with high or unclear risk of bias did not alter the results	- Poorer QOL was correlated with a higher incidence of psychological and gastrointestinal symptoms, greater reliance on maladaptive coping strategies, and poorer GFD adherence
Feeding and eating disorders				
Passananti (2013) [67]	Cross-sectional	CD, $n = 100$ (mean age 29 years, 72% females) HC, $n = 100$ (mean age 30 years, 68% females)	- BES > 17: 6% in CD vs. 0% controls ($p =$ NS) - Women with CD had significantly higher scores in pulse thinness, social insecurity, perfectionism, inadequacy, ascetisim, and interpersonal diffidence compared to HC women of the Eating Disorder Inventory - EAT-26 $\geq$ 20: 16% in CD vs. 4% in HC ($p = 0.01$) - SRDS > 44: 39% in CD vs. 6% in controls ($p < 0.001$) - SCL-90 pathological scores: 42% in CD vs. 6% in HC ($p < 0.0001$)	- EAT-26 demonstrated association between indices of diet-related disorders in both CD and the female gender after controlling for anxiety and depression
Satherley (2016) [68]	Cross-sectional	CD, $n = 157$ (mean age 38 years, sex NR) IBD, $n = 116$ (mean age 36 years, sex NR) DM-type 2, $n = 88$ (mean age 47 years, sex NR) HC, $n = 142$ (mean age 33 years, sex NR)	- EAT-26 > 20: 15.7% in CD vs. 8.8% in DM and 3.8% in HC ($p < 0.05$) - BES > 17: 19.4% in CD vs. 2.3% in controls ($p < 0.05$) - Mean EAT-26 and BES scores: 11.1 in CD vs. 7.7 in controls ($p < 0.05$) and 11.2 in CD vs. 3.9 in controls ($p < 0.05$), respectively - Significant associations between EAT-26 and BES scores with DASS-21 scores were reported ($p < 0.008$)	- Dietary-management and gastrointestinal symptoms were significantly associated with EAT scores in CD
Mårild (2017) [69]	Population-based cohort study	Group 1, $n = 17,959$ (median age 28 years); Matched controls, $n = 89,379$ Group 2, $n = 7455$ (median age 46 years); Matched controls, $n = 36,940$ Group 3, $n = 2307$ (median age 38 years); Matched controls, $n = 11,499$	- Risk of developing anorexia nervosa: Group 1: HR= 1.46 (95% CI: 1.08–1.98) Group 2: HR=2.12 (95% CI: 0.97–4.67) Group 3: HR=2.45 (95% CI: 1.10–5.45) - Adjustment for education level, socioeconomic status, and type 1 DM didn't affect conclusions in all groups	- There was no significantly increased risk for subsequent anorexia nervosa among males with CD

Table 4. *Cont.*

Author (Year)	Design	Sample Size and Demographic Characteristics	Summary of Outcomes	Associated Factors with Psychiatric Comorbidities and other Relevant Information
Sleep-Wake disorders				
Mårild (2015) [70]	Population-based cohort study	CD, n = 2933 (median age 28 years, 61.2% females) Controls, n = 14,571 (median age 28 years, 61.3 females)	- Poor sleep in CD vs. controls: 12.5% vs. 9.8% (HR = 1.36, 95% CI: 1.30–1.41) - Individuals with CD had a similar increased risk irrespective of age at CD diagnosis, sex and type of hypnotic used	- Overall, poor sleep was more prevalent in females than in males. However, differences in risk estimates for poor sleep were small between females and males with CD - Adjustment for sleep apnea and restless leg syndrome did not influence the risk of poor sleep in CD
Substance-related and addictive disorders				
Roos (2006) [71]	Cross-sectional	CD, n = 51 (age 45–64 years, 59% females) Controls, n = 182 (age 45–64 years, 57% females)	- PGWB index scores: 103 (95% CI: 99–107) in CD vs. 103 (95% CI: 100–106) in controls (p = NS)	- Males with CD tended to score higher on the PGWB domains than the male controls - CD women scored somewhat lower in the PGWB domains than the female controls - CD men tended to score higher than the CD women in all six domains of the PGWB
Gili 2013 [72]	Cross-sectional	CD, n = 3327 (mean age 49 years and 70% females). Controls, n = 5,471,988) (mean age 58 years and 54% females).	- Prevalence of alcohol disorders: 4.9% in CD vs. 6.3% in controls (p = 0.0009)	- The presence of alcohol disorders in CD increased the length of stay, costs and had an excess of mortality
Neurocognitive Disorders				
Lebwohl (2016) [73]	Population-based cohort	CD, n = 8846 (mean age 64 years ard 56% females). Control, n = 43,474 (mean age 64 years and 56% females).	- In a median follow-up period of 8.4 years: 4.3% of CD patients and 4.4% of controls had a diagnosis of dementia (HR 1.07; 95% CI 0.95–1.20) - A subgroup analysis showed an increased risk of vascular dementia (HR 1.28; 95% CI 1.00–1.64)	- A significant association between CD and dementia among the age group 60–69 was found, which was not present in the younger or older age groups - Increased risk of dementia was found in the first year following CD diagnosis
Various psychiatric conditions				
Fera (2003) [74]	Cross-sectional	CD, n = 100 (mean age 40 years, 75% females) DM, n = 100 (mean age 53 years, 74% females) HC, n = 100 (mean age 41 years, 68% females)	- CD, prevalence of OCD 28%, depressive disorder/dysthymia 19% - DM, prevalence of OCD 0%, depressive disorder/dysthymia 10% HC, anxiety and depression in 10% of subjects	- QOL was poorer in both CD and diabetic patients than in healthy controls and significantly correlated with anxiety
Sainsbury (2013) [75]	Study 1: cross-sectional	n = 390 (mean age 44 years, 82.8% females)	- Severe gastrointestinal symptoms at CD diagnosis were associated with: increased depression (r = 0.28, p <0.001), anxiety (r = 0.29, p <0.001), stress (r = 0.28, p <0.001), eating disorder (r = 0.15, p <0.01), and emotion-oriented coping (r = 0.17, p <0.01)	- Poorer QOL was significantly associated with a greater number and longer duration of CD symptoms prior to diagnosis - Higher number of symptoms was associated with poorer QOL - There were no gender differences in QOL, although females reported a greater number of symptoms - More severe gastrointestinal symptoms at diagnosis were also associated with increased psychological manifestations

Table 4. *Cont.*

Various psychiatric conditions

Author (Year)	Design	Sample Size and Demographic Characteristics	Summary of Outcomes	Associated Factors with Psychiatric Comorbidities and other Relevant Information
Sainsbury (2013) [75]	Study 2: cross-sectional	n = 189 (mean age 46.5 years, 87.3% females)	- Hierarchical regression analyses: Current psychological distress significantly contributed to poor QOL (accounting for 23.8% of the variance in QOL).	
Zylberberg (2017) [76]	Population-based cross-sectional	Diagnosed CD, n = 27 (age NR, 78% females) Undiagnosed CD, n = 79 (age NR, 58% females) PWAG; n = 213 (age NR, 55% females) Controls; n = 14,769 (demographic characteristics NR)	- Prevalence of depression: 8.2% of controls vs. 3.9% in CD (p = 0.18) and 2.9% in PWAGs (0.002) - Prevalence of sleep difficulty: 37.3% in CD, 34.1% in PWAGs vs. 27.4% in controls (p = NS) - Multivariate analysis adjusted for race/ethnicity, annual household income, number of healthcare visits: PWAGS, significantly lower odds of depression (OR = 0.25, 95% CI: 0.12–0.5, p = 0.0001) CD, OR = 0.30; 95% CI: 0.08–1.19, p = 0.09	- QOL: The presence of physical, mental, and emotional limitations was reported in 2.9% of controls vs. 13.8% diagnosed CD (p =0.004), 9.6% with undiagnosed CD (p = 0.02), and 5.1% in PWAGs (p = 0.18)

ADHD: Attention-Deficit Hyperactivity Disorder; ASD: Autistic Spectrum Disorders; BES: Binge Eating Scale; CD: celiac disease; CI: confidence interval; CPH: Chronic persistent hepatitis; DASS: Depression Anxiety Stress Scale; DM: Diabetes Mellitus; EAT: Eating Attitudes Test; EPDS: Edinburgh Postnatal Depression Scale; GFD: gluten-free diet; HC: healthy controls; HR: hazard ratio; IBD: Inflammatory Bowel Disease; IBS: Irritable Bowel Disease; MMPI: Minnesota Multiphasic Personality Inventory; M-SDS: Modified Zung Self-Rating Depression Scale; NCGS: non-celiac gluten sensitivity; NR: not reported; NS: not significant; OCD: Obsessive-Compulsive Disorder; OR: odd ratio; PGWB: Psychological General Well-being; PWAG: people who avoid gluten; QOL: quality of life; RR: relative risk; SCL: Symptom Check List; SRDS: Zung Self-Rating Depression Scale; vs: versus.

In two studies conducted by the same research group, the prevalence of state anxiety in patients with CD was substantially higher than in controls (62.5% vs. 31.3%, and 71.4% vs. 23.7%), although the difference was statistically significant in only one study [53,55]. Generalized anxiety disorder diagnosis in CD was not shown to be prevalent in CD compared to controls [57] and the overall prevalence of anxiety was not significantly higher compared to healthy adults in the meta-analysis conducted by Smith et al. [61]. The prevalence of social phobia in CD reached 70% in one cross-sectional study [59]; however, its lifetime prevalence in another study was only 8.3% [57]. Bipolar disorder and panic disorders were significantly more prevalent in patients with CD [57,58,63].

Three studies assessed the prevalence and risk of eating disorders in CD. Their prevalence was significantly higher in adults with CD compared to healthy controls as demonstrated via the elevated scores on the different assessment scales employed in two cross-sectional studies [67,68]. Elevated Eating Attitudes Test scores were seen in around 16% of patients with CD in both studies, whereas elevated Binge Eating Scale scores were only elevated in one study with 19.7% of adults with CD reporting high scores [68]. Moreover, severe gastrointestinal symptoms were linked to greater risk of eating disorders [75]. In the register-based cohort and case-control study conducted by Marild et al. [69], the likelihood of developing anorexia nervosa was significantly higher in women with CD (HR = 1.46, 95% CI: 1.08–1.98) and the likelihood was highest in women with normal mucosa and positive serology (HR = 2.45, 95% CI: 1.1–5.45).

While patients with CD were less likely to experience alcohol-related disorders [72], their risk of developing dementia was significantly higher as shown in a population-based cohort study [70,73]. The likelihood of developing poor sleep in CD based on the use of hypnotics was significantly elevated compared to controls HR = 1.36, 95% CI: 1.3–1.41) in the population-based case-control study conducted by Marild et al. [70]. On the other hand, sleep difficulty as measured with the Patient Health Questionnaire did not differ significantly between adults with CD and controls (37.3% vs. 27.4%, p = 0.15) in a population-based cross-sectional study [76].

While gender did not seem to affect the prevalence rates of ADHD in CD patients [45], males with CD were less likely to experience poor sleep problems [70] or subsequent anorexia nervosa [69] and they tended to score higher on the different Psychological General Well-being Index domains [71]. Conflicting results concerning the effect of the CD onset time on psychological symptomatology were obtained; on one hand, earlier onset of CD symptoms was linked to higher prevalence of major depressive disorder in one study [57] and on the other hand, depressive symptomatology scores did not differentiate between childhood or adulthood diagnosis of CD [54]. Finally, severe gastrointestinal symptomatology significantly correlated with increased psychological manifestations [68,75].

The risk of schizophrenia in patients with CD was assessed in three studies [47–49]. While one population-based case-control study showed no increased risk of schizophrenia in CD (OR = 0.75, 95% CI: 0.4–1.4) [47], its risk was shown to be significantly elevated in a population-based cohort study (Incidence rate ratio = 2.11, 95% CI: 1.1–3.6) and a cross-sectional study (adjusted incidence rate = 3.6, 95% CI: 1.2–10.6) [48,49]. In a meta-analysis including four studies, an increased risk of schizophrenia among patients with CD was found (OR = 2.03, 95% CI: 1.45–2.86) [50]. With respect to autistic spectrum disorders, its risk in a population-based cohort of CD appeared to be increased with the highest risk being present in patients with normal mucosa and positive serologic findings (HR = 3.09, 95% CI: 1.99–4.8) [46].

ADHD was assessed in one cross-sectional study that reported an increased prevalence of this disorder in adults with CD compared to controls (20.7% vs. 10.5%, p <0.01) [45]. The overall psychological status in adults with CD was evaluated in one study whereby no difference in the total Psychological General Well-Being Index was found between CD and controls [71].

In the two studies that evaluated the effects of gluten ingestion in adults with NCGS [62,64], significant worsening of depressive symptomatology [64] and increase in the depression subscale scores of Spielberger State Trait Personality Inventory [62] were reported.

4. Discussion

Our current review of the literature revealed the existence of an association between CD and other gluten-related disorders with psychiatric disorders across different age groups. CD is primarily an autoimmune disorder that is characterized by villous atrophy of the intestinal mucosa along with intraepithelial lymphocytosis and crypt hyperplasia [77]. Nevertheless, a major shift in clinical presentation with extraintestinal manifestations becoming more prevalent than classical gastrointestinal symptoms has been suggested [78]. The reviewed data demonstrate that a wide range of psychiatric disorders have been investigated in CD and NCGS including autism spectrum disorders, schizophrenia, attention-deficit disorder, depression and mood disorders, anxiety disorders, bipolar disorder, feeding and eating disorders, sleep disorders, substance-related and addictive disorders and neurocognitive disorders.

Most of the cross-sectional studies in the pediatric population did not find any significant differences in the point prevalence of depression or anxiety disorders [32,33,35–37], however, these studies had several methodological limitations which mainly included small sample size (ranging between 29 and 42 children with CD), the lack of specialized psychiatric clinical assessment, and the absence of adequate blinding measures to limit assessment bias. On the other hand, two population-based cohort studies including >9000 children each provided evidence for an increased likelihood of occurrence of depression and anxiety disorders in patients with CD [34,44]. In the cohort study conducted by Ludvigsson et al. [34], it was shown that adults and children with CD are at increased risk of being diagnosed with depression but not bipolar disorder later in life (i.e., during adulthood for children diagnosed with CD), whereas in the study conducted by Butwicka et al. [44], CD was identified as a risk factor for mood disorders, anxiety disorders, eating disorders, behavioral disorders, ADHD, ASD, and intellectual disability diagnosed prior to 18 years of age. Although the analyses in the two previous cohort studies were controlled for children's age, stratified analyses to identify the likelihood of occurrence of specific psychiatric disorders across the different age groups are worth evaluation taking into consideration the variation in clinical presentation across the developmental span between 0 and 15 years of age [79].

In adults, the point-prevalence of depression was significantly higher in patients with CD in the majority of published studies. These findings were ascertained by a population-based cohort study in which the HR of depression (in participants ≥16 years at diagnosis) was two folds higher than controls [34] and by a meta-analysis in which depression was shown to be more common and severe in CD than in healthy adults with an overall effect size of 0.97 [61]. A comprehensive review, evaluating the comorbidity of depression and anxiety in CD, concluded that these disorders are common disorders among patients with CD and contribute to a poorer quality of life [24]. Nevertheless, the lack of differences in the prevalence of depression when compared to patients with other physical disorders [61] raises a question about the existence of a specific underlying pathophysiological mechanism in patients with CD or whether depression represents a non-specific disorder affected by physical and psychosocial distress. The association between chronic medical diseases and depression is well-known and many different causes, including both genetic predisposition and environmental factors have been shown to be involved [80–82]. This association is frequently bidirectional, as the presence of physical illness often worsens the affective disorder and vice versa [81]. The current information relative to depression in patients with CD does not allow, at the present time, to ascertain the exact relationship and the predisposing factors involved between CD or NCGS and depressive symptomatology.

The association between CD and eating disorders has been investigated in a limited number of studies. Current findings reveal an elevated prevalence of eating disorders in CD among both children and adults with CD [39,40,44,67–69]. These disorders encompassed anorexia nervosa, bulimia nervosa and binge eating. Poor dietary management can occur as a result of physical dissatisfaction, which is not uncommon in patients with CD [83]. Moreover, evidence from the current literature suggests that young adults with chronic illnesses that require dietary modification are at higher risk of developing pathological eating practices [39]. The elevated lifetime comorbidity between depression and eating disorders [84] could be another explanatory mechanism of increased prevalence of eating disorders in CD patients who are more prone to developing depressive symptomatology.

Concerning psychotic disorders, the current evidence provided by solely two population-based cohort studies does not support the presence of an association between these disorders and CD in children [31,44]. However, children and young adults (≥16 years of age) with CD were 1.8-fold more likely to experience non-schizophrenic non-affective psychosis [31]. The authors of the latter cohort study yet did not rule out the presence of a potential association between CD and schizophrenia as the risk of the latter disorder was high despite the low number of individuals with schizophrenia. These findings were similar to another population-based case-control study conducted in adults in which no evidence of an increased risk of schizophrenia in CD was found [47]. In contrast, Benros et al. [49] demonstrated an increased incidence of schizophrenia in patients with prior CD in their population-based cohort study. Furthermore, Eaton et al. [48] showed also 3.8-fold increase in incidence rates of prior CD diagnosis in subjects with schizophrenia. However, in the latter study, data on parents' celiac status were also included in their analysis which might have led to biased findings. A meta-analysis including four studies demonstrated the presence of an increased risk of schizophrenia among patients with CD [50]. We believe that the pooled-effect estimate in the previous meta-analysis could be biased because their pooled analysis on one hand missed the negative findings reported by West et al. [47] and on the other hand included the findings of a study in which the prevalence of CD in patients with schizophrenia was investigated [85]. The objectives and outcome measures of the latter study [85] did not match the principal objective of the meta-analysis whereby the authors investigated the prevalence of autoimmune diseases (including CD) in patients with schizophrenia and not the other way around [85]. The association between CD and gluten-related disorders with schizophrenia has been under investigation for more than five decades but most studies evaluated the prevalence or risk of gluten-related disorders in patients already diagnosed with schizophrenia [86]. Current evidence suggests a two-fold increase in the prevalence of CD in schizophrenia patients [87] and an association between gluten ingestion and exacerbation of schizophrenia symptoms [88]; nonetheless, these findings are highly inconsistent across different clinical, immunological, and epidemiological studies [86] and have not been replicated in patients presenting with CD.

The underlying mechanisms behind the association between CD and psychiatric disorders are not well-known. Nevertheless, several potential biological and psychosocial explanations have been suggested: (i) Several psychiatric disorders such as depression, anxiety, and ADHD, among others have been linked to certain nutritional and vitamin deficiencies [89] and it is well-known that patients with CD often suffer from malnutrition prior to diagnosis or as a result of dietary non-compliance [90]; (ii) The immune-mediated processes underlying CD have been postulated as potential causative factors of the different psychiatric manifestations taking into consideration the involvement of chronic immune system activation in the etiology of various psychiatric conditions [91]; (iii) The bidirectional communication between the gastrointestinal tract [92] and the brain may suggest that alterations in the intestinal permeability, which is cardinal manifestation in CD [93], could be eventually involved in the pathophysiology of psychiatric manifestations in patients with CD; (iv) Finally, psychosocial aspects commonly seen in CD could place this population at an increased risk of developing psychiatric disorders, for instance, the introduction of GFD is associated with radical changes in daily life activities, eating habits and lifestyle which could be particularly stressful and difficult to accept [43,94]. In addition, effective adherence to GFD entails greater burden manifested via increased daily expenditure on more expensive products, social isolation and constant fear about dietary mistakes [95].

The studies included in this review provided limited data on potential factors associated with psychiatric comorbidity in patients with CD. Bearing in mind this limitation, none of the demographic factors has been consistently associated with the presence or occurrence of psychiatric comorbidities and the role of ethnicity in this context has not been studied. Regarding clinical factors, only severity of CD symptoms appears to be associated with the presence and/or severity of psychiatric disorders [33,51,52,68,75]. In this regard, the significant positive association between increased severity of gastrointestinal symptoms and worsening of psychiatric manifestations [75] and QOL [63] in CD indirectly demonstrates the importance of adherence to GFD. Nevertheless, few studies have documented the beneficial effects of GFD on psychiatric manifestations in patients with CD [27,66], with the majority of these studies suffering from several methodological flaws limiting our capacity of reaching definitive conclusions supporting the role of GFD in this context.

Only two studies in patients with NCGS supported the association between this relatively new entity and depressive symptomology [62,64]. It has not been until recently that standardized diagnostic criteria for NCGS were established [19], which might explain the limited number of studies investigating psychiatric comorbidities in NCGS. In our current review search, we could not find any study that investigated psychiatric comorbidities in patients with WA.

Limitations of our current review are essentially derived from the limited quality of the majority of the studies that have investigated psychiatric disorders in CD. Most of these studies are of cross-sectional design which does not allow establishing causal relationships and are of small sample size, whereas very few population-based studies have been published.

Evaluating psychiatric comorbidities in different age groups adds strength to our current review since up to the current date, none of the previous reviews had evaluated the evidence of psychiatric disorders in children and adults with CD separately. Interestingly, according to our review, the presence of CD in childhood seems to be associated with an increased risk of developing psychiatric disorders later during adulthood, but not with an increased prevalence of these disorders during childhood.

5. Conclusions

Our current comprehensive review ascertains the presence of an association between CD and psychiatric disorders with varying grades of evidence from one condition to another. In our view, there is enough evidence supporting an association of CD with depression and, to a lesser extent, with eating disorders. Some studies also point out to an association between CD and panic disorder, autism and ADHD, but the evidence is limited, and these potential associations should be further investigated. Finally, the data regarding the association of CD with schizophrenia or other anxiety disorders is conflicting. Overall, psychiatric symptomatology which could be perceived as part of the atypical manifestations of this chronic condition are linked to significant distortion in quality of life and moderately increased risk of suicide [96] and thus warrants further attention. Therefore, gastroenterologists and other healthcare professionals involved in the management of patients with CD should be aware of the increased risk of psychiatric disorders in these patients. Thus, routine surveillance of potential psychiatric manifestations, especially anxiety and/or depressive symptomatology that seem to be the most common forms of disturbances, should be carried out by the attending physician in order to refer the patient to the mental health services if necessary.

Supplementary Materials: The supplementary materials are available at: http://www.mdpi.com/2072-6643/10/7/875/s1. Table S1: Database specific search strategies.

Author Contributions: Conceptualization, E.P.C; Methodology, M.S., F.R.-V. and E.P.C.; Data extraction, F.R.-V. and M.S.; Writing—Original Draft Preparation, M.S., F.R.-V. and E.P.C.; Writing—Review and Editing, M.S., F.R.-V. and E.P.C.

Funding: This research received no external funding.

Conflicts of Interest: The authors declare no conflict of interest.

References

1. Sapone, A.; Bai, J.C.; Ciacci, C.; Dolinsek, J.; Green, P.H.; Hadjivassiliou, M.; Kaukinen, K.; Rostami, K.; Sanders, D.S.; Schumann, M.; et al. Spectrum of gluten-related disorders: Consensus on new nomenclature and classification. *BMC Med.* **2012**, *10*, 13. [CrossRef] [PubMed]

2. Guandalini, S.; Assiri, A. Celiac disease: A review. *JAMA Pediatr.* **2014**, *168*, 272–278. [CrossRef] [PubMed]

3. Green, P.H.; Lebwohl, B.; Greywoode, R. Celiac disease. *J. Allergy Clin. Immunol.* **2015**, *135*, 1099–1106, quiz 1107. [CrossRef] [PubMed]

4. Ludvigsson, J.F.; Bai, J.C.; Biagi, F.; Card, T.R.; Ciacci, C.; Ciclitira, P.J.; Green, P.H.; Hadjivassiliou, M.; Holdoway, A.; van Heel, D.A.; et al. Diagnosis and management of adult coeliac disease: Guidelines from the british society of gastroenterology. *Gut* **2014**, *63*, 1210–1228. [CrossRef] [PubMed]

5. Uibo, R.; Tian, Z.; Gershwin, M.E. Celiac disease: A model disease for gene-environment interaction. *Cell. Mol. Immunol.* **2011**, *8*, 93–95. [CrossRef] [PubMed]

6. Szajewska, H.; Shamir, R.; Chmielewska, A.; Piescik-Lech, M.; Auricchio, R.; Ivarsson, A.; Kolacek, S.; Koletzko, S.; Korponay-Szabo, I.; Mearin, M.L.; et al. Systematic review with meta-analysis: Early infant feeding and coeliac disease—Update 2015. *Aliment. Pharmacol. Ther.* **2015**, *41*, 1038–1054. [CrossRef] [PubMed]

7. Canova, C.; Zabeo, V.; Pitter, G.; Romor, P.; Baldovin, T.; Zanotti, R.; Simonato, L. Association of maternal education, early infections, and antibiotic use with celiac disease: A population-based birth cohort study in northeastern italy. *Am. J. Epidemiol.* **2014**, *180*, 76–85. [CrossRef] [PubMed]

8. Olivares, M.; Neef, A.; Castillejo, G.; Palma, G.D.; Varea, V.; Capilla, A.; Palau, F.; Nova, E.; Marcos, A.; Polanco, I.; et al. The hla-dq2 genotype selects for early intestinal microbiota composition in infants at high risk of developing coeliac disease. *Gut* **2015**, *64*, 406–417. [CrossRef] [PubMed]

9. Catassi, C.; Gatti, S.; Lionetti, E. World perspective and celiac disease epidemiology. *Dig. Dis.* **2015**, *33*, 141–146. [CrossRef] [PubMed]

10. Singh, P.; Arora, A.; Strand, T.A.; Leffler, D.A.; Catassi, C.; Green, P.H.; Kelly, C.P.; Ahuja, V.; Makharia, G.K. Global prevalence of celiac disease: Systematic review and meta-analysis. *Clin. Gastroenterol. Hepatol.* **2018**, *16*, 823–836.e2. [CrossRef] [PubMed]

11. Lauret, E.; Rodrigo, L. Celiac disease and autoimmune-associated conditions. *BioMed Res. Int.* **2013**, *2013*, 127589. [CrossRef] [PubMed]

12. Assa, A.; Frenkel-Nir, Y.; Tzur, D.; Katz, L.H.; Shamir, R. Large population study shows that adolescents with celiac disease have an increased risk of multiple autoimmune and nonautoimmune comorbidities. *Acta Paediatr.* **2017**, *106*, 967–972. [CrossRef] [PubMed]

13. Viljamaa, M.; Kaukinen, K.; Pukkala, E.; Hervonen, K.; Reunala, T.; Collin, P. Malignancies and mortality in patients with coeliac disease and dermatitis herpetiformis: 30-year population-based study. *Dig. Liver Dis.* **2006**, *38*, 374–380. [CrossRef] [PubMed]

14. Ilus, T.; Kaukinen, K.; Virta, L.J.; Pukkala, E.; Collin, P. Incidence of malignancies in diagnosed celiac patients: A population-based estimate. *Am. J. Gastroenterol.* **2014**, *109*, 1471–1477. [CrossRef] [PubMed]

15. Bai, J.C.; Fried, M.; Corazza, G.R.; Schuppan, D.; Farthing, M.; Catassi, C.; Greco, L.; Cohen, H.; Ciacci, C.; Eliakim, R.; et al. World gastroenterology organisation global guidelines on celiac disease. *J. Clin. Gastroenterol.* **2013**, *47*, 121–126. [CrossRef] [PubMed]

16. Pavlovic, M.; Berenji, K.; Bukurov, M. Screening of celiac disease in down syndrome—Old and new dilemmas. *World J. Clin. Cases* **2017**, *5*, 264–269. [CrossRef] [PubMed]

17. Jenkins, H.R.; Murch, S.H.; Beattie, R.M.; Coeliac Disease Working Group of British Society of Paediatric Gastroenterology, Hepatology and Nutrition. Diagnosing coeliac disease. *Arch. Dis. Child.* **2012**, *97*, 393–394. [CrossRef] [PubMed]

18. Elli, L.; Branchi, F.; Tomba, C.; Villalta, D.; Norsa, L.; Ferretti, F.; Roncoroni, L.; Bardella, M.T. Diagnosis of gluten related disorders: Celiac disease, wheat allergy and non-celiac gluten sensitivity. *World J. Gastroenterol.* **2015**, *21*, 7110–7119. [CrossRef] [PubMed]

19. Catassi, C.; Elli, L.; Bonaz, B.; Bouma, G.; Carroccio, A.; Castillejo, G.; Cellier, C.; Cristofori, F.; de Magistris, L.; Dolinsek, J.; et al. Diagnosis of non-celiac gluten sensitivity (ncgs): The salerno experts' criteria. *Nutrients* **2015**, *7*, 4966–4977. [CrossRef] [PubMed]

20. Nijeboer, P.; Bontkes, H.J.; Mulder, C.J.; Bouma, G. Non-celiac gluten sensitivity. Is it in the gluten or the grain? *J. Gastrointest. Liver Dis.* **2013**, *22*, 435–440.

21. Cianferoni, A. Wheat allergy: Diagnosis and management. *J. Asthma Allergy* **2016**, *9*, 13–25. [CrossRef] [PubMed]

22. Pietzak, M. Celiac disease, wheat allergy, and gluten sensitivity: When gluten free is not a fad. *JPEN J. Parenter. Enter. Nutr.* **2012**, *36*, 68s–75s. [CrossRef] [PubMed]

23. Jackson, J.R.; Eaton, W.W.; Cascella, N.G.; Fasano, A.; Kelly, D.L. Neurologic and psychiatric manifestations of celiac disease and gluten sensitivity. *Psychiatr. Q.* **2012**, *83*, 91–102. [CrossRef] [PubMed]

24. Zingone, F.; Swift, G.L.; Card, T.R.; Sanders, D.S.; Ludvigsson, J.F.; Bai, J.C. Psychological morbidity of celiac disease: A review of the literature. *United Eur. Gastroenterol. J.* **2015**, *3*, 136–145. [CrossRef] [PubMed]

25. Porcelli, B.; Verdino, V.; Bossini, L.; Terzuoli, L.; Fagiolini, A. Celiac and non-celiac gluten sensitivity: A review on the association with schizophrenia and mood disorders. *Auto Immun. Highlights* **2014**, *5*, 55–61. [CrossRef] [PubMed]

26. Cossu, G.; Carta, M.G.; Contu, F.; Mela, Q.; Demelia, L.; Elli, L.; Dell'Osso, B. Coeliac disease and psychiatric comorbidity: Epidemiology, pathophysiological mechanisms, quality-of-life, and gluten-free diet effects. *Int. Rev. Psychiatry* **2017**, *29*, 489–503. [CrossRef] [PubMed]

27. Brietzke, E.; Cerqueira, R.O.; Mansur, R.B.; McIntyre, R.S. Gluten related illnesses and severe mental disorders: A comprehensive review. *Neurosci. Biobehav. Rev.* **2018**, *84*, 368–375. [CrossRef] [PubMed]

28. Da Silva Kotze, L.M.; David Paiva, A.D.; Roberto Kotze, L. Emotional disturbances in children and adolescents with celiac disease. *Rev. Bras. Med. Psicossom.* **2000**, *4*, 9–15.

29. Horvath-Stolarczyk, A.; Sidor, K.; Dziechciarz, P.; Siemińska, J. Assessment of emotional status, selected personality traits and depression in young adults with celiac disease. *Pediatr. Wspolcz.* **2002**, *4*, 241–246.

30. Pavone, L.; Fiumara, A.; Bottaro, G.; Mazzone, D.; Coleman, M. Autism and celiac disease: Failure to validate the hypothesis that a link might exist. *Biol. Psychiatry* **1997**, *42*, 72–75. [CrossRef]

31. Ludvigsson, J.F.; Osby, U.; Ekbom, A.; Montgomery, S.M. Coeliac disease and risk of schizophrenia and other psychosis: A general population cohort study. *Scand. J. Gastroenterol.* **2007**, *42*, 179–185. [CrossRef] [PubMed]

32. Pynnönen, P.A.; Isometsä, E.T.; Aronen, E.T.; Verkasalo, M.A.; Savilahti, E.; Aalberg, V.A. Mental disorders in adolescents with celiac disease. *Psychosomatics* **2004**, *45*, 325–335. [CrossRef] [PubMed]

33. Accomando, S.; Fragapane, M.L.; Montaperto, D.; Trizzino, A.; Amato, G.M.; Calderone, F.; Accomando, I. Coeliac disease and depression: Two related entities? *Dig. Liver Dis.* **2005**, *37*, 298–299. [CrossRef] [PubMed]

34. Ludvigsson, J.F.; Reutfors, J.; Osby, U.; Ekbom, A.; Montgomery, S.M. Coeliac disease and risk of mood disorders—A general population-based cohort study. *J. Affect. Disord.* **2007**, *99*, 117–126. [CrossRef] [PubMed]

35. Fidan, T.; Ertekin, V.; Karabag, K. Depression-anxiety levels and the quality of life among children and adolescents with coeliac disease. *Dusunen Adam* **2013**, *26*, 232–238. [CrossRef]

36. Esenyel, S.; Unal, F.; Vural, P. Depression and anxiety in child and adolescents with follow-up celiac disease and in their families. *Turk. J. Gastroenterol.* **2014**, *25*, 381–385. [CrossRef] [PubMed]

37. Simsek, S.; Baysoy, G.; Gencoglan, S.; Uluca, U. Effects of gluten-free diet on quality of life and depression in children with celiac disease. *J. Pediatr. Gastroenterol. Nutr.* **2015**, *61*, 303–306. [CrossRef] [PubMed]

38. Smith, L.B.; Lynch, K.F.; Kurppa, K.; Koletzko, S.; Krischer, J.; Liu, E.; Johnson, S.B.; Agardh, D.; Rewers, M.; Bautista, K.; et al. Psychological manifestations of celiac disease autoimmunity in young children. *Pediatrics* **2017**, *139*, e20162848. [CrossRef] [PubMed]

39. Wagner, G.; Zeiler, M.; Berger, G.; Huber, W.D.; Favaro, A.; Santonastaso, P.; Karwautz, A. Eating disorders in adolescents with celiac disease: Influence of personality characteristics and coping. *Eur. Eat. Disord. Rev.* **2015**, *23*, 361–370. [CrossRef] [PubMed]

40. Babio, N.; Alcázar, M.; Castillejo, G.; Recasens, M.; Martínez-Cerezo, F.; Gutiérrez-Pensado, V.; Vaqué, C.; Vila-Martí, A.; Torres-Moreno, M.; Sánchez, E.; et al. Risk of eating disorders in patients with celiac disease. *J. Pediatr. Gastroenterol. Nutr.* **2018**, *66*, 53–57. [CrossRef] [PubMed]

41. Terrone, G.; Parente, I.; Romano, A.; Auricchio, R.; Greco, L.; Del Giudice, E. The pediatric symptom checklist as screening tool for neurological and psychosocial problems in a paediatric cohort of patients with coeliac disease. *Acta Paediatr. Int. J. Paediatr.* **2013**, *102*, e325–e328. [CrossRef] [PubMed]

42. Ruggieri, M.; Incorpora, G.; Polizzi, A.; Parano, E.; Spina, M.; Pavone, P. Low prevalence of neurologic and psychiatric manifestations in children with gluten sensitivity. *J. Pediatr.* **2008**, *152*, 244–249. [CrossRef] [PubMed]

43. Mazzone, L.; Reale, L.; Spina, M.; Guarnera, M.; Lionetti, E.; Martorana, S.; Mazzone, D. Compliant gluten-free children with celiac disease: An evaluation of psychological distress. *BMC Pediatr.* **2011**, *11*, 46. [CrossRef] [PubMed]

44. Butwicka, A.; Lichtenstein, P.; Frisen, L.; Almqvist, C.; Larsson, H.; Ludvigsson, J.F. Celiac disease is associated with childhood psychiatric disorders: A population-based study. *J. Pediatr.* **2017**, *184*, 87–93.e81. [CrossRef] [PubMed]

45. Zelnik, N.; Pacht, A.; Obeid, R.; Lerner, A. Range of neurologic disorders in patients with celiac disease. *Pediatrics* **2004**, *113*, 1672–1676. [CrossRef] [PubMed]

46. Ludvigsson, J.F.; Reichenberg, A.; Hultman, C.M.; Murray, J.A. A nationwide study of the association between celiac disease and the risk of autistic spectrum disorders. *JAMA Psychiatry* **2013**, *70*, 1224–1230. [CrossRef] [PubMed]

47. West, J.; Logan, R.F.; Hubbard, R.B.; Card, T.R. Risk of schizophrenia in people with coeliac disease, ulcerative colitis and crohn's disease: A general population-based study. *Aliment. Pharmacol. Ther.* **2006**, *23*, 71–74. [CrossRef] [PubMed]

48. Eaton, W.W.; Byrne, M.; Ewald, H.; Mors, O.; Chen, C.Y.; Agerbo, E.; Mortensen, P.B. Association of schizophrenia and autoimmune diseases: Linkage of danish national registers. *Am. J. Psychiatry* **2006**, *163*, 521–528. [CrossRef] [PubMed]

49. Benros, M.E.; Nielsen, P.R.; Nordentoft, M.; Eaton, W.W.; Dalton, S.O.; Mortensen, P.B. Autoimmune diseases and severe infections as risk factors for schizophrenia: A 30-year population-based register study. *Am. J. Psychiatry* **2011**, *168*, 1303–1310. [CrossRef] [PubMed]

50. Wijarnpreecha, K.; Jaruvongvanich, V.; Cheungpasitporn, W.; Ungprasert, P. Association between celiac disease and schizophrenia: A meta-analysis. *Eur. J. Gastroenterol. Hepatol.* **2018**, *30*, 442–446. [CrossRef] [PubMed]

51. Hallert, C.; Aström, J. Psychic disturbances in adult coeliac disease. II. Psychological findings. *Scand. J. Gastroenterol.* **1982**, *17*, 21–24. [CrossRef] [PubMed]

52. Hallert, C.; Aström, J.; Walan, A. Reversal of psychopathology in adult coeliac disease with the aid of pyridoxine (vitamin b6). *Scand. J. Gastroenterol.* **1983**, *18*, 299–304. [CrossRef] [PubMed]

53. Addolorato, G.; Stefanini, G.F.; Capristo, E.; Caputo, F.; Gasbarrini, A.; Gasbarrini, G. Anxiety and depression in adult untreated celiac subjects and in patients affected by inflammatory bowel disease: A personality "trait" or a reactive illness? *Hepato-Gastroenterology* **1996**, *43*, 1513–1517. [PubMed]

54. Ciacci, C.; Iavarone, A.; Mazzacca, G.; De Rosa, A. Depressive symptoms in adult coeliac disease. *Scand. J. Gastroenterol.* **1998**, *33*, 247–250. [CrossRef] [PubMed]

55. Addolorato, G.; Capristo, E.; Ghittoni, G.; Valeri, C.; Masciana, R.; Ancona, C.; Gasbarrini, G. Anxiety but not depression decreases in coeliac patients after one-year gluten-free diet: A longitudinal study. *Scand. J. Gastroenterol.* **2001**, *36*, 502–506. [CrossRef] [PubMed]

56. Cicarelli, G.; Della Rocca, G.; Amboni, M.; Ciacci, C.; Mazzacca, G.; Filla, A.; Barone, P. Clinical and neurological abnormalities in adult celiac disease. *Neurol. Sci.* **2003**, *24*, 311–317. [CrossRef] [PubMed]

57. Carta, M.G.; Hardoy, M.C.; Boi, M.F.; Mariotti, S.; Carpiniello, B.; Usai, P. Association between panic disorder, major depressive disorder and celiac disease: A possible role of thyroid autoimmunity. *J. Psychosom. Res.* **2002**, *53*, 789–793. [CrossRef]

58. Carta, M.G.; Hardoy, M.C.; Usai, P.; Carpiniello, B.; Angst, J. Recurrent brief depression in celiac disease. *J. Psychosom. Res.* **2003**, *55*, 573–574. [CrossRef]

59. Addolorato, G.; Mirijello, A.; D'Angelo, C.; Leggio, L.; Ferrulli, A.; Vonghia, L.; Cardone, S.; Leso, V.; Miceli, A.; Gasbarrini, G. Social phobia in coeliac disease. *Scand. J. Gastroenterol.* **2008**, *43*, 410–415. [CrossRef] [PubMed]

60. Garud, S.; Leffler, D.; Dennis, M.; Edwards-George, J.; Saryan, D.; Sheth, S.; Schuppan, D.; Jamma, S.; Kelly, C.P. Interaction between psychiatric and autoimmune disorders in coeliac disease patients in the northeastern united states. *Aliment. Pharmacol. Ther.* **2009**, *29*, 898–905. [CrossRef] [PubMed]

61. Smith, D.F.; Gerdes, L.U. Meta-analysis on anxiety and depression in adult celiac disease. *Acta Psychiatr. Scand.* **2012**, *125*, 189–193. [CrossRef] [PubMed]

62. Peters, S.L.; Biesiekierski, J.R.; Yelland, G.W.; Muir, J.G.; Gibson, P.R. Randomised clinical trial: Gluten may cause depression in subjects with non-coeliac gluten sensitivity—An exploratory clinical study. *Aliment. Pharmacol. Ther.* **2014**, *39*, 1104–1112. [CrossRef] [PubMed]

63. Carta, M.G.; Conti, A.; Lecca, F.; Sancassiani, F.; Cossu, G.; Carruxi, R.; Boccone, A.; Cadoni, M.; Pisanu, A.; Moro, M.F.; et al. The burden of depressive and bipolar disorders in celiac disease. *Clin. Pract. Epidemiol. Ment. Health* **2015**, *11*, 180–185. [CrossRef] [PubMed]

64. Di Sabatino, A.; Volta, U.; Salvatore, C.; Biancheri, P.; Caio, G.; De Giorgio, R.; Di Stefano, M.; Corazza, G.R. Small amounts of gluten in subjects with suspected nonceliac gluten sensitivity: A randomized, double-blind, placebo-controlled, cross-over trial. *Clin. Gastroenterol. Hepatol.* **2015**, *13*, 1604–1612.e1603. [CrossRef] [PubMed]

65. Tortora, R.; Imperatore, N.; Ciacci, C.; Zingone, F.; Capone, P.; Leo, M.; Pellegrini, L.; De Stefano, G.; Caporaso, N.; Rispo, A. High prevalence of post-partum depression in coeliac women. *Dig. Liver Dis.* **2013**, *45*, S120. [CrossRef]

66. Sainsbury, K.; Marques, M.M. The relationship between gluten free diet adherence and depressive symptoms in adults with coeliac disease: A systematic review with meta-analysis. *Appetite* **2018**, *120*, 578–588. [CrossRef] [PubMed]

67. Passananti, V.; Siniscalchi, M.; Zingone, F.; Bucci, C.; Tortora, R.; Iovino, P.; Ciacci, C. Prevalence of eating disorders in adults with celiac disease. *Gastroenterol. Res. Pract.* **2013**, *2013*, 491657. [CrossRef] [PubMed]

68. Satherley, R.M.; Howard, R.; Higgs, S. The prevalence and predictors of disordered eating in women with coeliac disease. *Appetite* **2016**, *107*, 260–267. [CrossRef] [PubMed]

69. Marild, K.; Størdal, K.; Bulik, C.M.; Rewers, M.; Ekbom, A.; Liu, E.; Ludvigsson, J.F. Celiac disease and anorexia nervosa: A nationwide study. *Pediatrics* **2017**, *139*, e20164367. [CrossRef] [PubMed]

70. Marild, K.; Morgenthaler, T.I.; Somers, V.K.; Kotagal, S.; Murray, J.A.; Ludvigsson, J.F. Increased use of hypnotics in individuals with celiac disease: A nationwide case-control study. *BMC Gastroenterol.* **2015**, *15*, 10. [CrossRef] [PubMed]

71. Roos, S.; Karner, A.; Hallert, C. Psychological well-being of adult coeliac patients treated for 10 years. *Dig. Liver Dis.* **2006**, *38*, 177–180. [CrossRef] [PubMed]

72. Gili, M.; Béjar, L.; Ramirez, G.; Lopez, J.; Cabanillas, J.L.; Sharp, B. Celiac disease and alcohol use disorders: Increased length of hospital stay, overexpenditures and attributable mortality. *Rev. Esp. Enferm. Dig.* **2013**, *105*, 537–543. [CrossRef] [PubMed]

73. Lebwohl, B.; Luchsinger, J.A.; Freedberg, D.E.; Green, P.H.; Ludvigsson, J.F. Risk of dementia in patients with celiac disease: A population-based cohort study. *J. Alzheimer's Dis.* **2016**, *49*, 179–185. [CrossRef] [PubMed]

74. Fera, T.; Cascio, B.; Angelini, G.; Martini, S.; Guidetti, C.S. Affective disorders and quality of life in adult coeliac disease patients on a gluten-free diet. *Eur. J. Gastroenterol. Hepatol.* **2003**, *15*, 1287–1292. [CrossRef] [PubMed]

75. Sainsbury, K.; Mullan, B.; Sharpe, L. Reduced quality of life in coeliac disease is more strongly associated with depression than gastrointestinal symptoms. *J. Psychosom. Res.* **2013**, *75*, 135–141. [CrossRef] [PubMed]

76. Zylberberg, H.M.; Demmer, R.T.; Murray, J.A.; Green, P.H.R.; Lebwohl, B. Depression and insomnia among individuals with celiac disease or on a gluten-free diet in the United States: Results from the national health and nutrition examination survey (nhanes) 2009–2014. *Gastroenterology* **2017**, *152*, S482–S483. [CrossRef]

77. Dickson, B.C.; Streutker, C.J.; Chetty, R. Coeliac disease: An update for pathologists. *J. Clin. Pathol.* **2006**, *59*, 1008–1016. [CrossRef] [PubMed]

78. Leffler, D.A.; Green, P.H.; Fasano, A. Extraintestinal manifestations of coeliac disease. *Nat. Rev. Gastroenterol. Hepatol.* **2015**, *12*, 561–571. [CrossRef] [PubMed]

79. Scott, J.G.; Mihalopoulos, C.; Erskine, H.E.; Roberts, J.; Rahman, A. Childhood mental and developmental disorders. In *Mental, Neurological, and Substance Use Disorders: Disease Control Priorities*, 3rd ed.; Patel, V., Chisholm, D., Dua, T., Laxminarayan, R., Medina-Mora, M.E., Eds.; The World Bank: Washington, DC, USA, 2016; Volume 4.

80. Egede, L.E. Major depression in individuals with chronic medical disorders: Prevalence, correlates and association with health resource utilization, lost productivity and functional disability. *Gen. Hosp. Psychiatry* **2007**, *29*, 409–416. [CrossRef] [PubMed]

81. Katon, W.J. Epidemiology and treatment of depression in patients with chronic medical illness. *Dialog. Clin. Neurosci.* **2011**, *13*, 7–23.

82. Kang, H.J.; Kim, S.Y.; Bae, K.Y.; Kim, S.W.; Shin, I.S.; Yoon, J.S.; Kim, J.M. Comorbidity of depression with physical disorders: Research and clinical implications. *Chonnam Med. J.* **2015**, *51*, 8–18. [CrossRef] [PubMed]

83. Karwautz, A.; Wagner, G.; Berger, G.; Sinnreich, U.; Grylli, V.; Huber, W.D. Eating pathology in adolescents with celiac disease. *Psychosomatics* **2008**, *49*, 399–406. [CrossRef] [PubMed]

84. Hudson, J.I.; Hiripi, E.; Pope, H.G., Jr.; Kessler, R.C. The prevalence and correlates of eating disorders in the national comorbidity survey replication. *Biol. Psychiatry* **2007**, *61*, 348–358. [CrossRef] [PubMed]

85. Chen, S.J.; Chao, Y.L.; Chen, C.Y.; Chang, C.M.; Wu, E.C.; Wu, C.S.; Yeh, H.H.; Chen, C.H.; Tsai, H.J. Prevalence of autoimmune diseases in in-patients with schizophrenia: Nationwide population-based study. *Br. J. Psychiatry* **2012**, *200*, 374–380. [CrossRef] [PubMed]

86. Ergun, C.; Urhan, M.; Ayer, A. A review on the relationship between gluten and schizophrenia: Is gluten the cause? *Nutr. Neurosci.* **2017**. [CrossRef] [PubMed]

87. Cascella, N.G.; Kryszak, D.; Bhatti, B.; Gregory, P.; Kelly, D.L.; Mc Evoy, J.P.; Fasano, A.; Eaton, W.W. Prevalence of celiac disease and gluten sensitivity in the united states clinical antipsychotic trials of intervention effectiveness study population. *Schizophr. Bull.* **2011**, *37*, 94–100. [CrossRef] [PubMed]

88. Kalaydjian, A.E.; Eaton, W.; Cascella, N.; Fasano, A. The gluten connection: The association between schizophrenia and celiac disease. *Acta Psychiatr. Scand.* **2006**, *113*, 82–90. [CrossRef] [PubMed]

89. Kaplan, B.J.; Crawford, S.G.; Field, C.J.; Simpson, J.S. Vitamins, minerals, and mood. *Psychol. Bull.* **2007**, *133*, 747–760. [CrossRef] [PubMed]

90. Wierdsma, N.J.; van Bokhorst-de van der Schueren, M.A.; Berkenpas, M.; Mulder, C.J.; van Bodegraven, A.A. Vitamin and mineral deficiencies are highly prevalent in newly diagnosed celiac disease patients. *Nutrients* **2013**, *5*, 3975–3992. [CrossRef] [PubMed]

91. Najjar, S.; Pearlman, D.M.; Alper, K.; Najjar, A.; Devinsky, O. Neuroinflammation and psychiatric illness. *J. Neuroinflam.* **2013**, *10*, 43. [CrossRef] [PubMed]

92. Grenham, S.; Clarke, G.; Cryan, J.F.; Dinan, T.G. Brain-gut-microbe communication in health and disease. *Front. Physiol.* **2011**, *2*, 94. [CrossRef] [PubMed]

93. Heyman, M.; Abed, J.; Lebreton, C.; Cerf-Bensussan, N. Intestinal permeability in coeliac disease: Insight into mechanisms and relevance to pathogenesis. *Gut* **2012**, *61*, 1355–1364. [CrossRef] [PubMed]

94. Leffler, D.A.; Edwards-George, J.; Dennis, M.; Schuppan, D.; Cook, F.; Franko, D.L.; Blom-Hoffman, J.; Kelly, C.P. Factors that influence adherence to a gluten-free diet in adults with celiac disease. *Dig. Dis. Sci.* **2008**, *53*, 1573–1581. [CrossRef] [PubMed]

95. Lebwohl, B.; Ludvigsson, J.F.; Green, P.H. Celiac disease and non-celiac gluten sensitivity. *BMJ* **2015**, *351*, h4347. [CrossRef] [PubMed]

96. Ludvigsson, J.F.; Sellgren, C.; Runeson, B.; Langstrom, N.; Lichtenstein, P. Increased suicide risk in coeliac disease—A Swedish nationwide cohort study. *Dig. Liver Dis.* **2011**, *43*, 616–622. [CrossRef] [PubMed]

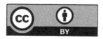

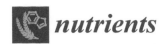

Review

Celiac Disease and Liver Disorders: From Putative Pathogenesis to Clinical Implications

Iva Hoffmanová [1,2,*], Daniel Sánchez [3], Ludmila Tučková [3] and Helena Tlaskalová-Hogenová [3]

1   Centre for Research on Nutrition, Metabolism and Diabetes, Third Faculty of Medicine, Charles University, Ruska 87, 100 00 Prague, Czech Republic
2   Second Department of Internal Medicine, Third Faculty of Medicine, Charles University, Ruska 87, 100 00 Prague, Czech Republic
3   Laboratory of Cellular and Molecular Immunology, Institute of Microbiology of the Czech Academy of Sciences, v.v.i., Videnska 1083, 142 20 Prague, Czech Republic; sanchez@biomed.cas.cz (D.S.); ltuckova@gmail.com (L.T.); tlaskalo@biomed.cas.cz (H.T.-H.)
*   Correspondence: iva.hoffmanova@fnkv.cz; Tel.: +420-723-705-493

Received: 24 May 2018; Accepted: 10 July 2018; Published: 12 July 2018

Abstract: Immunologically mediated liver diseases belong to the common extraintestinal manifestations of celiac disease. We have reviewed the current literature that addresses the association between celiac disease and liver disorders. We searched relevant articles on MEDLINE/PubMed up to 15 June 2018. The objective of the article is to provide a comprehensive and up-to-date review on the latest hypotheses explaining the pathogenetic relationship between celiac disease and liver injury. Besides the involvement of gut–liver axis, tissue transglutaminase antibodies, and impairment of intestinal barrier, we integrate the latest achievements made in elucidation of the role of gut microbiota in celiac disease and liver disorders, that has not yet been sufficiently discussed in the literature in this context. The further objective is to provide a complete clinical overview on the types of liver diseases frequently found in celiac disease. In conclusion, the review highlights the clinical implication, recommend a rational approach for managing elevated transaminases in celiac patients, and underscore the importance of screening for celiac disease in patients with associated liver disease.

Keywords: autoimmunity; celiac hepatitis; gut–liver axis; liver immunity; non-alcoholic fatty liver disease; tolerance; intestinal barrier

---

1. Introduction

The liver is an organ playing a regulatory role in innate and adaptive immunity. Constituents in portal blood circulating from the intestine to the liver, such as food antigens (including peptides derived from gluten and related cereals), bacterial components and products, can under specific conditions (e.g., impaired intestinal barrier and/or dysregulation of gut–liver axis) trigger the hepatic immune response, which is connected to liver inflammation and fibrosis.

During the past four decades a vast number of papers documented the clinical relationship between celiac disease and liver disorders. Although immunologically mediated liver diseases are the most common extraintestinal manifestations of celiac disease [1–8], there are still many scientific and clinical question to be answered.

This narrative review attempts to summarize the current status of knowledge regarding (1) the pathogenetic relationship between celiac disease and liver injury, (2) the types of liver diseases frequently found in celiac disease, (3) recommendation for a rational approach for managing elevated transaminases in celiac patients, and (4) *vice versa* for screening for celiac disease in patients with liver diseases. A search for English written articles was performed using MEDLINE/PubMed (from 1977 up to 15 June 2018). We included scientific papers regarding liver immunology to emphasize liver as an organ with unique immune function, and to summarize hypotheses explaining connection between celiac diseases and liver disorders. Especially, we highlight the gut microbiota as further possible link clarifying the relationship between liver injury and celiac disease. In addition, number of observational studies and meta-analyses were used to document the current clinical approach to the liver disorders in celiac patients.

2. Immune Reactivity in the Liver

The liver, traditionally viewed as the central organ engaged in metabolism, nutrient storage, and detoxification, is also an immune organ, having an important regulatory role in innate and adaptive immunity. From an immunological point of view, the liver is exposed to large numbers of foreign molecules coming from the gastrointestinal tract via the portal vein. These non-self-antigens are derived from food (including peptides derived from gluten and related cereals), and from the microbiota (i.e., bacterial components and products) that have breached the intestinal barrier. The liver must tolerate these gut–derived molecules, while still providing immunosurveillance for pathogenic infections and malignant cells. The liver sinusoids and the sub-endothelial compartment (the space of Disse) are populated with various resident immune cells (of the innate and adaptive immune system) capable of dynamic interaction, antigen sensing, phagocytosis, antigen presentation, cytokine and chemokine production, cytotoxicity, T cells programing, and communication with circulating immune cells passing through the liver. The diversity of immune interplay determines the balance between tolerance, protective immunity against infection, tissue damage, and metastases, and autoimmunity in the liver. Variety of antigen-presenting cells (APCs), such as liver-resident macrophages, called Kupffer cells, liver-resident dendritic cells, and liver sinusoidal endothelial cells, play a central role in creating the tolerogenic environment of the liver. Kupffer cells act as the primary filter, constantly removing antigens from the circulation. The liver is particularly enriched with populations of resident innate lymphoid cells (natural killer (NK) cells, natural killer T (NKT) cells, mucosal-associated invariant T cells, and $\gamma\delta$ T cells), which recognize conserved antigens (expressed by microbial pathogens, pathogen-infected cells, and tumor cells), and respond by killing target cells, or selectively activating and regulating the diverse arms of both the innate and adaptive immune responses in the liver, including T helper (Th)1, (Th)2, (Th)17, T_{reg} cells, and antibody responses. Lymphoid cells of adaptive immunity comprise the classic major histocompatibility complex (MHC)-restricted CD4+ and CD8+ T cells, activated T cells, memory T cells, as well as B cells. Besides the above mentioned professional APCs, parenchymal cells and hepatic stellate cells act as semi-professional APCs, which can work as sensors or triggers of immune responses and assist in local or systemic immune regulation and inflammation. All types of liver cells, including resident immune cells, hepatocytes, cholangiocytes, sinusoidal endothelial cells, and hepatic stellate cells express a range of pattern recognition receptors (PRRs), such as toll-like receptors (TLRs), NOD-like receptors (NLRs), RIG-like receptors, carbohydrate receptors, and scavenger receptors, which bind to microbial-associated molecular patterns (MAMPs) and damage-associated molecular patterns (DAMPs) that may be present in portal blood. Kupffer cells, liver sinusoidal endothelial cells, and hepatocytes also express variable numbers of class II MHC molecules and are capable of presenting antigens to classic T cells [9,10].

The liver is a highly immunotolerant organ with many mechanisms to actively prevent the induction of immunity. While maintaining an overall tolerogenic setting, the hepatic immune system must be capable of rapidly activating immune responses to "dangerous" antigens or to liver tissue damage (of any origin). Immune tolerance to self-antigens in the liver can be impaired, which can lead to autoimmune liver diseases, such as autoimmune hepatitis (AIH), primary biliary cholangitis (PBC), and primary sclerosing cholangitis (PSC). The hepatic immune system plays an important role in responding to hepatic injury, and in the initiation and progression of liver diseases. Thus, chronic liver diseases of infectious, toxic, metabolic, cholestatic, and autoimmune origin are characterized by persistent activation of innate immune pathways, which are usually associated with cytopathic effects on liver parenchymal cells [9,10].

About 1–2% of food antigens are translocated into the circulation in an immunogenic form [11]. The liver is able to suppress immunity to many antigens, including dietary antigens. Additionally, various dietary constituents and metabolites can influence hepatic APCs and other liver cells (mainly by activating specific receptors, leading to altered intracellular signaling, gene expression, and release of cytokines) and therefore modulate physiological immune maintenance in the liver. Dietary constituents and metabolites can also increase pathological activation of liver immune cells. Liver metabolic processes are linked to hepatic inflammation through the inflammatory effects of metabolites such as saturated fatty acids, cholesterol, or succinate, which promote TLRs signaling and inflammasome activation on dendritic cells and macrophages [9,10]. Data sets published on the potential influence of dietary components, such as branch-chain amino acids, arginine, tryptophan, vitamins, and various types of lipids, on hepatic immunity show equivocal or conflicting results in terms of whether they induce tolerance or initiate an immune response [10]. Similarly, the role of dietary gluten and other immunogenic wheat proteins, in the modulation of hepatic immunity, has not been elucidated.

3. Gut–Liver Axis and Celiac Disease

Although the relationship between celiac disease (CD) and liver disorders have been clinically evident for more than 40 years [1], its pathophysiology is far from being fully understood with many explanations being hypothetical. In addition to a probable genetic relationship, the interplay of the many aspects of the gut–liver axis may also contribute to the explanation of this link (Figure 1).

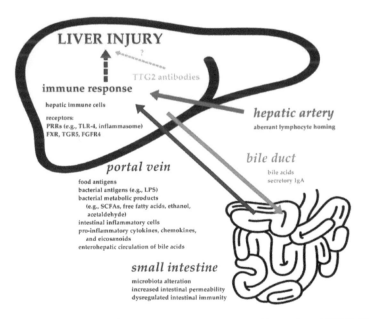

Figure 1. Putative pathogenesis of liver injury in celiac disease. Abbreviations: FGFR4, fibroblast growth factor receptor 4; FXR, farnesoid X receptor; LPS, lipopolysacharide; NLRs, NOD like receptors; PRRs, pattern-recognition receptors; SCFAs, short chain fatty acids; TGR5, Takeda G-protein receptor 5; TLR-4, toll like receptor 4; TTG2, tissue transglutaminase 2.

The term gut–liver axis describes a close anatomical, metabolic, and immunologic connection between the gut and liver. The liver and intestine are tightly linked via the portal circulation, which supplies the liver not only with nutrients but also with gut–derived food and bacterial antigens, and bacterial metabolic products. The liver portal and liver arterial circulation are the afferent part of the gut–liver axis, while the biliary tree is the efferent part of the gut–liver axis. Intestinal and biliary epithelia share many properties, including expression of PRRs and tight junction (TJs) proteins, as well as the ability to release secretory IgA. The secretion of bile (especially bile acids, and IgA) affects the gut–liver axis and modulates the composition of the intestinal microbiota [12]. Moreover, both organs are characterized by shared lymphocyte homing and recruitment pathways. Gut-derived T-lymphocytes may also contribute to hepato-biliary inflammation [13].

The gut–liver axis is a complex system involving multiple components—the intestinal barrier, gut microbiota, bile, shared lymphocyte homing, and several hepatic receptors, such as PRRs, or farnesoid X receptor (FXR), Takeda G-protein receptor 5 (TGR5), fibroblast growth factor receptor 4 (FGFR4)—that connect metabolic pathways to inflammation. Dysregulation or impairment of the gut–liver axis can activate the hepatic innate immune response leading to induction of liver injury, or contribute to the progression of liver damage (of any origin) [12,14] (Table 1).

Table 1. A role of the components of gut–liver axis in putative pathogenesis of liver injury in celiac disease.

Components of Gut-Liver Axis	Initial Pathogenetic Mechanism	Pathogenetic Consequences in the Intestine	Impact on Liver Immune Cells and Receptors	Consequent Liver Pathology and Altered Liver Physiology
Intestinal barrier	dysregulated intestinal immunity	stimulation of GALT, and entry of intestinal inflammatory cells, cytokines, chemokines, eicosanoids to the liver via the portal vein	triggering immune response via the interaction with liver resident immune cells	liver inflammation and injury
	increased intestinal permeability (e.g., up-regulation of chemokine CXCR3)	increased entry of - food antigens - bacterial antigens (LPS, etc.) - bacterial metabolites (SCFAs, etc.) to the liver via the portal vein	triggering immune response via: - CXCR3 up-regulation - via activation PRRs (CD14/TLR-4 complex, inflammasome, etc.)	liver inflammation and injury altered metabolic regulation (nutrient storage)
Microbiota	dysbiosis	increase of intestinal permeability and inflammation		
		proteolytic activity that can modify the immunogenicity of gliadin peptides		
		enhancement of celiac-disease-associated immunopathology		
		altered bile acid signatures	impact on liver bile salt receptors (FXR, TGR5) and receptor FGFR4	liver and biliary inflammation altered regulation of hepatic bile acids metabolism, and hepatic triglyceride, glucose, and energy homeostasis
Bile	altered bile acid signatures	changes in microbiota composition (dysbiosis)		
	secretion of IgA	changes in microbiota composition (dysbiosis)		
		Aberrant lymphocyte homing from the intestine to the liver		liver and biliary inflammation and injury

Abbreviations: FGFR4, fibroblast growth factor receptor 4; FXR, farnesoid X receptor; GALT, gut–associated lymphatic tissue; LPS, lipopolysaccharide; PRRs, pattern-recognition receptors; SCFAs, short chain fatty acids; TGR5, Takeda G-protein receptor 5; TLR-4, toll like receptor 4.

When the intestinal barrier is impaired (i.e., during increased intestinal permeability or dysregulated intestinal immunity), food antigens and bacterial antigens with strong immune-activating properties (e.g., lipopolysaccharide (LPS), peptidoglycans, super-antigens, bacterial DNA, flagellin, and heat shock proteins) can cross the intestinal epithelium in greater numbers than under healthy conditions, which can stimulate gut–associated lymphatic tissue (GALT) to release pro-inflammatory cytokines (TNF, IL-1, IL-6, etc.), chemokines, and eicosanoids. The load of antigens is not eliminated by GALT and together with intestinal inflammatory cells, cytokines, chemokines, and bacterial metabolites (such as ethanol, acetaldehyde, trimethylamine, short chain fatty acids (SCFAs), and free fatty acids) are transported to the liver via the portal vein. In the liver, the massive influx of these components activates the hepatic immune response thus promoting liver damage, inflammation, and fibrogenesis. Increased intestinal permeability as well as plasma levels of inflammatory cytokines has been demonstrated in both the pathophysiology and progression of chronic liver diseases. Similarly, increased levels of bacterial LPS have been documented in the portal and/or systemic circulation (endotoxemia) in several chronic liver diseases [12,13,15,16].

Among the compounds that can disrupt the function of the intestinal barrier are known dietary items or eating habits (e.g., alcohol use, high-fat, or high-carbohydrate diets), intestinal mucosal inflammation (regardless of etiology), infections, toxins, medications (e.g., non-steroidal antirheumatic drugs, proton-pump-inhibitors), and intestinal hypoperfusion [12]. It is also hypothesized that industrial food additives (such as gluten, microbial transglutaminase, glucose, salt, emulsifiers, organic solvents) that are commonly used in dough, may have a negative impact on the function of the intestinal barrier [17]. Another leading factor influencing intestinal permeability is the microbiota [18].

In CD, increased intestinal permeability is thought to be an early feature in the pathogenesis. Dietary gluten drives inflammation and impairs the function of the small intestinal barrier [19,20]. Using markers of epithelial apoptosis (cytokeratin 18 caspase-cleaved fragment) and enterocyte damage (intestinal fatty acid-binding protein), we found an impairment of small intestinal mucosal barrier integrity in patients with active celiac disease and also in patients with diabetes mellitus [21]. It has been demonstrated that patients having active CD with elevated serum transaminases have a more severely compromised intestinal barrier and greater intestinal permeability than those having active CD with normal liver tests; and both intestinal permeability and transaminases normalize when patients follow a gluten-free diet (GFD) [20,22].

In CD, gliadin *per se* has been shown to increase intestinal permeability by releasing zonulin—a modulator of small-intestinal TJs [13,23]. Luminal gliadin binds to the chemokine receptor, CXCR3, expressed on intestinal epithelium, and induces an MyD88-dependent zonulin release, which leads to an opening of enterocyte TJs. CXCR3 is over-expressed in CD patients, where it is co-localized with gliadin. CXCR3 is predominantly expressed on immune cells, but its expression has also been reported on non-immune cells, including hepatic parenchymal cells. Resident hepatic immune cells and hepatocytes express CXCR3 in both the normal and injured liver. While the role of these receptors in the homeostatic liver environment is not understood, during injury, they are engaged in cellular survival, activation, proliferation, apoptosis, inflammatory cell infiltration, fibrogenesis, angiogenesis, and expression of additional chemokines and growth factors [24]. Up-regulated production of CXCR3 ligands under inflammatory gut–liver interactions was recently demonstrated using an integrative multi-organ platform comprising human liver (hepatocytes and Kupffer cells) and intestinal (enterocytes, goblet cells, and dendritic cells) models [25].

It is not known, if gluten can affect intestinal permeability and hepatic immunity in healthy individuals. But, studies in murine monocytes/macrophages have demonstrated that gluten peptides activate the arginase metabolic pathway and increase intestinal permeability in vitro (on Caco-2 epithelial monolayers) [26]. Gliadin activated monocytes/macrophages contribute to the innate immune response in CD [27] by releasing inflammatory cytokines and nitric oxide (NO). Arginine is an obligatory substrate of inducible NO synthase, an enzyme that produces large amounts of NO. Moreover, it has been recently demonstrated that in both celiac subjects and healthy individuals, gluten peptides exert the same level of activation of arginine metabolism and cell polarization in human monocytes; therefore, ingested gluten might elicit innate activation of human monocytes even in healthy people [28].

4. Involvement of Microbiota in Celiac Disease and Liver Disorders

Dysbiosis (i.e., a reduction in bacterial diversity of beneficial bacterial species, and an increase in potentially pathogenic species relative to a healthy microbiome) is a feature of CD as well as both early and advanced liver disease.

CD is strongly associated with intestinal dysbiosis that is not completely restored by a GFD. Although, no distinct celiac microbiota pattern has yet to be found, an altered composition of fecal and duodenal microbiota has been identified in individuals with active celiac disease: e.g., an abundance of Firmicutes and Proteobacteria, or of Gram-negative bacteria (such as *Bacteroides* and *E. coli*), or *Staphylococcus* and *Clostridium*. This is accompanied by a related reduction in protective, anti-inflammatory bacteria (such as *Bifidobacterium* and Lactobacillus), and Gram-positive bacteria [19,29]. Microbiota might contribute to the pathogenesis and manifestation of CD via proteolytic activity that can modify the immunogenicity of gliadin peptides or by influencing intestinal permeability and inflammation [30].

There is also growing evidence that perturbations in the microbiota composition (dysbiosis or bacterial overgrowth) contribute to the pathogenesis (manifestation and/or maintenance and progression) of certain liver diseases, such as non-alcoholic fatty liver disease (NAFLD) (and its progressive variant, non-alcoholic steatohepatitis (NASH)), alcohol-related liver disease, primary sclerosing cholangitis (PSC), primary biliary cholangitis (PBC), and even liver cirrhosis and its complications including hepatocellular carcinoma [31,32]. The mechanism by which the microbiota affects intestinal permeability and TJs function is unknown. Several studies have shown that dysbiosis contributes to intestinal inflammation, bacterial translocation, and liver fibrosis [33].

The MAMPs are recognized by PRRs, such as TLRs or NLRs, which are expressed on intestinal epithelial and antigen presenting cells, and on liver resident immune and parenchymal cells. The CD14/TLR-4 complex (which is involved in the recognition and signal transduction of bacterial LPS) plays a central role in the initiation or maintenance of innate immune responses in the small intestine and in the liver and contributes to impairment of intestinal barrier [30].

In active celiac disease, increased TLR4 (and TLR2) expression in the duodenum has been documented [34]. In addition, our group reported increased sCD14 protein seropositivity in active CD. Soluble CD14 (sCD14) is considered to be an indicator of innate immunity activation in response to mucosal translocation of LPS. So, in CD, circulating LPS might contribute to innate immune activation of extraintestinal organs, including the liver [21].

In experimental models, the evaluation of specific bacteria isolated from celiac patients suggests that some commensal bacteria might promote an adverse response to dietary gluten, whereas others can be protective [35], and that gut microbiota can enhance or reduce celiac-disease-associated immunopathology (such as modifying T_{reg} induction, epithelial cell stress, and activation of intraepithelial lymphocytes, maturation of dendritic cells, pro-inflammatory cytokine production, intestinal permeability, and the induction of CD4+ T cell responses) [29]. Gut microbiota promotes chronic liver inflammation and fibrogenesis through the activation of TLR4 (on Kupffer cells and hepatic stellate cells). It has been demonstrated in mice, that bacterial LPS enhance TGF-β signaling in hepatic stellate cells, via the TLR4-MyD88-NF-κB pathway, subsequently leading to liver fibrogenesis [36]. Intestinal dysbiosis is associated with increased levels of LPS in the portal and/or systemic blood (endotoxemia) and propagates liver injury in several types of chronic liver diseases [12].

In addition to TLR4, inflammasome activation contributes to the pathogenesis of most acute and chronic liver disease. Inflammasomes are multiprotein complexes (involving NLRs) that can recognize a diverse range of MAMPs and DAMPs. Inflammasome-mediated dysbiosis enhances liver inflammation through activation of caspase-1 cascade and production of various proinflammatory cytokines (such as IL-1, IL-18, IL-6, TNF-α), enhances hepatocyte dysfunction, necrosis, apoptosis, and the generation of extracellular fibrosis [37].

Moreover, the activation of TLRs and inflammasome in hepatocytes seems to also be involved in metabolic regulation, since dysbiosis may alter nutritional absorption and storage [38].

Dysbiosis may also influence bile acid signatures in the gut and in enterohepatic circulation. Gut microbial enzymes (bile salt hydrolase, or bile acid-inducible enzymes) deconjugate and dehydroxylate primary bile acids in the intestine into unconjugated secondary bile acids. Bile acids (besides their well-known role in nutrient absorption and biliary secretion of lipids, toxic metabolites, and xenobiotics) are ligands for liver bile salt receptors, such as the nuclear FXR and membrane TGR5 [14]. Hepatic FXR plays a key role not only in regulation of hepatic bile acids metabolism, but also in the coordination of hepatic triglyceride, glucose, and energy homeostasis [39]. TGR5 is localized on various non-parenchymal liver cells (sinusoidal endothelial cells, Kupffer cells, hepatic stellate cells) and in cholangiocytes. Activation of TGR5 mediates choleretic, cell-protective, anti-inflammatory, and proliferative effects in cholangiocytes. A disturbance in the bile acids signaling mechanisms can contribute to the development or progression of biliary diseases, such as primary biliary cholangitis (PBC) and primary sclerosing cholangitis (PSC) [40]. Moreover, bile acids also influence hepatic inflammation and regeneration (via the intestinal bile acids-intestinal FXR-fibroblast growth factor (FGF) 15/19 and liver FGF receptor 4 axis). The alteration in the bile acid profile might provide signals that connect bile acid, lipid, and glucose metabolism in the liver to hepatic and biliary inflammation. Bile acids also have antimicrobial properties and therefore can modulate gut microbiota composition, intestinal immunity, and barrier integrity [14].

5. The Role of Tissue Tranglutaminase Antibodies and Vitamin D in a Pathogenetic Link between Celiac Disease and Hepatic Disorders

Beside the contribution of the gut–liver axis to hepatic injury in CD, it has also been suggested that tissue transglutaminase 2 (TTG2) (a key enzyme and part of target autoantigen involved in the pathogenesis of celiac disease [19]) may play a role in celiac-associated liver damage. This hypothesis is supported by observation that chronic unexplained hypertransaminasemia is frequently present in active CD, but not in other small intestinal diseases associated with dysbiosis and an increased inflammatory mucosal response, such as tropical sprue or diarrhea predominant-irritable bowel syndrome [41].

TTG2 is a ubiquitous cellular and extracellular enzyme, participating in important biological processes such as wound healing, tissue repair, fibrogenesis, apoptosis, inflammation, and cell-cycle control. In the extracellular space, TTG2 is involved in cell-extracellular matrix interactions as well as in remodeling and stabilization of the extracellular matrix [42]. It is also known to modulate inflammation and fibrosis in chronic liver diseases, although the mechanism appears to be quite complex and is not completely understood [43]. TTG2 is overexpressed in the liver (mainly in endothelial cells and periportal hepatocytes) of patients suffering from chronic liver diseases. Our group documented that overexpression of TTG2 is more pronounced in the liver tissue of patients suffering simultaneously from both liver disease (such as toxic hepatitis, primary sclerosing cholangitis, or autoimmune hepatitis type I) and active CD [44].

There is also evidence that enhanced TTG2 enzymatic activity seems to protect the liver from acute and chronic injury [43]. In CD, the presence of celiac antibodies has been shown to inhibit TTG2 enzymatic activity, which can lead to a decrease in the availability of active transforming growth factor (TGF)-β [45]. IgA antibodies targeted against TTG2 (IgA-TTG2 deposits), which have been found in liver biopsy specimens from patients with active CD and elevated liver transaminase values, and also in skeletal muscle, the appendix, and lymph nodes, suggest that alteration in TTG2 bioactivity (i.e., inhibition by anti-TTG2 antibodies) might play a role in celiac extra-intestinal manifestations, including liver injury [46]. We described that also another autoantigen, calcium binding protein calreticulin, could be involved in putative pathogenesis of liver injury and celiac disease [16,47].

Moreover, vitamin D deficiency, which is commonly found in active celiac disease [48], could also contribute to a proinflammatory state in the liver. Vitamin D is known for its anti-inflammatory effects on immune cells, which might be particularly relevant to the liver's immune response. For instance, vitamin D inhibits the inflammatory maturation of dendritic cells, influences the responsiveness of macrophages to LPS and other MAMPs, and facilitates homing of activated T cells [10].

6. Celiac Disease and Liver Disorders in the Clinical Context

Although CD is associated with a wide spectrum of liver disorders, two distinct forms can be distinguished: (1) cryptogenic hypertransaminasaemia (celiac hepatitis), and (2) associated autoimmune liver diseases (AILD), such as autoimmune hepatitis (AIH), autoimmune cholangitis, primary biliary cholangitis (PBC), primary sclerosing cholangitis (PSC). Cryptogenic hypertransaminasaemia (celiac hepatitis), a common extraintestinal presentation of CD, is closely related to gluten intake. Additionally, CD can simply coexist as a coincidental finding with several liver diseases, such as non-alcoholic fatty liver disease (NAFLD) (and its subgroup termed non-alcoholic steatohepatitis (NASH)), chronic viral hepatitis B or C, alcoholic liver disease, hemochromatosis, Wilson's disease, and other hereditary hepatic diseases [3,44,49–51]. Swedish epidemiological studies have revealed that patients with CD have an increased risk of both prior and subsequent liver disease, four-times and six-times, respectively [52], and an eight-times increased risk of mortality from liver cirrhosis [53]; however, no increased risk of liver transplantation was found (HR, 1.07; 95% CI, 0.12–9.62; $p = 0.954$) [52]. Similarly, in the large-scale screening study, we observed that seropositivity for IgA anti-TTG antibodies in patients with various liver diseases is higher (3%) [44] then prevalence of celiac disease in the general population [54].

6.1. Celiac Hepatitis

Isolated elevation of serum transaminases (alanine aminotransferase (ALT) and aspartate aminotransferase (AST)) is often present in newly diagnosed, active CD. The liver injury in CD, when other concomitant hepatic disease is absent, and that completely resolves after GFD, has been termed "celiac hepatitis" [55]. The reported prevalence of elevated serum transaminase levels in active celiac diseases varies from 10–50% [2–6].

Elevated transaminases do not correlate with sex, weight, height, or body mass index [4–6]. Some studies found no correlation with CD symptoms at diagnosis and found that patients were usually asymptomatic [5,6,56]. While others have reported an association between hypertransaminasemia and malabsorption and diarrhea, or poor growth in children [4,6]. In a study performed by Aarela et al., factors associated with increased ALT were poor growth and severe villous atrophy. There was a moderate statistically significant correlation between ALT and endomysial antibodies ($r = 0.334$, $p < 0.001$), TTG2 antibodies ($r = 0.264$, $p = 0.002$), and ferritin ($r = -0.225$, $p = 0.03$), but not with other laboratory values [6]. Similarly, in adult celiac patients, one study found a correlation between hypertransaminasemia and malabsorption (odds ratio (OR), 2.22; $p = 0.004$), diarrhea (OR, 1.72; $p = 0.005$), and increasing severity of mucosal lesions (OR, 1.46; $p = 0.001$) [4]. By contrast, another study reported that the severity of intestinal histological changes did not correlate with transaminases levels [57]. Hypertransaminasaemia has been shown to correlate with intestinal permeability. In active CD, the intestinal permeability index (% lactulose/% mannitol in a 5 h urine collection) is statistically significantly ($p < 0.0001$) higher in patients with elevated transaminases and is correlated with AST (tau = 0.34; $p < 0.0001$) and ALT (tau = 0.32; $p < 0.0001$) [22].

Generally, hypertransaminasaemia is mild. Values greater than 5-time the ULN (upper limit of normal) are seen in a minority of patients [4,5]. The clinical presentation of celiac hepatitis is often asymptomatic but can vary up to advanced liver disease. Chronic untreated CD may also lead to chronic hepatitis and consequent liver cirrhosis, including, although seldom, end-stage liver cirrhosis requiring liver transplantation [58,59]. Acute cryptogenic liver failure, which resolved after a GFD without the necessity for liver transplantation, has been, although rarely, described in untreated CD [58,60], or CD that was diagnosed long after liver transplantation due to "cryptogenic" liver cirrhosis [61]. In childhood CD, six cases of severe liver disease (two of them needing liver transplantation) have been reported [62].

No histologic findings are pathognomonic for celiac hepatitis. Non-specific reactive hepatitis is the mostly described lesion, but the histologic picture varies from normal liver architecture, or minimal lymphocytic infiltrates of portal tracts, to mild or moderate reactive hepatitis, steatosis, fibrosis, and rarely to late morphological changes, such as advanced fibrosis or cirrhosis. Inflammatory alterations of the bile ducts have not been found [1,44,56,63].

Celiac hepatitis is characterized by the presence of liver injury that resolves after introduction of a GFD. In the majority patients, a GFD leads to normalization of previously elevated transaminases levels within 1 year [2–6,60]. This suggests that gluten intake (that is responsible for small intestinal damage and the autoimmune reaction) drives the pathogenesis of celiac hepatitis.

Only a small percentage of patients with celiac hepatitis will need longer periods for complete normalization of liver tests. The time needed probably reflects the time required for complete intestinal mucosal recovery, which has been shown to take up to 3–5 years after the initiation of a GFD [64,65].

The relationship between hypertransaminasemia and gluten intake in celiac hepatitis has also been documented in other observations: (1) liver transaminases remained elevated during GFD non-compliance [66], (2) even normal transaminase levels decreased significantly on a GFD, and (3) a gluten challenge can lead to mild but transient hypertransaminasemia [67]. Several other observations have shown histologic improvement of liver injury (i.e., a decrease in steatosis, portal and lobular inflammation, and fibrosis score) on a GFD [63].

6.2. Associated Autoimmune Liver Diseases

The association between CD and AILD is more uncommon than celiac hepatitis, although it has been widely demonstrated. According to systematic reviews, the prevalence of CD in AIH is 6.3% in children [2] and about 4% in adults [7]. The prevalence of CD in PBC varies from 3–7%, and in PSC from 2–3% [8].

The pathophysiology of CD associated AILD is not driven directly by gluten, since good adherence to a GFD alone usually does not lead to an improvement in liver tests or in the course of hepatic disease [3,8,44,49,50]. Patients with AILD and CD require both specific immunosuppressive therapy for the liver disorder as well as a GFD. GFD only improves symptoms related to CD while decreasing the risk of long-term CD complications. It is unknown if the prognosis of patients with AILD associated with CD is different from patients with AILD alone. The clinical impact of a GFD on the progression of AILD, therefore, remains uncertain [68,69]. Although, studies carried out on a small number of pediatric patients with AIH showed that children with AIH and CD on a GFD achieved treatment-free sustained remission in a significantly higher proportion compared to those without CD [70,71]. Another study reported that several children with CD and AIH developed relapses during a spontaneous gluten challenge [72]. So, a GFD may prevent an early relapse of AIH in patients having AIH associated with CD.

Moreover, in several patients with newly diagnosed CD and suffering simultaneously from liver failure due to AILD, GFD was able to reverse hepatic dysfunction, even in cases where liver transplantation was being considered [58,60]. The mechanisms underlying the association between CD and AILD are poorly understood. The most important feature is likely a shared genetic predisposition to autoimmunity [68,69]. Like other autoimmune diseases, CD is a polygenic disorder. In CD, genetic susceptibility is largely associated with specific human leucocyte antigen (HLA) class II molecules on antigen-presenting cells. About 90% of CD patients carry a particular HLA variant (HLA-DQ2.5) that encodes the DQ2.5 molecule, the rest carry HLA-DQ8 or HLA-DQ2.2 [73]. The main genetic marker of CD, HLA-DQ2.5, has a strong linkage disequilibrium with HLA-DR4, HLA-DR52, and HLA-DR3, being the major HLA risk factor for autoimmune liver disease (AIH, PSC, PBC) [74]. Additionally, gene polymorphisms outside the HLA contribute to the genetic susceptibility to both CD and AILD. There are 39 well-established non-HLA loci, including a greater number of independent genetic variants that are associated with CD risk [73]. Many of these loci are related to immune regulations, particularly to B cell and T cell function, and are also shared with other autoimmune diseases, including AILD. The sharing of genetic loci between CD and AILD suggests that there are also shared dysregulated immune responses contributing to the relationship between the two diseases.

Moreover, epigenetics, microbiota, and intestinal barrier dysfunction are emerging as potent factors modulating genetic susceptibility and affecting disease manifestation [32,73].

It remains an open question, whether recently described gluten/wheat-related disorders, such as non-celiac gluten sensitivity and wheat-sensitive irritable bowel syndrome have any link to liver diseases [75].

6.3. Non-Alcoholic Fatty Liver Disease and Celiac Disease

NAFLD is currently a major cause of chronic liver disease with an estimated global prevalence of approximately 25% [76]. Its occurrence in CD patients is likely a coincidence rather than a true relationship, due to the high frequency of both diseases in the general population [51].

Patients with NAFLD are at increased risk for a later diagnosis of CD [77]. The reported prevalence of CD in patients with NAFLD is 2–14% [78]. Conversely, individuals with CD seem to be at increased risk (4–6-times) of NAFLD compared to the general population [52,77]. The relative risk of NAFLD development after a CD diagnosis is higher in the first five years (probably because of excessive weight gain on a GFD) but remained statistically significant even 15 years after a CD diagnosis [77]. GFD could be connected with some dietetic imbalances (such as slightly increased calories, lipid and cholesterol intake, or decreased fiber intake) [79], so patients on GFD are prone to develop NAFLD.

Besides lipotoxicity of specific lipid classes that are stored in hepatocytes, the pathogenesis for NAFLD/NASH may also involve changes in gut permeability, gut microbiota, and other components of gut–liver axis [80]. It has been demonstrated (using the ^{51}Cr-EDTA test, by immunohistochemical analysis of zonula occludens protein-1 expression in duodenal biopsy specimens, by the lactulose/mannitol ratio, and by increased levels of circulating zonulin) that NAFLD patients have increased intestinal permeability [81,82]. Moreover, increased intestinal permeability and increased levels of circulating zonulin correlate with the severity of steatosis [82].

NAFLD frequently occurs in type 2 diabetes mellitus and obesity. However, when metabolic syndrome is absent, NAFLD may be related to concomitant CD. Therefore, in the absence of type 2 diabetes mellitus or obesity, and when other causes of liver disease are excluded, patients with NAFLD should be screened for CD [50].

Conversely, NAFLD/NASH in patients with CD may also occur as a metabolic sequel of malabsorption and long-standing malnutrition [51]. Malnutrition generates mitochondrial dysfunction in hepatocytes and a reduction in mitochondrial fatty acid β-oxidation, which subsequently leads to abnormal hepatic fat deposition [83]. A GFD usually leads to resolution of liver steatosis and even steatofibrosis in these CD patients [84]. Beyond the mere improvement in nutritional status, a GFD may contribute to restoration of innate immune liver function via harmonization of the gut–liver axis. Luckily, CD disease presenting with severe malabsorption is now uncommon [85].

7. Clinical Implications: Hepatic Manifestation of Celiac Disease

Liver tests should be routinely checked in all patients with newly diagnosed CD. Hepatic manifestation of CD (i.e., hypertransaminasemia in active CD) deserves specific clinical attention. When a patient's history and physical and/or ultrasonographic evaluation shows no signs of concomitant hepatic disorder, there is a higher probability of celiac hepatitis than of associated autoimmune liver disease or other coexisting liver disease. Asymptomatic hypertransaminasemia (<5-time the ULN and an AST/ALT < 1) together with a normal physical and ultrasound examination strongly suggests celiac hepatitis. Instead of initial extensive (and expensive) investigations for other causes of liver injury, a "treat-first then re-evaluate" approach is recommended. Liver enzymes should be re-checked after 6–12 months on a strict GFD. If the elevated transaminases return to normal after gluten exclusion, a diagnosis of celiac hepatitis is confirmed, and only follow-ups are recommended, which should optimally include a physical examination, abdominal ultrasound, and liver tests once a year. Because of the nonspecific nature of the findings, liver biopsies are not useful in celiac hepatitis [49,70].

However, lack of normalization of liver enzymes within one year despite adherence to a GFD increases the probability of another concomitant liver disease (of autoimmune, viral, metabolic, or toxic origin). In such cases, a thorough hepatologic examination is necessary [49,70].

Furthermore, patients with elevated liver tests at the time of a CD diagnosis require an extended search for other liver disease, i.e., when the clinical evaluation is not consistent with celiac hepatitis, such as: (1) elevated transaminases levels >5-time the ULN and/or AST/ALT > 1, (2) laboratory signs of cholestasis (i.e., elevated gamma glutamyl transferase, alkaline phosphatase of liver origin, and/or bilirubin), (3) symptomatic liver disorder and/or (4) physical and ultrasonographic signs suggesting a liver disorder. Additionally, abnormal liver tests during follow-up of CD patients who are strictly adhering to a GFD should raise suspicion of other liver disease [49].

8. Clinical Implications: Screening of Celiac Disease in Liver Diseases

Screening for CD is recommended in groups of patients with associated AILD (AIH, PBC, PSC), as well as in patients with chronic unexplained hypertransaminasemia, hepatitis or cirrhosis of unknown etiology, and in patients with NAFLD (particularly in those without metabolic syndrome) [8,44,50,58,63,68].

Although the magnitude of the benefit from gluten avoidance relative to reversing autoimmune liver disease in CD patients is controversial, a theoretical context (balance in gut–liver axis and subsequent decline in liver innate immune response) and several of the above-mentioned clinical observations suggest the importance of a GFD. Early detection and treatment of CD may mitigate progression to end-stage liver disease and liver failure [8,58,69].

The first steps in CD screening should include serological testing of TTG2 IgA, together with total serum IgA, followed by subsequent endomysial antibody (EMA) testing in questionable cases (i.e., low titers, possibly false-positive result of TTG2 IgA, which can occur in other autoimmune diseases, etc.). EMA has very high specificity (>99%) for CD. Serologic positivity needs to be confirm with a distal duodenal biopsy [86]. Screening for CD in the context of liver disease deserves special attention in terms of the interpretation of celiac serologic tests, since their accuracy is significantly lower than in individuals without liver disease; especially the guinea pig based anti-TTG2 ELISA testing, which has been shown to have higher rate of false positive results in patients with liver fibrosis. [49]. Thus, in patients with chronic liver disease, EMA evaluation is an important test that can increase diagnostic accuracy. Moreover, immunosuppression (in AILD or after liver transplantation) in the absence of gluten withdrawal can normalize both EMA and TTG2 antibodies. Therefore, in AILD or in end-stage liver cirrhosis, screening for CD must be performed before the start of immunosuppressive therapy or before liver transplantation [49,50].

9. Conclusions and Recommendation

The liver is a highly immunologically active organ that must simultaneously induce and maintain tolerance while being able to trigger immune responses leading to both protective immunity as well as liver inflammation and fibrosis. An impaired intestinal barrier, dysbiosis, and translocation of bacterial antigens are characteristics of both CD and chronic liver diseases. Disturbances in the gut–liver axis, inhibition of liver TTG2 enzymatic activity, and vitamin D deficiency probably all contribute to liver injury associated with CD. The intestinal microbiome influences the composition of nutrients delivered to the liver and affects metabolic liver functions connected with inflammation.

A simultaneous clinical presentation of CD with a wide spectrum of liver disorders is well-documented and common. In celiac hepatitis, gluten intake drives liver injury, and a gluten-free diet is the only widely used treatment. Patients with AILD associated with CD can (in addition to specific immunosuppressive treatment) also benefit from a GFD. Overlooked CD can cause chronic hepatitis and rarely liver cirrhosis. Screening for CD should be integrated into the diagnostic routine not only in AIH, PSC, and PBD, but also in unexplained hypertransaminasaemia, chronic hepatitis or cirrhosis of unknown origin, and NAFLD presenting without metabolic syndrome.

Nutrients **2018**, *10*, 892

A better understanding of the link between gluten-related immunity and liver injury could contribute to prevention and offer new approaches to the treatment of liver diseases of different etiologies.

Author Contributions: I.H. wrote the manuscript. D.S., L.T., and H.T.-H. had contributions to the manuscript conception, and substantially revised the manuscript.

Funding: The work was supported by projects 13-14608S and 16-06326S of the Czech Science Foundation, TH03010019 of Technology Agency of the Czech Republic, Institutional Research Concept RVO: 61388971, and COST Action 1402, Programme Progres Q36/64 (Initial Stages of Diabetes Mellitus, Metabolic and Nutritional Disorders) of Charles University, Czech Republic, and Strategy AV21-8 (The Czech Academy of Sciences).

Acknowledgments: Michal Anděl and Michal Kršek (Third Faculty of Medicine, Charles University, Czech Republic) for supporting of our work; and Thomas Secrest for the English Language Editing.

Conflicts of Interest: The authors declare no conflict of interest.

Abbreviations

AIH	autoimmune hepatitis
AILD	autoimmune liver disease
APCs	antigen presenting cells
CD	celiac disease
DAMPs	damage-associated molecular patterns
DCs	dendritic cells
DNA	deoxyribonucleic acid
FGFR4	fibroblast growth factor receptor 4
FXR	farnesoid X receptor
GALT	gut–associated lymphatic tissue
GFD	gluten free diet
GIT	gastrointestinal tract
HLA	human leucocyte antigen
IFN-γ	interferon γ
IL	interleukin
LPS	lipopolysacharide
MAMPs	microbial-associated molecular patterns
MDSC	myeloid-derived suppressor cells
MHC	major histocompatibility complex
NAFLD	non-alcoholic fatty liver disease
NASH	non-alcoholic steatohepatitis
NK cells	natural killer cells
NKT cells	natural killer T cells NKT cells
NLRs	NOD like receptors
PBC	primary biliary cholantitis
PRRs	pattern-recognition receptors
PSC	primary sclerosing cholangitis
SCFAs	short chain fatty acids
T_{reg} cells	regulatory T cells
TGF-β	transforming growth factor β
TGR5	Takeda G-protein receptor 5
Th cells	T helper cells
TJs	tight junctions
TLRs	toll like receptors
TNF	tumor necrosis factor
TTG2	tissue transglutaminase 2
ULN	upper limit of normal

References

1. Hagander, B.; Berg, N.O.; Brandt, L.; Norden, A.; Sjolund, K.; Stenstam, M. Hepatic injury in adult coeliac disease. *Lancet* **1977**, *2*, 270–272. [CrossRef]
2. Vajro, P.; Paolella, G.; Maggiore, G.; Giordano, G. Pediatric celiac disease, cryptogenic hypertransaminasemia, and autoimmune hepatitis. *J. Pediatr. Gastroenterol. Nutr.* **2013**, *56*, 663–670. [CrossRef] [PubMed]
3. Sainsbury, A.; Sanders, D.S.; Ford, A.C. Meta-analysis: Coeliac disease and hypertransaminasaemia. *Aliment. Pharmacol. Ther.* **2011**, *34*, 33–40. [CrossRef] [PubMed]
4. Zanini, B.; Basche, R.; Ferraresi, A.; Pigozzi, M.G.; Ricci, C.; Lanzarotto, F.; Villanacci, V.; Lanzini, A. Factors that contribute to hypertransaminasemia in patients with celiac disease or functional gastrointestinal syndromes. *Clin. Gastroenterol. Hepatol.* **2014**, *12*, 804–810. [CrossRef] [PubMed]
5. Lee, G.J.; Boyle, B.; Ediger, T.; Hill, I. Hypertransaminasemia in Newly Diagnosed Pediatric Patients with Celiac Disease. *J. Pediatr. Gastroenterol. Nutr.* **2016**, *63*, 340–343. [CrossRef] [PubMed]
6. Aarela, L.; Nurminen, S.; Kivela, L.; Huhtala, H.; Maki, M.; Viitasalo, A.; Kaukinen, K.; Lakka, T.; Kurppa, K. Prevalence and associated factors of abnormal liver values in children with celiac disease. *Dig. Liver Dis.* **2016**, *48*, 1023–1029. [CrossRef] [PubMed]
7. Mirzaagha, F.; Azali, S.H.; Islami, F.; Zamani, F.; Khalilipour, E.; Khatibian, M.; Malekzadeh, R. Coeliac disease in autoimmune liver disease: A cross-sectional study and a systematic review. *Dig. Liver Dis.* **2010**, *42*, 620–623. [CrossRef] [PubMed]
8. Volta, U.; Caio, G.; Tovoli, F.; De Giorgio, R. Gut-liver axis: An immune link between celiac disease and primary biliary cirrhosis. *Expert Rev. Gastroenterol. Hepatol.* **2013**, *7*, 253–261. [CrossRef] [PubMed]
9. Robinson, M.W.; Harmon, C.; O'Farrelly, C. Liver immunology and its role in inflammation and homeostasis. *Cell. Mol. Immunol.* **2016**, *13*, 267–276. [CrossRef] [PubMed]
10. Carambia, A.; Herkel, J. Dietary and metabolic modulators of hepatic immunity. *Semin. Immunopathol.* **2018**, *40*, 175–188. [CrossRef] [PubMed]
11. Husby, S. Normal immune responses to ingested foods. *J. Pediatr. Gastroenterol. Nutr.* **2000**, *30*, S13–S19. [CrossRef] [PubMed]
12. Wiest, R.; Albillos, A.; Trauner, M.; Bajaj, J.S.; Jalan, R. Targeting the gut–liver axis in liver disease. *J. Hepatol.* **2017**, *67*, 1084–1103. [CrossRef] [PubMed]
13. Sturgeon, C.; Fasano, A. Zonulin, a regulator of epithelial and endothelial barrier functions, and its involvement in chronic inflammatory diseases. *Tissue Barriers* **2016**, *4*, e1251384. [CrossRef] [PubMed]
14. Schneider, K.M.; Albers, S.; Trautwein, C. Role of bile acids in the gut–liver axis. *J. hepatol.* **2018**, *68*, 1083–1085. [CrossRef] [PubMed]
15. Pekarikova, A.; Sanchez, D.; Palova-Jelinkova, L.; Simsova, M.; Benes, Z.; Hoffmanova, I.; Drastich, P.; Janatkova, I.; Mothes, T.; Tlaskalova-Hogenova, H.; et al. Calreticulin is a B cell molecular target in some gastrointestinal malignancies. *Clin. Exp. Immunol.* **2010**, *160*, 215–222. [CrossRef] [PubMed]
16. Sanchez, D.; Tuckova, L.; Mothes, T.; Kreisel, W.; Benes, Z.; Tlaskalova-Hogenova, H. Epitopes of calreticulin recognised by IgA autoantibodies from patients with hepatic and coeliac disease. *J. Autoimmun.* **2003**, *21*, 383–392. [CrossRef]
17. Lerner, A.; Aminov, R.; Matthias, T. Transglutaminases in Dysbiosis As Potential Environmental Drivers of Autoimmunity. *Front. Microbiol.* **2017**, *8*, 66. [CrossRef] [PubMed]
18. Federico, A.; Dallio, M.; Caprio, G.G.; Ormando, V.M.; Loguercio, C. Gut microbiota and the liver. *Minerva Gastroenterol. Dietol.* **2017**, *63*, 385–398. [PubMed]
19. De Re, V.; Magris, R.; Cannizzaro, R. New Insights into the Pathogenesis of Celiac Disease. *Front. Med.* **2017**, *4*, 137. [CrossRef] [PubMed]
20. Spadoni, I.; Zagato, E.; Bertocchi, A.; Paolinelli, R.; Hot, E.; Di Sabatino, A.; Caprioli, F.; Bottiglieri, L.; Oldani, A.; Viale, G.; et al. A gut–vascular barrier controls the systemic dissemination of bacteria. *Science* **2015**, *350*, 830–834. [CrossRef] [PubMed]
21. Hoffmanova, I.; Sanchez, D.; Habova, V.; Andel, M.; Tuckova, L.; Tlaskalova-Hogenova, H. Serological markers of enterocyte damage and apoptosis in patients with celiac disease, autoimmune diabetes mellitus and diabetes mellitus type 2. *Physiol. Res.* **2015**, *64*, 537–546. [PubMed]

22. Novacek, G.; Miehsler, W.; Wrba, F.; Ferenci, P.; Penner, E.; Vogelsang, H. Prevalence and clinical importance of hypertransaminasaemia in coeliac disease. *Eur. J. Gastroenterol. Hepatol.* **1999**, *11*, 283–288. [CrossRef] [PubMed]
23. Fasano, A. Zonulin, regulation of tight junctions, and autoimmune diseases. *Ann. N. Y. Acad. Sci.* **2012**, *1258*, 25–33. [CrossRef] [PubMed]
24. Saiman, Y.; Friedman, S.L. The role of chemokines in acute liver injury. *Front. Physiol.* **2012**, *3*, 213. [CrossRef] [PubMed]
25. Chen, W.L.K.; Edington, C.; Suter, E.; Yu, J.; Velazquez, J.J.; Velazquez, J.G.; Shockley, M.; Large, E.M.; Venkataramanan, R.; Hughes, D.J.; et al. Integrated gut/liver microphysiological systems elucidates inflammatory inter-tissue crosstalk. *Biotechnol. Bioeng.* **2017**, *114*, 2648–2659. [CrossRef] [PubMed]
26. Barilli, A.; Rotoli, B.M.; Visigalli, R.; Ingoglia, F.; Cirlini, M.; Prandi, B.; Dall'Asta, V. Gliadin-mediated production of polyamines by RAW264.7 macrophages modulates intestinal epithelial permeability in vitro. *Biochim. Biophys. Acta* **2015**, *1852*, 1779–1786. [CrossRef] [PubMed]
27. Cinova, J.; Palova-Jelinkova, L.; Smythies, L.E.; Cerna, M.; Pecharova, B.; Dvorak, M.; Fruhauf, P.; Tlaskalova-Hogenova, H.; Smith, P.D.; Tuckova, L. Gliadin peptides activate blood monocytes from patients with celiac disease. *J. Clin. Immunol.* **2007**, *27*, 201–209. [CrossRef] [PubMed]
28. Barilli, A.; Gaiani, F.; Prandi, B.; Cirlini, M.; Ingoglia, F.; Visigalli, R.; Rotoli, B.M.; de'Angelis, N.; Sforza, S.; de'Angelis, G.L.; et al. Gluten peptides drive healthy and celiac monocytes toward an M2-like polarization. *J. Nutr. Bioch.* **2018**, *54*, 11–17. [CrossRef] [PubMed]
29. Verdu, E.F.; Galipeau, H.J.; Jabri, B. Novel players in coeliac disease pathogenesis: Role of the gut microbiota. *Nat. Rev. Gastroenterol. Hepatol.* **2015**, *12*, 497–506. [CrossRef] [PubMed]
30. Cenit, M.C.; Olivares, M.; Codoner-Franch, P.; Sanz, Y. Intestinal Microbiota and Celiac Disease: Cause, Consequence or Co-Evolution? *Nutrients* **2015**, *7*, 6900–6923. [CrossRef] [PubMed]
31. Woodhouse, C.A.; Patel, V.C.; Singanayagam, A.; Shawcross, D.L. Review article: The gut microbiome as a therapeutic target in the pathogenesis and treatment of chronic liver disease. *Aliment. Pharmacol. Ther.* **2018**, *47*, 192–202. [CrossRef] [PubMed]
32. Sabino, J.; Vieira-Silva, S.; Machiels, K.; Joossens, M.; Falony, G.; Ballet, V.; Ferrante, M.; van Assche, G.; Van der Merwe, S.; Vermeire, S.; et al. Primary sclerosing cholangitis is characterised by intestinal dysbiosis independent from IBD. *Gut* **2016**, *65*, 1681–1689. [CrossRef] [PubMed]
33. Grander, C.; Adolph, T.E.; Wieser, V.; Lowe, P.; Wrzosek, L.; Gyongyosi, B.; Ward, D.V.; Grabherr, F.; Gerner, R.R.; Pfister, A.; et al. Recovery of ethanol-induced Akkermansia muciniphila depletion ameliorates alcoholic liver disease. *Gut* **2018**, *67*, 891–901. [CrossRef] [PubMed]
34. Szebeni, B.; Veres, G.; Dezsofi, A.; Rusai, K.; Vannay, A.; Bokodi, G.; Vasarhelyi, B.; Korponay-Szabo, I.R.; Tulassay, T.; Arato, A. Increased mucosal expression of Toll-like receptor (TLR)2 and TLR4 in coeliac disease. *J. Pediatr. Gastroenterol. Nutr.* **2007**, *45*, 187–193. [CrossRef] [PubMed]
35. Cenit, M.C.; Codoner-Franch, P.; Sanz, Y. Gut Microbiota and Risk of Developing Celiac Disease. *J. Clin. Gastroenterol.* **2016**, *50* (Suppl. 2), S148–S152. [CrossRef] [PubMed]
36. Fukui, H. Gut Microbiota and Host Reaction in Liver Diseases. *Microorganisms* **2015**, *3*, 759–791. [CrossRef] [PubMed]
37. Del Campo, J.A.; Gallego, P.; Grande, L. Role of inflammatory response in liver diseases: Therapeutic strategies. *World J. Hepatol.* **2018**, *10*, 1–7. [CrossRef] [PubMed]
38. Schnabl, B.; Brenner, D.A. Interactions between the intestinal microbiome and liver diseases. *Gastroenterology* **2014**, *146*, 1513–1524. [CrossRef] [PubMed]
39. Hartmann, P.; Hochrath, K.; Horvath, A.; Chen, P.; Seebauer, C.T.; Llorente, C.; Wang, L.; Alnouti, Y.; Fouts, D.E.; Starkel, P.; et al. Modulation of the intestinal bile acid/farnesoid X receptor/fibroblast growth factor 15 axis improves alcoholic liver disease in mice. *Hepatology* **2018**, *67*, 2150–2166. [CrossRef] [PubMed]
40. Deutschmann, K.; Reich, M.; Klindt, C.; Droge, C.; Spomer, L.; Haussinger, D.; Keitel, V. Bile acid receptors in the biliary tree: TGR5 in physiology and disease. *Biochim. Biophys. Acta* **2018**, *1864*, 1319–1325. [CrossRef] [PubMed]
41. Pelaez-Luna, M.; Schmulson, M.; Robles-Diaz, G. Intestinal involvement is not sufficient to explain hypertransaminasemia in celiac disease? *Med. Hypotheses* **2005**, *65*, 937–941. [CrossRef] [PubMed]
42. Griffin, M.; Casadio, R.; Bergamini, C.M. Transglutaminases: Nature's biological glues. *Biochim. J.* **2002**, *368*, 377–396. [CrossRef] [PubMed]

43. Elli, L.; Bergamini, C.M.; Bardella, M.T.; Schuppan, D. Transglutaminases in inflammation and fibrosis of the gastrointestinal tract and the liver. *Dig. Liver Dis.* **2009**, *41*, 541–550. [CrossRef] [PubMed]
44. Drastich, P.; Honsova, E.; Lodererova, A.; Jaresova, M.; Pekarikova, A.; Hoffmanova, I.; Tuckova, L.; Tlaskalova-Hogenova, H.; Spicak, J.; Sanchez, D. Celiac disease markers in patients with liver diseases: A single center large scale screening study. *World J. Gastroenterol.* **2012**, *18*, 6255–6262. [CrossRef] [PubMed]
45. Esposito, C.; Paparo, F.; Caputo, I.; Rossi, M.; Maglio, M.; Sblattero, D.; Not, T.; Porta, R.; Auricchio, S.; Marzari, R.; et al. Anti-tissue transglutaminase antibodies from coeliac patients inhibit transglutaminase activity both in vitro and in situ. *Gut* **2002**, *51*, 177–181. [CrossRef] [PubMed]
46. Korponay-Szabo, I.R.; Halttunen, T.; Szalai, Z.; Laurila, K.; Kiraly, R.; Kovacs, J.B.; Fesus, L.; Maki, M. In vivo targeting of intestinal and extraintestinal transglutaminase 2 by coeliac autoantibodies. *Gut* **2004**, *53*, 641–648. [CrossRef] [PubMed]
47. Sanchez, D.; Tuckova, L.; Sebo, P.; Michalak, M.; Whelan, A.; Sterzl, I.; Jelinkova, L.; Havrdova, E.; Imramovska, M.; Benes, Z.; et al. Occurrence of IgA and IgG autoantibodies to calreticulin in coeliac disease and various autoimmune diseases. *J. Autoimmun.* **2000**, *15*, 441–449. [CrossRef] [PubMed]
48. Hoffmanova, I.; Sanchez, D.; Dzupa, V. Bone and Joint Involvement in Celiac Disease. *Acta Chir. Orthop. Traumatol. Cech.* **2015**, *82*, 308–312. [PubMed]
49. Rubio-Tapia, A.; Murray, J.A. Liver involvement in celiac disease. *Minerva Med.* **2008**, *99*, 595–604. [PubMed]
50. Narciso-Schiavon, J.L.; Schiavon, L.L. To screen or not to screen? Celiac antibodies in liver diseases. *World J. Gastroenterol.* **2017**, *23*, 776–791. [CrossRef] [PubMed]
51. Freeman, H.J. Hepatic manifestations of celiac disease. *Clin. Exp. Gastroenterol.* **2010**, *3*, 33–39. [CrossRef] [PubMed]
52. Ludvigsson, J.F.; Elfstrom, P.; Broome, U.; Ekbom, A.; Montgomery, S.M. Celiac disease and risk of liver disease: A general population-based study. *Clin. Gastroenterol. Hepatol.* **2007**, *5*, 63–69. [CrossRef] [PubMed]
53. Peters, U.; Askling, J.; Gridley, G.; Ekbom, A.; Linet, M. Causes of death in patients with celiac disease in a population-based Swedish cohort. *Arch. Intern. Med.* **2003**, *163*, 1566–1572. [CrossRef] [PubMed]
54. Vancikova, Z.; Chlumecky, V.; Sokol, D.; Horakova, D.; Hamsikova, E.; Fucikova, T.; Janatkova, I.; Ulcova-Gallova, Z.; Stepan, J.; Limanova, Z.; et al. The serologic screening for celiac disease in the general population (blood donors) and in some high-risk groups of adults (patients with autoimmune diseases, osteoporosis and infertility) in the Czech Republic. *Folia Microbiol.* **2002**, *47*, 753–758. [CrossRef]
55. Maggiore, G.; Caprai, S. The liver in celiac disease. *J. Pediatr. Gastroenterol. Nutr.* **2003**, *37*, 117–119. [CrossRef] [PubMed]
56. Volta, U.; De Franceschi, L.; Lari, F.; Molinaro, N.; Zoli, M.; Bianchi, F.B. Coeliac disease hidden by cryptogenic hypertransaminasaemia. *Lancet* **1998**, *352*, 26–29. [CrossRef]
57. Bardella, M.T.; Fraquelli, M.; Quatrini, M.; Molteni, N.; Bianchi, P.; Conte, D. Prevalence of hypertransaminasemia in adult celiac patients and effect of gluten-free diet. *Hepatology* **1995**, *22*, 833–836. [PubMed]
58. Kaukinen, K.; Halme, L.; Collin, P.; Farkkila, M.; Maki, M.; Vehmanen, P.; Partanen, J.; Hockerstedt, K. Celiac disease in patients with severe liver disease: Gluten-free diet may reverse hepatic failure. *Gastroenterology* **2002**, *122*, 881–888. [CrossRef] [PubMed]
59. Rubio-Tapia, A.; Murray, J.A. The liver in celiac disease. *Hepatology* **2007**, *46*, 1650–1658. [CrossRef] [PubMed]
60. Stevens, F.M.; McLoughlin, R.M. Is coeliac disease a potentially treatable cause of liver failure? *Eur. J. Gastroenterol. Hepatol.* **2005**, *17*, 1015–1017. [CrossRef] [PubMed]
61. Ecevit, C.; Karakoyun, M.; Unal, F.; Yuksekkaya, H.A.; Doganavsargil, B.; Yagci, R.V.; Aydogdu, S. An autoimmune disease refractory to immunosuppressive regimens: Celiac disease diagnosed long after liver transplantation. *Pediatr. Transpl.* **2013**, *17*, E156–E160. [CrossRef] [PubMed]
62. Casswall, T.H.; Papadogiannakis, N.; Ghazi, S.; Nemeth, A. Severe liver damage associated with celiac disease: Findings in six toddler-aged girls. *Eur. J. Gastroenterol. Hepatol.* **2009**, *21*, 452–459. [CrossRef] [PubMed]
63. Majumdar, K.; Sakhuja, P.; Puri, A.S.; Gaur, K.; Haider, A.; Gondal, R. Coeliac disease and the liver: spectrum of liver histology, serology and treatment response at a tertiary referral centre. *J. Clin. Pathol.* **2018**, *71*, 412–419. [CrossRef] [PubMed]

64. Rubio-Tapia, A.; Rahim, M.W.; See, J.A.; Lahr, B.D.; Wu, T.-T.; Murray, J.A. Mucosal recovery and mortality in adults with celiac disease after treatment with a gluten-free diet. *Am. J. Gastroenterol.* **2010**, *105*, 1412–1420. [CrossRef] [PubMed]

65. Newnham, E.D.; Shepherd, S.J.; Strauss, B.J.; Hosking, P.; Gibson, P.R. Adherence to the gluten-free diet can achieve the therapeutic goals in almost all patients with coeliac disease: A 5-year longitudinal study from diagnosis. *J. Gastroenterol. Hepatol.* **2016**, *31*, 342–349. [CrossRef] [PubMed]

66. Dickey, W.; McMillan, S.A.; Collins, J.S.; Watson, R.G.; McLoughlin, J.C.; Love, A.H. Liver abnormalities associated with celiac sprue. How common are they, what is their significance, and what do we do about them? *J. Clin. Gastroenterol.* **1995**, *20*, 290–292. [CrossRef] [PubMed]

67. Korpimaki, S.; Kaukinen, K.; Collin, P.; Haapala, A.-M.; Holm, P.; Laurila, K.; Kurppa, K.; Saavalainen, P.; Haimila, K.; Partanen, J.; et al. Gluten-sensitive hypertransaminasemia in celiac disease: An infrequent and often subclinical finding. *Am. J. Gastroenterol.* **2011**, *106*, 1689–1696. [CrossRef] [PubMed]

68. Rubio-Tapia, A.; Murray, J.A. Celiac disease beyond the gut. *Clin. Gastroenterol. Hepatol.* **2008**, *6*, 722–723. [CrossRef] [PubMed]

69. Marciano, F.; Savoia, M.; Vajro, P. Celiac disease-related hepatic injury: Insights into associated conditions and underlying pathomechanisms. *Dig. Liver Dis.* **2016**, *48*, 112–119. [CrossRef] [PubMed]

70. Nastasio, S.; Sciveres, M.; Riva, S.; Filippeschi, I.P.; Vajro, P.; Maggiore, G. Celiac disease-associated autoimmune hepatitis in childhood: Long-term response to treatment. *J. Pediatr. Gastroenterol. Nutr.* **2013**, *56*, 671–674. [CrossRef] [PubMed]

71. Di Biase, A.R.; Colecchia, A.; Scaioli, E.; Berri, R.; Viola, L.; Vestito, A.; Balli, F.; Festi, D. Autoimmune liver diseases in a paediatric population with coeliac disease—A 10-year single-centre experience. *Aliment. Pharmacol. Ther.* **2010**, *31*, 253–260. [PubMed]

72. Caprai, S.; Vajro, P.; Ventura, A.; Sciveres, M.; Maggiore, G. Autoimmune liver disease associated with celiac disease in childhood: A multicenter study. *Clin. Gastroenterol. Hepatol.* **2008**, *6*, 803–806. [CrossRef] [PubMed]

73. Ricano-Ponce, I.; Wijmenga, C.; Gutierrez-Achury, J. Genetics of celiac disease. *Best Pract. Res. Clin. Gastroenterol.* **2015**, *29*, 399–412. [CrossRef] [PubMed]

74. Williamson, K.D.; Chapman, R.W. Primary sclerosing cholangitis: A clinical update. *Br. Med. Bull.* **2015**, *114*, 53–64. [CrossRef] [PubMed]

75. Catassi, C.; Alaedini, A.; Bojarski, C.; Bonaz, B.; Bouma, G.; Carroccio, A.; Castillejo, G.; de Magistris, L.; Dieterich, W.; Di Liberto, D.; et al. The Overlapping Area of Non-Celiac Gluten Sensitivity (NCGS) and Wheat-Sensitive Irritable Bowel Syndrome (IBS): An Update. *Nutrients* **2017**, *9*, 1268. [CrossRef] [PubMed]

76. Araujo, A.R.; Rosso, N.; Bedogni, G.; Tiribelli, C.; Bellentani, S. Global epidemiology of non-alcoholic fatty liver disease/non-alcoholic steatohepatitis: What we need in the future. *Liver Int.* **2018**, *38* (Suppl. 1), 47–51. [CrossRef] [PubMed]

77. Reilly, N.R.; Lebwohl, B.; Hultcrantz, R.; Green, P.H.R.; Ludvigsson, J.F. Increased risk of non-alcoholic fatty liver disease after diagnosis of celiac disease. *J. Hepatol.* **2015**, *62*, 1405–1411. [CrossRef] [PubMed]

78. Abenavoli, L.; Milic, N.; de Lorenzo, A.; Luzza, F. A pathogenetic link between non-alcoholic fatty liver disease and celiac disease. *Endocrine* **2013**, *43*, 65–67. [CrossRef] [PubMed]

79. Barone, M.; Della Valle, N.; Rosania, R.; Facciorusso, A.; Trotta, A.; Cantatore, F.P.; Falco, S.; Pignatiello, S.; Viggiani, M.T.; Amoruso, A.; et al. A comparison of the nutritional status between adult celiac patients on a long-term, strictly gluten-free diet and healthy subjects. *Eur. J. Clin. Nutr.* **2016**, *70*, 23–27. [CrossRef] [PubMed]

80. Marra, F.; Svegliati-Baroni, G. Lipotoxicity and the gut–liver axis in NASH pathogenesis. *J. Hepatol.* **2018**, *68*, 280–295. [CrossRef] [PubMed]

81. Hendy, O.M.; Elsabaawy, M.M.; Aref, M.M.; Khalaf, F.M.; Oda, A.M.A.; El Shazly, H.M. Evaluation of circulating zonulin as a potential marker in the pathogenesis of nonalcoholic fatty liver disease. *APMIS* **2017**, *125*, 607–613. [CrossRef] [PubMed]

82. Pacifico, L.; Bonci, E.; Marandola, L.; Romaggioli, S.; Bascetta, S.; Chiesa, C. Increased circulating zonulin in children with biopsy-proven nonalcoholic fatty liver disease. *World J. Gastroenterol.* **2014**, *20*, 17107–17114. [CrossRef] [PubMed]

83. Bjorndal, B.; Alteras, E.K.; Lindquist, C.; Svardal, A.; Skorve, J.; Berge, R.K. Associations between fatty acid oxidation, hepatic mitochondrial function, and plasma acylcarnitine levels in mice. *Nutr. Metab.* **2018**, *15*, 10. [CrossRef] [PubMed]

84. Gaur, K.; Sakhuja, P.; Puri, A.S.; Majumdar, K. Gluten-Free hepatomiracle in "celiac hepatitis": A case highlighting the rare occurrence of nutrition-induced near total reversal of advanced steatohepatitis and cirrhosis. *Saudi J. Gastroenterol.* **2016**, *22*, 461–464. [PubMed]

85. Newnham, E.D. Coeliac disease in the 21st century: Paradigm shifts in the modern age. *J. Gastroenterol. Hepatol.* **2017**, *32* (Suppl. 1), 82–85. [CrossRef] [PubMed]

86. Parzanese, I.; Qehajaj, D.; Patrinicola, F.; Aralica, M.; Chiriva-Internati, M.; Stifter, S.; Elli, L.; Grizzi, F. Celiac disease: From pathophysiology to treatment. *World J. Gastrointest. Pathophysiol.* **2017**, *8*, 27–38. [CrossRef] [PubMed]

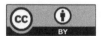

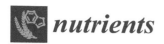

Review

Extraintestinal Manifestations of Celiac Disease: Early Detection for Better Long-Term Outcomes

Pilvi Laurikka [1,2], Samuli Nurminen [3], Laura Kivelä [3] and Kalle Kurppa [3,*]

1   Celiac Disease Research Center, Faculty of Medicine and Life Sciences, University of Tampere, 33014 Tampere, Finland; laurikka.pilvi.l@student.uta.fi
2   Department of Internal Medicine, Hospital District of South Ostrobothnia, 60200 Seinäjoki, Finland
3   Tampere Center for Child Health Research, Tampere University Hospital and University of Tampere, 33014 Tampere, Finland; nurminen.samuli.j@student.uta.fi (S.N.); laura.kivela@fimnet.fi (L.K.)
*   Correspondence: kalle.kurppa@uta.fi; Tel.: +358-50-318-6316

Received: 1 July 2018; Accepted: 31 July 2018; Published: 3 August 2018

Abstract: Population-based screening studies have shown celiac disease to be one of the most common chronic gastrointestinal diseases. Nevertheless, because of the diverse clinical presentation, the great majority of patients remain unrecognized. Particularly difficult to identify are the multifaceted extraintestinal symptoms that may appear at variable ages. Although the pathogenesis and long-term outcome of these manifestations are still poorly established, there is some evidence that unrecognized celiac disease predisposes to severe complications if not diagnosed and prevented with an early-initiated gluten-free diet. Therefore, it is of utmost importance that physicians of different disciplines learn to recognize celiac disease in individuals with non-gastrointestinal symptoms. In the future, more studies are needed to clarify the factors affecting development and prognosis of the extraintestinal manifestations.

Keywords: celiac disease; extraintestinal; recognition; diagnosis; clinical presentation; gluten-free diet; prognosis

1. Introduction

During the past few decades, we have come to recognize that celiac disease is among the most common gastrointestinal diseases, both in children and adults. The true prevalence of the disease in many Western countries is estimated to be as high as 1–3% and is increasing [1]. At the same time, modern sensitive and specific transglutaminase 2 (TG2) antibody based serological tests have made non-invasive case finding and screening of celiac disease considerably easier. In theory, the simplified diagnostics should have also increased the proportion of clinically detected cases, and this has indeed been the case in some, particularly Northern European, countries [2,3]. However, even in these areas, let alone globally, celiac disease remains seriously underdiagnosed. For example, it is estimated that in the United States, more than 90% of all affected patients are unrecognized [4]. It must also be emphasized that, instead of clinical case finding, a substantial proportion of patients in the aforesaid countries are found by at-risk group screening [5].

The evident difficulty in identifying celiac disease may be explained by in part by the heterogeneous and often vague clinical presentations. While the characteristic malabsorptive disease and gastrointestinal symptoms are relatively well known, the majority of celiac disease patients may in fact suffer from extraintestinal manifestations. These may affect almost every organ of the body, including the nervous system, liver, skin, and reproductive and musculoskeletal system [6–9]. Furthermore, some of these manifestations appear in early childhood, while the rest are not seen until adulthood, including in the elderly. Although evidence is limited, some extraintestinal presentations may lead to permanent complications if not recognized and treated early enough.

Therefore, extraintestinal celiac disease needs to be recognized by physicians of various specialities, including gastroenterologists, internists, pediatricians, neurologists, dermatologists, gynecologists, and particularly general practitioners and family doctors.

In this review, we will provide an overview about current understanding of the pathogenesis and age-related clinical outcomes of the variable extraintestinal manifestations of celiac disease. In particular, we aim to improve the early recognition and diagnostic yield of this multifaceted condition, and subsequently reduce the risk of ill health and long-term complications.

2. Changes in Clinical Presentation

Celiac disease was long considered as a rare malabsorptive disease affecting mainly infants and toddlers. Classical symptoms included failure to thrive, chronic diarrhea, and abdominal distention. In the 1970s, the incidence of 'typical' celiac disease patients seemed to decrease and concurrently, older patients with milder symptoms were identified. When screening for celiac disease with sensitive and specific endomysium and transglutaminase antibodies from serum became possible in the 1980s and 1990s, respectively, the high prevalence and wide clinical presentation of celiac disease started to become evident [5,10].

Gastrointestinal related symptoms and signs such as anemia, impaired growth, decreased bone mineral density, and micronutrient deficiencies were recognized from early on to be associated with untreated celiac disease. Although these were initially thought to be present only in connection with malabsorption, it was later understood that they could also be a sole manifestation [11–13]. Dermatitis herpetiformis was among the first extra-intestinal symptoms of celiac disease recognized [14]. Later, other organ systems were found to be affected, when, for example, patients with earlier unexplained neurological and articular symptoms were diagnosed. In addition, as a result of the increased screening, the symptoms common in the general population, such as headache and tiredness, were often recognized in celiac disease patients. However, their true association to the disease and especially the response to the dietary treatment remains controversial [15]. Altogether, it is important to remember the unspecificity and complexity of the above-mentioned symptoms, as they may be present also in many other common disorders, such as irritable bowel syndrome (IBS), chronic fatigue syndrome, and migraine.

3. Variable Definitions for Symptoms and Findings

Clinical features of celiac disease are often classified categorically as 'typical' and 'atypical'. However, the definition for these terms is heterogeneous, which likely reflects the above-described historical background. Extra-intestinal manifestations are particularly difficult to classify, even though they may actually be even more common than the 'typical' symptoms. Consequently, a few years ago, a group of experts encouraged the alternate terminology of 'classical' and 'non-classical' celiac disease [16].

Another challenge in celiac disease is to discriminate the symptoms from the complications and from the independently associated diseases. Celiac disease symptoms should be reversible with the gluten free diet, whereas complications may be permanent and irreversible, especially if the initiation of treatment is delayed (Figure 1). Well-known associated conditions with an increased risk for celiac disease are for example type 1 diabetes, autoimmune thyroidal disease, and Down's syndrome [17]. Whether the early diagnosis and treatment of celiac disease could prevent some of these conditions has been debated [18,19]. Again, these conditions should not be confused with totally unrelated disorders with often overlapping symptoms, such as IBS.

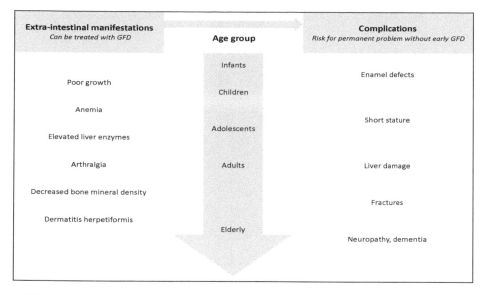

Figure 1. Extra-intestinal manifestations and complications of celiac disease classified based on their response to early initiated gluten-free diet (GFD) and typical age of development.

4. Epidemiology and Pathogenesis of Extraintestinal Manifestations

Although the existence of extraintestinal manifestations in celiac disease has been known for decades, their prevalence remains poorly established. This issue is complicated by the variable definitions and considerable age-related variations in the appearance of these symptoms (Table 1). For example, poor growth and delayed puberty are evidently exclusively pediatric presentations, whereas osteoporosis, infertility, and dermatitis herpetiformis are typical adulthood findings. Anemia, liver abnormalities, and joint problems are seen in both pediatric and adult patients (Table 1). Although celiac disease is known to be more common in females, the gender distribution of the extraintestinal symptoms is currently mostly obscure [20].

The pathogenesis of most extraintestinal manifestations is also obscure. There is some evidence that their presence is associated with an overall more severe clinical and histological presentation [20], but neither the appearance nor severity seems to be just a direct consequence of intestinal damage [21–26]. Another intriguing question is the balance between genetic and environmental factors, as even identical twins with celiac disease may have completely different phenotype [27]. The at least partially different pathogenic background of the variable presentations of celiac disease is further supported by the peculiar appearance of serological markers in some of these conditions [6,22,24]. The clinical features and plausible pathophysiological mechanisms of the best-characterized extraintestinal manifestations are further discussed below.

Table 1. Prevalence of the best-characterized extraintestinal manifestations of untreated celiac disease in children and adults.

	Children	Adults	
	%	%	References
Poor growth [1]	11–70	-	[20,28,29]
Short stature [1]	4–33	3	[15,30–33]
Anemia	12–40	23–48	[12,15,20,28,30,32–34]
Neurological symptoms	4–52	24	[15,20,28,29,31]
Enamel defects	0–15	1–83	[20,29,32,33,35,36]
Liver abnormalities	1–57	2–5	[8,15,32]
Joint manifestations	1–10	2–9	[15,20,29,30,32,33]
Dermatitis herpetiformis	2–3	10–20	[20,30,32,37]
Osteoporosis	0	4–23	[15,32]
Infertility	-	5	[9,15]

[1] Definitions of poor growth and short stature have varied between the studies.

4.1. Poor Growth

Poor growth is likely one of the most common extraintestinal manifestations in pediatric celiac disease, although defining its true prevalence is complicated by its variable definitions (Table 1). We recently observed that impaired growth might be particularly common in children with a younger age at diagnosis and a more severe overall presentation of the disease [11]. For example, the malabsorption of nutrients and abnormalities in growth hormone-insulin-like growth factor axis and/or in thyroid function have been suggested as pathogenic mechanisms [26,38,39], but further studies are needed to confirm these findings.

4.2. Anemia

Anemia is a common extraintestinal manifestation of untreated celiac disease in all age groups (Table 1). Like poor growth, the presence of anemia seems to be associated with a more severe disease presentation [12,34]. Its prevalence could be expected to decrease over time as a result of an earlier diagnosis and the generally improved nutritional status of children. Regardless, celiac disease is still increasingly found in subjects with unexplained anemia [5]. With regards to pathogenesis, malabsorption/deficiencies of iron, vitamin B12, and folic acid may be implicated [40]. However, the etiology of anemia in celiac disease might be more complex, as it may be present in autoantibody positive individuals even before the development of enteropathy [41].

4.3. Neurologic Manifestations

Approximately one-fifth of celiac disease patients suffer from neurological manifestations (Table 1). The most common of these are gluten ataxia and peripheral neuropathy [42], which often present without accompanying gastrointestinal symptoms [43]. The pathogenesis of neurological manifestations is still somewhat obscure. In gluten ataxia, gluten-dependent transglutaminase 6 (TG6) autoantibodies targeted against the cerebellar cells may play a role and might be useful in the diagnostics of this condition [6,22]. However, TG6 antibodies have also been detected in children with celiac disease without association to neurological symptoms [23]. It remains to be proven whether this could predict the later adult onset of neurological symptoms.

4.4. Dental Enamel Defects

Disturbances in the amelogenesis of permanent teeth is a well-defined finding in celiac disease, but there are considerable variations in its reported prevalence (Table 1). Enamel defects have been particularly common in older studies together with severe infant celiac disease and lower general health [36]. It is possible that this manifestation is disappearing as, for example, is rickets related to celiac disease. However, for an accurate diagnosis the dental enamel should be evaluated by an expert dentist. Malnutrition, hypocalcemia, and immunologic disturbances have been suggested as causative factors of enamel defects [35], and the severity seems to be associated with the duration of gluten-exposure [44].

4.5. Liver Abnormalities

Prevalence of hypertransaminasemia has been reported in older studies up to 57%, while more recent studies report only 9–14% (Table 1), possibly again reflecting earlier diagnosis and milder presentation of celiac disease. Usually the hepatic injury is mild and easily reversible, but in rare occasions, celiac disease may lead even to liver failure [45]. The severity of hypertransaminasemia seems to be associated with the presence of malabsorption, high values of celiac autoantibodies, and advanced duodenal lesion [8,46], and the suggested mechanisms include altered gut permeability leading to an increased exposure to hepatotoxins in the portal circulation [47]. Interestingly, TG2 autoantibody deposits have been found in liver biopsies from affected patients and could contribute to the hepatocellular damage [21]. It is also important to keep in mind that celiac patients have overrepresentation of coexisting liver diseases such as autoimmune hepatitis, primary biliary cholangitis, and primary sclerosing cholangitis [48].

4.6. Joint Manifestations

Variable joint symptoms are quite often, although again inconsistently, reported in celiac disease (Table 1). The observed symptoms are usually described vaguely as arthralgia rather than objective synovitis [20,49]. However, subclinical synovial effusion and sacroiliitis have also been reported [50–52]. Differential diagnosis is challenging and includes, for example, growing pains in children and variable musculoskeletal complaints and arthrosis in adults. Once again, it should be remembered that celiac disease is associated with many autoimmune conditions, including rheumatologic diseases such as Sjögren's syndrome [53], juvenile rheumatoid/idiopathic arthritis [54], and systemic lupus erythematosus [55]. At present, the pathogenesis of the joint symptoms in celiac disease remains entirely speculative.

4.7. Dermatitis Herpetiformis

Dermatitis herpetiformis is a dermatological manifestation of celiac disease that usually appears in adulthood (Table 1). The characteristic itching and blistering rash appears mostly on elbows, knees, and buttocks. In contrast to intestinal celiac disease, dermatitis herpetiformis is more common in males than females [7]. The diagnosis is based on skin biopsy showing characteristic IgA deposits in the papillary dermis next to the lesion [56]. Interestingly, besides TG2, dermatitis herpetiformis patients can also develop autoantibodies targeted against epidermal transglutaminase 3 [24]. Even though the characteristic rash is the primary manifestation, up to 72% of the patients also have enteropathy [57]. Interestingly, the incidence of dermatitis herpetiformis seems to be decreasing in contrast to other forms of celiac disease [7]. Furthermore, 'classical' celiac disease patients with poor dietary adherence can change their phenotype to dermatitis herpetiformis over time [58].

4.8. Bone Disease

Rickets is a classical finding in children with celiac disease, but it is nowadays rarely seen in developed countries. On the contrary, osteoporosis is common in adult celiac disease patients (Table 1), particularly in elderly patients and in postmenopausal women. The malabsorption of calcium and vitamin D may lead to secondary hyperparathyroidism and subsequently a high bone turnover and osteoporosis [59]. Increasing the circulating cytokines and an altered balance of bone turnover have also been suggested to play a role [60,61]. Neutralizing autoantibodies against osteoprotegerin have been detected in celiac disease patients [25], but their true role in the development of osteoporosis remains contradictory [62]. Decreased bone mineral density can also be seen in screen-detected patients [63], even before the development of enteropathy [64]. These observations emphasize the importance of early diagnosis of celiac disease to prevent advanced bone disease and subsequent fractures.

4.9. Problems in Reproductive and Endocrine Systems

Delayed puberty can be observed in children with untreated celiac disease [15,32], and various problems in reproductive health, such as infertility, recurrent miscarriages, and intrauterine growth restriction, have been reported in adult female patients [9,15]. The pathogenesis of delayed puberty in celiac disease is unknown, although it is a common finding also in many other chronic diseases during adolescence. However, there are several hypotheses for the pathogenesis of reproductive system's maladies. Untreated celiac disease may lead to deficiencies of micronutrients such as zinc, selenium, and folic acid which are important during pregnancy and fetal development, anemia may also have a role [9]. Celiac disease may affect other hormonal systems, for example, TG2 autoantibodies are able to bind to TG2 in thyroid tissue and the celiac autoantibody titers have been shown to correlate with the antithyroperoxidase antibody titers [65]. However, this should not be confused with the overrepresentation of celiac disease among children with autoimmune thyroid disease due to a shared genetic background [66].

4.10. Other Extraintestinal Manifestations

Besides the above-mentioned, several other extraintestinal manifestations have been suggested to be associated with celiac disease. Aphtous ulcers, headache, and fatigue are frequently reported but unspecific clinical findings [15,31,35]. Several neuropsychiatric conditions including learning disorders, developmental delay, and attention deficit hyperactivity disorder have also been associated with celiac disease [31], as well as are psychiatric disorders including depression, anxiety, and even schizophrenia [15,67]. In addition, there are reports about possible associations between celiac disease and uveitis, eczema, psoriasis, asthma, and various cardiovascular symptoms [68–71]. However, because of the common and non-specific nature of these conditions, a true pathogenic relationship to celiac disease requires further evidence [15,72].

5. Effects of Dietary Treatment to the Extraintestinal Manifestations

In general, a gluten-free diet is an effective treatment for celiac disease. However, the dietary response might be faster and more complete in children than in adults [73,74]. Extraintestinal manifestations also have a good prognosis in children if appropriately treated with a gluten-free diet (Table 2) [8,73,75], but in adults and in a subgroup of children, the dietary response might be incomplete [12]. In such cases, the possibility of coexisting conditions should be remembered. Dapsone medication is often needed as an additional therapy in dermatitis herpetiformis for some time [75].

A gluten-free diet has also been shown to be beneficial for more advanced extraintestinal manifestations, such as a low bone mineral density, liver failure, and infertility [9,13,46,76–78], but here, the timing of the diagnosis is crucial (Table 2). Early developing complications such as dental enamel defects should actually be treated even before their appearance [44]. In children with poor growth, a significant catch-up growth is usually achieved after the beginning of dietary treatment and thus reduced adult height is uncommon [78,79]. However, growth problems should likely be treated at latest in puberty, in order to avoid suboptimal height development [80–82]. With regards to bone health, patients diagnosed in childhood seem to have no increased risk for osteoporotic fractures [83], but again, in order to achieve optimal bone accrual, an early diagnosis is beneficial [84].

Table 2. Response of extraintestinal manifestations in celiac disease to a gluten-free diet (GFD).

Manifestation	Response	Comments	References
Anemia	Yes	Sometimes slow or incomplete response	[12,15]
Dermatitis herpetiformis	Yes	Dietary response may be slow and require additional Dapsone medication	[15,75]
Transaminasemia	Usually	Often mild and reversible; in rare cases may lead to liver failure	[8,45]
Poor growth	Variable	May lead to reduced adulthood height if not treated before puberty	[15,82]
Neurological symptoms	Variable	In children, usually good response, but in adults, possibly irreversible	[6,43]
Decreased bone mineral density	Variable	Initiation of GFD before school age may be needed for optimal bone accrual	[13,76,84]
Joint problems	Variable	Coexisting musculoskeletal disease should be excluded if poor response	[15]
Enamel defects	Infrequently	Early appearance and irreversible in permanent teeth	[44]
Infertility	Unclear	Conflicting results	[9,77,85]

Non-adherence is the most common reason for an unsatisfactory treatment response [15,73]. Nevertheless, some extraintestinal manifestations may not improve entirely despite an apparently strict diet, which may reflect their more complex etiology [15,72,73], but it is also possible that at least a part of them are in fact related to disorders other than celiac disease. Accordingly, Jericho et al. found that almost 30% of the children with a failure of catch-up growth on a gluten-free diet to have some co-existing condition [15]. Therefore, additional reasons for poor response should be sought in cases with proven adherence. True pediatric refractory celiac disease is almost non-existent and one should be very cautious before making such a diagnosis [86].

6. Importance of Early Diagnosis

As discussed, it seems that most of the advanced extraintestinal manifestations might be preventable by the early diagnosis of celiac disease. One way to increase the diagnostic yield would be screening of at-risk groups. Counterweighting this approach is the burden of a gluten-free diet, which is challenging to maintain, socially restrictive, and expensive. This may lead to reduced quality of life particularly in patients with negligible symptoms. There is, however, some evidence that even apparently asymptomatic adults may already have advanced histological disease and benefit from the diet [63,87]. Furthermore, a long diagnostic delay may increase the risk of poor clinical response [73,88,89]. This issue is less well defined in screen-detected children, but there is data showing that they may also experience unrecognized symptoms, including extraintestinal manifestations [90,91], and benefit from an early diagnosis [91–94].

An unsolved question is that a part of screened individuals may have a so-called potential celiac disease with positive celiac autoantibodies but normal villi, and thus do not fulfil the current diagnostic criteria [95]. This might be an early stage of developing celiac disease, but at present, more evidence about the natural history of this condition is warranted [96].

Population-based mass screening would be a very effective approach to finding unrecognized celiac patients, but is currently not recommended because of the lack of scientific evidence [95,97,98]. Major open questions concerning such a wide-scale screening are the above-mentioned challenges in the diagnostics of patients with early or potential celiac disease, and the balance of the benefits and harms of the treatment for asymptomatic patients. Furthermore, the cost-effectiveness of screening is particularly important in these circumstances, but, unfortunately, this issue is currently very scarcely studied.

All in all, the current recommendations about screening for celiac disease have been varying between countries and between children and adults [95,98,99]. However, most organizations recommend a targeted at-risk group screening, this usually including first-degree relatives of celiac disease patients and those suffering from type 1 diabetes [95,99]. Meanwhile, before further evidence about screening is provided, active case finding is especially important. By carrying this out efficiently, at least part a of the patients with extraintestinal manifestations could be diagnosed before appearance of permanent complications.

7. Conclusions

In recent years, we have witnessed an upsurge of interest towards different gluten-related conditions, demonstrated, for example, by the rapid increase of the popularity of self-adopted gluten-free lifestyle. This notwithstanding, the clinical prevalence of officially diagnosed celiac disease, is all but satisfactory. This is worrisome, as the condition is proven to be associated with an increased risk of long-term complications that could very likely be prevented by timely diagnosis and initiation of a gluten-free diet.

As wide-scale serological screening is currently not recommended, we should aim to improve the physicians' and other allied health professionals' knowledge of the diverse presentations of celiac disease. For pediatricians, this especially means the identification of the manifestations that can present already at early childhood and may lead to permanent problems if undetected. Then again, many extraintestinal symptoms may appear later in life and should thus be known by physicians of relevant adult subspecialties. It is important to acknowledge the critical role of primary healthcare in these circumstances, as only effective first-line case finding can lessen the ill-health caused by untreated celiac disease at the population level. Therefore, we should educate particularly the primary care providers, in order to understand the value of the early detection of this multifaceted condition.

In the future, we need more information on the prevalence, age of appearance, dietary response, and long-term prognosis of the variable extraintestinal features of celiac disease. Moreover, at present, the details of the pathogenesis and reasons for the substantial phenotype heterogeneity in celiac disease remain mostly obscure. This information could, besides improving the diagnostics of celiac disease, also provide novel insight of the development of autoimmune diseases in general.

Author Contributions: Writing (original draft preparation), P.L., S.N., and L.K.; writing (review and editing), K.K. All of the authors have accepted the final version of the manuscript.

Funding: This research received no external funding.

Conflicts of Interest: The authors declare no conflict of interest.

References

1. Singh, P.; Arora, A.; Strand, T.A.; Leffler, D.A.; Catassi, C.; Green, P.H.; Kelly, C.P.; Ahuja, V.; Makharia, G.K. Global prevalence of celiac disease: Systematic review and meta-analysis. *Clin. Gastroenterol. Hepatol.* **2018**, *16*, 823–836. [CrossRef] [PubMed]
2. Virta, L.J.; Kaukinen, K.; Collin, P. Incidence and prevalence of diagnosed coeliac disease in Finland: Results of effective case finding in adults. *Scand. J. Gastroenterol.* **2009**, *44*, 933–938. [CrossRef] [PubMed]
3. Mårild, K.; Kahrs, C.R.; Tapia, G.; Stene, L.C.; Størdal, K. Infections and risk of celiac disease in childhood: A prospective nationwide cohort study. *Am. J. Gastroenterol.* **2015**, *110*, 1475–1484. [CrossRef] [PubMed]
4. Liu, E.; Dong, F.; Barón, A.E.; Taki, I.; Norris, J.M.; Frohnert, B.I.; Hoffenberg, E.J.; Rewers, M. High incidence of celiac disease in a long-term study of adolescents with susceptibility genotypes. *Gastroenterology* **2017**, *152*, 1329–1336. [CrossRef] [PubMed]

5. Kivelä, L.; Kaukinen, K.; Lähdeaho, M.-L.; Huhtala, H.; Ashorn, M.; Ruuska, T.; Hiltunen, P.; Visakorpi, J.; Mäki, M.; Kurppa, K. Presentation of celiac disease in Finnish children is no longer changing: A 50-year perspective. *J. Pediatr.* **2015**, *167*, 1109–1115. [CrossRef] [PubMed]
6. Hadjivassiliou, M.; Mäki, M.; Sanders, D.S.; Williamson, C.A.; Grünewald, R.A.; Woodroofe, N.M.; Korponay-Szabó, I.R. Autoantibody targeting of brain and intestinal transglutaminase in gluten ataxia. *Neurology* **2006**, *66*, 373–377. [CrossRef] [PubMed]
7. Salmi, T.T.; Hervonen, K.; Kautiainen, H.; Collin, P.; Reunala, T. Prevalence and incidence of dermatitis herpetiformis: A 40-year prospective study from Finland. *Br. J. Dermatol.* **2011**, *165*, 354–359. [CrossRef] [PubMed]
8. Äärelä, L.; Nurminen, S.; Kivelä, L.; Huhtala, H.; Mäki, M.; Viitasalo, A.; Kaukinen, K.; Lakka, T.; Kurppa, K. Prevalence and associated factors of abnormal liver values in children with celiac disease. *Dig. Liver Dis.* **2016**, *48*, 1023–1029. [CrossRef] [PubMed]
9. Tersigni, C.; Castellani, R.; De Waure, C.; Fattorossi, A.; De Spirito, M.; Gasbarrini, A.; Scambia, G.; Di Simone, N. Celiac disease and reproductive disorders: Meta-analysis of epidemiologic associations and potential pathogenic mechanisms. *Hum. Reprod. Update* **2014**, *20*, 582–593. [CrossRef] [PubMed]
10. McGowan, K.E.; Castiglione, D.A.; Butzner, J.D. The changing face of childhood celiac disease in North America: Impact of serological testing. *Pediatrics* **2009**, *124*, 1572–1578. [CrossRef] [PubMed]
11. Nurminen, S.; Kivelä, L.; Taavela, J.; Huhtala, H.; Mäki, M.; Kaukinen, K.; Kurppa, K. Factors associated with growth disturbance at celiac disease diagnosis in children: A retrospective cohort study. *BMC Gastroenterol.* **2015**, *15*, 125. [CrossRef] [PubMed]
12. Rajalahti, T.; Repo, M.; Kivelä, L.; Huhtala, H.; Mäki, M.; Kaukinen, K.; Lindfors, K.; Kurppa, K. Anemia in pediatric celiac disease: Association with clinical and histological features and response to gluten-free diet. *J. Pediatr. Gastroenterol. Nutr.* **2017**, *64*, e1–e6. [CrossRef] [PubMed]
13. Björck, S.; Brundin, C.; Karlsson, M.; Agardh, D. Reduced bone mineral density in children with screening-detected celiac disease. *J. Pediatr. Gastroenterol. Nutr.* **2017**, *65*, 526–532. [CrossRef] [PubMed]
14. Weinstein, W.; Brow, J.; Parker, F.; Rubin, C. The small intestinal mucosa in dermatitis herpetiformis. *Gastroenterology* **1971**, *60*, 362–369. [PubMed]
15. Jericho, H.; Sansotta, N.; Guandalini, S. Extraintestinal manifestations of celiac disease: Effectiveness of the gluten-free diet. *J. Pediatr. Gastroenterol. Nutr.* **2017**, *65*, 75–79. [CrossRef] [PubMed]
16. Ludvigsson, J.F.; Leffler, D.A.; Bai, J.C.; Biagi, F.; Fasano, A.; Green, P.H.R.; Hadjivassiliou, M.; Kaukinen, K.; Kelly, C.P.; Leonard, J.N.; et al. The Oslo definitions for coeliac disease and related terms. *Gut* **2013**, *62*, 43–52. [CrossRef] [PubMed]
17. Elli, L.; Bonura, A.; Garavaglia, D.; Rulli, E.; Floriani, I.; Tagliabue, G.; Contiero, P.; Bardella, M.T. Immunological comorbity in coeliac disease: Associations, risk factors and clinical implications. *J. Clin. Immunol.* **2012**, *32*, 984–990. [CrossRef] [PubMed]
18. Sategna Guidetti, C.; Solerio, E.; Scaglione, N.; Aimo, G.; Mengozzi, G. Duration of gluten exposure in adult coeliac disease does not correlate with the risk for autoimmune disorders. *Gut* **2001**, *49*, 502–505. [CrossRef] [PubMed]
19. Ventura, A.; Magazzù, G.; Greco, L. Duration of exposure to gluten and risk for autoimmune disorders in patients with celiac disease. SIGEP Study Group for Autoimmune Disorders in Celiac Disease. *Gastroenterology* **1999**, *117*, 297–303. [CrossRef] [PubMed]
20. Nurminen, S.; Kivelä, L.; Huhtala, H.; Kaukinen, K.; Kurppa, K. Extraintestinal manifestations were common in children with celiac disease and were more prevalent in patients with more severe clinical and histological presentation. *Acta Paediatr.* **2018**. [CrossRef] [PubMed]
21. Korponay-Szabó, I.R.; Halttunen, T.; Szalai, Z.; Laurila, K.; Király, R.; Kovács, J.B.; Fésüs, L.; Mäki, M. In vivo targeting of intestinal and extraintestinal transglutaminase 2 by coeliac autoantibodies. *Gut* **2004**, *53*, 641–648. [CrossRef] [PubMed]
22. Hadjivassiliou, M.; Aeschlimann, P.; Sanders, D.S.; Mäki, M.; Kaukinen, K.; Grünewald, R.A.; Bandmann, O.; Woodroofe, N.; Haddock, G.; Aeschlimann, D.P. Transglutaminase 6 antibodies in the diagnosis of gluten ataxia. *Neurology* **2013**, *80*, 1740–1745. [CrossRef] [PubMed]

23. De Leo, L.; Aeschlimann, D.; Hadjivassiliou, M.; Aeschlimann, P.; Salce, N.; Vatta, S.; Ziberna, F.; Cozzi, G.; Martelossi, S.; Ventura, A.; et al. Anti-transglutaminase 6 antibody development in children with celiac disease correlates with duration of gluten exposure. *J. Pediatr. Gastroenterol. Nutr.* **2018**, *66*, 64–68. [CrossRef] [PubMed]

24. Sárdy, M.; Kárpáti, S.; Merkl, B.; Paulsson, M.; Smyth, N. Epidermal transglutaminase (TGase 3) is the autoantigen of dermatitis herpetiformis. *J. Exp. Med.* **2002**, *195*, 747–757. [CrossRef] [PubMed]

25. Riches, P.L.; McRorie, E.; Fraser, W.D.; Determann, C.; van't Hof, R.; Ralston, S.H. Osteoporosis associated with neutralizing autoantibodies against osteoprotegerin. *N. Engl. J. Med.* **2009**, *361*, 1459–1465. [CrossRef] [PubMed]

26. Street, M.E.; Volta, C.; Ziveri, M.A.; Zanacca, C.; Banchini, G.; Viani, I.; Rossi, M.; Virdis, R.; Bernasconi, S. Changes and relationships of IGFS and IGFBPS and cytokines in coeliac disease at diagnosis and on gluten-free diet. *Clin. Endocrinol. (Oxf.)* **2008**, *68*, 22–28. [CrossRef] [PubMed]

27. Hervonen, K.; Karell, K.; Holopainen, P.; Collin, P.; Partanen, J.; Reunala, T. Concordance of dermatitis herpetiformis and celiac disease in monozygous twins. *J. Investig. Dermatol.* **2000**, *115*, 990–993. [CrossRef] [PubMed]

28. Savilahti, E.; Kolho, K.L.; Westerholm-Ormio, M.; Verkasalo, M. Clinics of coeliac disease in children in the 2000s. *Acta Paediatr. Int. J. Paediatr.* **2010**, *99*, 1026–1030. [CrossRef] [PubMed]

29. Rashid, M. Celiac Disease: Evaluation of the diagnosis and dietary compliance in Canadian children. *Pediatrics* **2005**, *116*, e754–e759. [CrossRef] [PubMed]

30. Roma, E.; Panayiotou, J.; Karantana, H.; Constantinidou, C.; Siakavellas, S.I.; Krini, M.; Syriopoulou, V.P.; Bamias, G. Changing pattern in the clinical presentation of pediatric celiac disease: A 30-year study. *Digestion* **2009**, *80*, 185–191. [CrossRef] [PubMed]

31. Zelnik, N.; Pacht, A.; Obeid, R.; Lerner, A. Range of neurologic disorders in patients with celiac disease. *Pediatrics* **2004**, *113*, 1672–1676. [CrossRef] [PubMed]

32. Bottaro, G.; Cataldo, F.; Rotolo, N.; Spina, M.; Corazza, G.R. The clinical pattern of subclinical/silent celiac disease: An analysis on 1026 consecutive cases. *Am. J. Gastroenterol.* **1999**, *94*, 691–696. [CrossRef] [PubMed]

33. Mubarak, A.; Spierings, E.; Wolters, V.M.; Otten, H.G.; ten Kate, F.J.W.; Houwen, R.H.J. Children with celiac disease and high tTGA are genetically and phenotypically different. *World J. Gastroenterol.* **2013**, *19*, 7114–7120. [CrossRef] [PubMed]

34. Abu Daya, H.; Lebwohl, B.; Lewis, S.K.; Green, P.H. Celiac disease patients presenting with anemia have more severe disease than those presenting with diarrhea. *Clin. Gastroenterol. Hepatol.* **2013**, *11*, 1472–1477. [CrossRef] [PubMed]

35. Cheng, J.; Malahias, T.; Brar, P.; Minaya, M.T.; Green, P.H.R. The Association between celiac disease, dental enamel defects, and aphthous ulcers in a United States cohort. *J. Clin. Gastroenterol.* **2010**, *44*, 191–194. [CrossRef] [PubMed]

36. Aine, L.; Maki, M.; Collin, P.; Keyrilainen, O. Dental enamel defects in celiac disease. *J. Oral Pathol. Med.* **1990**, *19*, 241–245. [CrossRef] [PubMed]

37. Green, P.H.; Stavropoulos, S.N.; Panagi, S.G.; Goldstein, S.L.; Mcmahon, D.J.; Absan, H.; Neugut, A.I. Characteristics of adult celiac disease in the USA: Results of a national survey. *Am. J. Gastroenterol.* **2001**, *96*, 126–131. [CrossRef] [PubMed]

38. Jansson, U.H.G.; Kristiansson, B.; Magnusson, P.; Larsson, L.; Albertsson-Wikland, K.; Bjarnason, R. The decrease of IGF-I, IGF-binding protein-3 and bone alkaline phosphatase isoforms during gluten challenge correlates with small intestinal inflammation in children with coeliac disease. *Eur. J. Endocrinol.* **2001**, *144*, 417–423. [CrossRef] [PubMed]

39. Ferrante, E.; Giavoli, C.; Elli, L.; Redaelli, A.; Novati, E.; De Bellis, A.; Ronchi, C.L.; Bergamaschi, S.; Lania, A.; Bardella, M.T.; et al. Evaluation of GH-IGF-I axis in adult patients with coeliac disease. *Horm. Metab. Res.* **2010**, *42*, 45–49. [CrossRef] [PubMed]

40. Wierdsma, N.; van Bokhorst-de van der Schueren, M.A.; Berkenpas, M.; Mulder, C.; van Bodegraven, A. Vitamin and mineral deficiencies are highly prevalent in newly diagnosed celiac disease patients. *Nutrients* **2013**, *5*, 3975–3992. [CrossRef] [PubMed]

41. Repo, M.; Lindfors, K.; Mäki, M.; Huhtala, H.; Laurila, K.; Lähdeaho, M.-L.; Saavalainen, P.; Kaukinen, K.; Kurppa, K. Anemia and iron deficiency in children with potential celiac disease. *J. Pediatr. Gastroenterol. Nutr.* **2017**, *64*, 56–62. [CrossRef] [PubMed]
42. Luostarinen, L.; Pirttilä, T.; Collin, P. Coeliac disease presenting with neurological disorders. *Eur. Neurol.* **1999**, *42*, 132–135. [CrossRef] [PubMed]
43. Hadjivassiliou, M.; Grünewald, R.; Sharrack, B.; Sanders, D.; Lobo, A.; Williamson, C.; Woodroofe, N.; Wood, N.; Davies-Jones, A. Gluten ataxia in perspective: Epidemiology, genetic susceptibility and clinical characteristics. *Brain* **2003**, *126*, 685–691. [CrossRef] [PubMed]
44. Majorana, A.; Bardellini, E.; Ravelli, A.; Plebani, A.; Pol, A.; Campus, G. Implications of gluten exposure period, CD clinical forms, and HLA typing in the association between celiac disease and dental enamel defects in children. A case-control study. *Int. J. Paediatr. Dent.* **2010**, *20*, 119–124. [CrossRef] [PubMed]
45. Kaukinen, K.; Halme, L.; Collin, P.; Färkkilä, M.; Mäki, M.; Vehmanen, P.; Partanen, J.; Höckerstedt, K. Celiac disease in patients with severe liver disease: Gluten-free diet may reverse hepatic failure. *Gastroenterology* **2002**, *122*, 881–888. [CrossRef] [PubMed]
46. Zanini, B.; Baschè, R.; Ferraresi, A.; Pigozzi, M.G.; Ricci, C.; Lanzarotto, F.; Villanacci, V.; Lanzini, A. Factors that contribute to hypertransaminasemia in patients with celiac disease or functional gastrointestinal syndromes. *Clin. Gastroenterol. Hepatol.* **2014**, *12*, 804–810. [CrossRef] [PubMed]
47. Novacek, G.; Miehsler, W.; Wrba, F.; Ferenci, P.; Penner, E.; Vogelsang, H. Prevalence and clinical importance of hypertransaminasaemia in coeliac disease. *Eur. J. Gastroenterol. Hepatol.* **2000**, *11*, 283–288. [CrossRef]
48. Marciano, F.; Savoia, M.; Vajro, P. Celiac disease-related hepatic injury: Insights into associated conditions and underlying pathomechanisms. *Dig. Liver Dis.* **2016**, *48*, 112–119. [CrossRef] [PubMed]
49. Daron, C.; Soubrier, M.; Mathieu, S. Occurrence of rheumatic symptoms in celiac disease: A meta-analysis: Comment on the article "Osteoarticular manifestations of celiac disease and non-celiac gluten hypersensitivity" by Dos Santos and Lioté. Joint Bone Spine 2016. *Jt. Bone Spine* **2017**, *84*, 645–646. [CrossRef] [PubMed]
50. Usai, P.; Francesa, M.; Piga, M.; Cacace, E.; Antonia Lai, M.; Beccaris, A.; Piras, E.; La Nasa, G.; Mulargia, M.; Balestrieri, A. Adult celiac disease is frequently associated with sacroiliitis. *Dig. Dis. Sci.* **1995**, *40*, 1906–1908. [CrossRef] [PubMed]
51. Lubrano, E.; Ciacci, C.; Ames, P.R.; Mazzacca, G.; Oriente, P.; Scarpa, R. The arthritis of coeliac disease: Prevalence and pattern in 200 adult patients. *Br. J. Rheumatol.* **1996**, *35*, 1314–1318. [CrossRef] [PubMed]
52. Iagnocco, A.; Ceccarelli, F.; Mennini, M.; Rutigliano, I.M.; Perricone, C.; Nenna, R.; Petrarca, L.; Mastrogiorgio, G.; Valesini, G.; Bonamico, M. Subclinical synovitis detected by ultrasound in children affected by coeliac disease: A frequent manifestation improved by a gluten-free diet. *Clin. Exp. Rheumatol.* **2014**, *32*, 137–142. [PubMed]
53. Iltanen, S.; Collin, P.; Korpela, M.; Holm, K. Celiac disease and markers of celiac disease latency in patients with primary Sjogren's syndrome. *Am. J. Gastroenterol.* **1999**, *94*, 1042–1046. [CrossRef] [PubMed]
54. Stagi, S.; Giani, T.; Simonini, G.; Falcini, F. Thyroid function, autoimmune thyroiditis and coeliac disease in juvenile idiopathic arthritis. *Rheumatology* **2005**, *44*, 517–520. [CrossRef] [PubMed]
55. Dahan, S.; Shor, D.B.A.; Comaneshter, D.; Tekes-Manova, D.; Shovman, O.; Amital, H.; Cohen, A.D. All disease begins in the gut: Celiac disease co-existence with SLE. *Autoimmun. Rev.* **2016**, *15*, 848–853. [CrossRef] [PubMed]
56. Zone, J.J.; Meyer, L.J.; Petersen, M.J. Deposition of granular IgA relative to clinical lesions in dermatitis herpetiformis. *Arch. Dermatol.* **1996**, *132*, 912–918. [CrossRef] [PubMed]
57. Mansikka, E.; Hervonen, K.; Kaukinen, K.; Collin, P.; Huhtala, H.; Reunala, T.; Salmi, T. Prognosis of dermatitis herpetiformis patients with and without villous atrophy at diagnosis. *Nutrients* **2018**, *10*, 641. [CrossRef] [PubMed]
58. Salmi, T.T.; Hervonen, K.; Kurppa, K.; Collin, P.; Kaukinen, K.; Reunala, T. Celiac disease evolving into dermatitis herpetiformis in patients adhering to normal or gluten-free diet. *Scand. J. Gastroenterol.* **2015**, *50*, 387–392. [CrossRef] [PubMed]

59. Mautalen, C.; Gonzalez, D.; Mazure, R.; Vazquez, H.; Lorenzetti, M.P.; Maurino, E.; Niveloni, S.; Pedreira, S.; Smecuol, E.; Boerr, L.A.; et al. Effect of treatment on bone mass, mineral metabolism, and body composition in untreated celiac disease patients. *Am. J. Gastroenterol.* **1997**, *92*, 313–318. [PubMed]
60. Fornari, M.C.; Pedreira, S.; Niveloni, S.; González, D.; Diez, R.A.; Vázquez, H.; Mazure, R.; Sugai, E.; Smecuol, E.; Boerr, L.; et al. Pre- and post-treatment serum levels of cytokines IL-1beta, IL-6, and IL-1 receptor antagonist in celiac disease. Are they related to the associated osteopenia? *Am. J. Gastroenterol.* **1998**, *93*, 413–418. [CrossRef] [PubMed]
61. Fiore, C.E.; Pennisi, P.; Ferro, G.; Ximenes, B.; Privitelli, L.; Mangiafico, R.A.; Santoro, F.; Parisi, N.; Lombardo, T. Altered osteoprotegerin/RANKL ratio and low bone mineral density in celiac patients on long-term treatment with gluten-free diet. *Horm. Metab. Res.* **2006**, *38*, 417–422. [CrossRef] [PubMed]
62. Larussa, T.; Suraci, E.; Nazionale, I.; Leone, I.; Montalcini, T.; Abenavoli, L.; Imeneo, M.; Pujia, A.; Luzza, F. No evidence of circulating autoantibodies against osteoprotegerin in patients with celiac disease. *World J. Gastroenterol.* **2012**, *18*, 1622–1627. [CrossRef] [PubMed]
63. Mustalahti, K.; Collin, P.; Sievänen, H.; Salmi, J.; Mäki, M. Osteopenia in patients with clinically silent coeliac disease warrants screening. *Lancet* **1999**, *354*, 744–745. [CrossRef]
64. Kurppa, K.; Collin, P.; Sievänen, H.; Huhtala, H.; Mäki, M.; Kaukinen, K. Gastrointestinal symptoms, quality of life and bone mineral density in mild enteropathic coeliac disease: A prospective clinical trial. *Scand. J. Gastroenterol.* **2010**, *45*, 305–314. [CrossRef] [PubMed]
65. Naiyer, A.J.; Shah, J.; Hernandez, L.; Kim, S.-Y.; Ciaccio, E.J.; Cheng, J.; Manavalan, S.; Bhagat, G.; Green, P.H.R. Tissue transglutaminase antibodies in individuals with celiac disease bind to thyroid follicles and extracellular matrix and may contribute to thyroid dysfunction. *Thyroid* **2008**, *18*, 1171–1178. [CrossRef] [PubMed]
66. Larizza, D.; Calcaterra, V.; De Giacomo, C.; De Silvestri, A.; Asti, M.; Badulli, C.; Autelli, M.; Coslovich, E.; Martinetti, M. Celiac disease in children with autoimmune thyroid disease. *J. Pediatr.* **2001**, *139*, 738–740. [CrossRef] [PubMed]
67. Wijarnpreecha, K.; Jaruvongvanich, V.; Cheungpasitporn, W.; Ungprasert, P. Association between celiac disease and schizophrenia: A meta-Analysis. *Eur. J. Gastroenterol. Hepatol.* **2018**, *30*, 442–446. [CrossRef] [PubMed]
68. Mollazadegan, K.; Kugelberg, M.; Tallstedt, L.; Ludvigsson, J.F. Increased risk of uveitis in coeliac disease: A nationwide cohort study. *Br. J. Ophthalmol.* **2012**, *96*, 857–861. [CrossRef] [PubMed]
69. De Bastiani, R.; Gabrielli, M.; Lora, L.; Napoli, L.; Tosetti, C.; Pirrotta, E.; Ubaldi, E.; Bertolusso, L.; Zamparella, M.; De Polo, M.; et al. Association between coeliac disease and psoriasis: Italian primary care multicentre study. *Dermatology* **2015**, *230*, 156–160. [CrossRef] [PubMed]
70. Wei, L.; Spiers, E.; Reynolds, N.; Walsh, S.; Fahey, T.; MacDonald, T.M. The association between coeliac disease and cardiovascular disease. *Aliment. Pharmacol. Ther.* **2008**, *27*, 514–519. [CrossRef] [PubMed]
71. Canova, C.; Pitter, G.; Ludvigsson, J.F.; Romor, P.; Zanier, L.; Zanotti, R.; Simonato, L. Coeliac disease and asthma association in children: The role of antibiotic consumption. *Eur. Respir. J.* **2015**, *46*, 115–122. [CrossRef] [PubMed]
72. Smith, D.F.; Gerdes, L.U. Meta-analysis on anxiety and depression in adult celiac disease. *Acta Psychiatr. Scand.* **2012**, *125*, 189–193. [CrossRef] [PubMed]
73. Sansotta, N.; Amirikian, K.; Guandalini, S.; Jericho, H. Celiac disease symptom resolution: Effectiveness of the gluten-free diet. *J. Pediatr. Gastroenterol. Nutr.* **2018**, *66*, 48–52. [CrossRef] [PubMed]
74. Laurikka, P.; Salmi, T.; Collin, P.; Huhtala, H.; Mäki, M.; Kaukinen, K.; Kurppa, K. Gastrointestinal symptoms in celiac disease patients on a long-term gluten-free diet. *Nutrients* **2016**, *8*, 429. [CrossRef] [PubMed]
75. Hervonen, K.; Salmi, T.T.; Kurppa, K.; Kaukinen, K.; Collin, P.; Reunala, T. Dermatitis herpetiformis in children: A long-term follow-up study. *Br. J. Dermatol.* **2014**, *171*, 1242–1243. [CrossRef] [PubMed]
76. Kalayci, A.G.; Kansu, A.; Girgin, N.; Kucuk, O.; Aras, G. Bone mineral density and importance of a gluten-free diet in patients with celiac disease in childhood. *Pediatrics* **2001**, *108*, E89. [CrossRef] [PubMed]
77. Santonicola, A.; Iovino, P.; Cappello, C.; Capone, P.; Andreozzi, P.; Ciacci, C. From menarche to menopause: The fertile life span of celiac women. *Menopause* **2011**, *18*, 1125–1130. [CrossRef] [PubMed]

78. Bode, S.H.; Bachmann, E.H.; Gudmand-Hoyer, E.; Jensen, G.B. Stature of adult coeliac patients: No evidence for decreased attained height. *Eur. J. Clin. Nutr.* **1991**, *45*, 145–149. [PubMed]

79. Pärnänen, A.; Kaukinen, K.; Helakorpi, S.; Uutela, A.; Lähdeaho, M.-L.; Huhtala, H.; Collin, P.; Mäki, M.; Kurppa, K. Symptom-detected and screen-detected celiac disease and adult height. *Eur. J. Gastroenterol. Hepatol.* **2012**, *24*, 1066–1070. [CrossRef] [PubMed]

80. Bardella, M.T.; Fredella, C.; Prampolini, L.; Molteni, N.; Giunta, A.M.; Bianchi, P.A. Body composition and dietary intakes in adult celiac disease patients consuming a strict gluten-free diet. *Am. J. Clin. Nutr.* **2000**, *72*, 937–939. [CrossRef] [PubMed]

81. Cosnes, J.; Cosnes, C.; Cosnes, A.; Contou, J.-F.; Reijasse, D.; Carbonnel, F.; Beaugerie, L.; Gendre, J.-P. Undiagnosed celiac disease in childhood. *Gastroenterol. Clin. Biol.* **2002**, *26*, 616–623. [PubMed]

82. Weiss, B.; Skourikhin, Y.; Modan-Moses, D.; Broide, E.; Fradkin, A.; Bujanover, Y. Is adult height of patients with celiac disease influenced by delayed diagnosis? *Am. J. Gastroenterol.* **2008**, *103*, 1770–1774. [CrossRef] [PubMed]

83. Canova, C.; Pitter, G.; Zanier, L.; Simonato, L.; Michaelsson, K.; Ludvigsson, J.F. Risk of fractures in youths with celiac disease—A population-based study. *J. Pediatr.* **2018**, *198*, 117–120. [CrossRef] [PubMed]

84. Tau, C.; Mautalen, C.; De Rosa, S.; Roca, A.; Valenzuela, X. Bone mineral density in children with celiac disease. Effect of a Gluten-free diet. *Eur. J. Clin. Nutr.* **2006**, *60*, 358–363. [CrossRef] [PubMed]

85. Moleski, S.M.; Lindenmeyer, C.C.; Jon Veloski, J.; Miller, R.S.; Miller, C.L.; Kastenberg, D.; Dimarino, A.J. Increased rates of pregnancy complications in women with celiac disease. *Ann. Gastroenterol.* **2015**, *28*, 236–240. [PubMed]

86. Rawal, N. Remission of refractory celiac disease with infliximab in a pediatric patient. *ACG Case Rep. J.* **2015**, *2*, 121–123. [CrossRef] [PubMed]

87. Kurppa, K.; Paavola, A.; Collin, P.; Sievänen, H.; Laurila, K.; Huhtala, H.; Saavalainen, P.; Mäki, M.; Kaukinen, K. Benefits of a gluten-free diet for asymptomatic patients with serologic markers of celiac disease. *Gastroenterology* **2014**, *147*, 610.e1–617.e1. [CrossRef] [PubMed]

88. Paarlahti, P.; Kurppa, K.; Ukkola, A.; Collin, P.; Huhtala, H.; Mäki, M.; Kaukinen, K. Predictors of persistent symptoms and reduced quality of life in treated coeliac disease patients: A large cross-sectional study. *BMC Gastroenterol.* **2013**, *13*, 75. [CrossRef] [PubMed]

89. Ukkola, A.; Mäki, M.; Kurppa, K.; Collin, P.; Huhtala, H.; Kekkonen, L.; Kaukinen, K. Changes in body mass index on a gluten-free diet in coeliac disease: A nationwide study. *Eur. J. Intern. Med.* **2012**, *23*, 384–388. [CrossRef] [PubMed]

90. Agardh, D.; Lee, H.-S.; Kurppa, K.; Simell, V.; Aronsson, C.A.; Jorneus, O.; Hummel, M.; Liu, E.; Koletzko, S. Clinical features of celiac disease: A prospective birth cohort. *Pediatrics* **2015**, *135*, 627–634. [CrossRef] [PubMed]

91. Kivelä, L.; Kaukinen, K.; Huhtala, H.; Lähdeaho, M.L.; Mäki, M.; Kurppa, K. At-risk screened children with celiac disease are comparable in disease severity and dietary adherence to those found because of clinical suspicion: A large cohort study. *J. Pediatr.* **2017**, *183*, 115–121. [CrossRef] [PubMed]

92. Kinos, S.; Kurppa, K.; Ukkola, A.; Collin, P.; Lähdeaho, M.L.; Huhtala, H.; Kekkonen, L.; Mäki, M.; Kaukinen, K. Burden of illness in screen-detected children with celiac disease and their families. *J. Pediatr. Gastroenterol. Nutr.* **2012**, *55*, 412–416. [CrossRef] [PubMed]

93. Mattila, E.; Kurppa, K.; Ukkola, A.; Collin, P.; Huhtala, H.; Forma, L.; Lähdeaho, M.L.; Kekkonen, L.; Mäki, M.; Kaukinen, K. Burden of illness and use of health care services before and after celiac disease diagnosis in children. *J. Pediatr. Gastroenterol. Nutr.* **2013**, *57*, 53–56. [CrossRef] [PubMed]

94. Kivelä, L.; Popp, A.; Arvola, T.; Huhtala, H.; Kaukinen, K.; Kurppa, K. Long-term health and treatment outcomes in adult coeliac disease patients diagnosed by screening in childhood. *United Eur. Gastroenterol. J.* **2018**, 205064061877838. [CrossRef]

95. Husby, S.; Koletzko, S.; Korponay-Szabó, I.R.; Mearin, M.L.; Phillips, A.; Shamir, R.; Troncone, R.; Giersiepen, K.; Branski, D.; Catassi, C.; et al. European Society for Pediatric Gastroenterology, Hepatology, and Nutrition European Society for Pediatric Gastroenterology, Hepatology, and Nutrition guidelines for the diagnosis of coeliac disease. *J. Pediatr. Gastroenterol. Nutr.* **2012**, *54*, 136–160. [CrossRef] [PubMed]

96. Tosco, A.; Salvati, V.M.; Auricchio, R.; Maglio, M.; Borrelli, M.; Coruzzo, A.; Paparo, F.; Boffardi, M.; Esposito, A.; D'Adamo, G.; et al. Natural history of potential celiac disease in children. *Clin. Gastroenterol. Hepatol.* **2011**, *9*, 320–325. [CrossRef] [PubMed]

97. Ludvigsson, J.F.; Card, T.R.; Kaukinen, K.; Bai, J.; Zingone, F.; Sanders, D.S.; Murray, J.A. Screening for celiac disease in the general population and in high-risk groups. *United Eur. Gastroenterol. J.* **2015**, *3*, 106–120. [CrossRef] [PubMed]

98. US Preventive Services Task Force; Bibbins-Domingo, K.; Grossman, D.C.; Curry, S.J.; Barry, M.J.; Davidson, K.W.; Doubeni, C.A.; Ebell, M.; Epling, J.W.; Herzstein, J.; et al. Screening for celiac disease: US Preventive Services Task Force recommendation statement. *JAMA* **2017**, *317*, 1252–1257. [CrossRef] [PubMed]

99. Rubio-Tapia, A.; Hill, I.D.; Kelly, C.P.; Calderwood, A.H.; Murray, J.A. American College of Gastroenterology ACG Clinical Guidelines: Diagnosis and management of celiac disease. *Am. J. Gastroenterol.* **2013**, *108*, 656–676. [CrossRef] [PubMed]

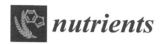

Review

Movement Disorders Related to Gluten Sensitivity: A Systematic Review

Ana Vinagre-Aragón *, Panagiotis Zis, Richard Adam Grunewald and Marios Hadjivassiliou

Academic Department of Neurosciences, Sheffield Teaching Hospitals NHS Foundation Trust, Sheffield S10 2JF, South Yorkshire, UK; takiszis@gmail.com (P.Z.); Richard.Grunewald@sth.nhs.uk (R.A.G); m.hadjivassiliou@sth.nhs.uk (M.H.)
* Correspondence: anavinara@gmail.com; Tel.: +34-606-706-294

Received: 24 July 2018; Accepted: 6 August 2018; Published: 8 August 2018

Abstract: Gluten related disorders (GRD) represent a wide spectrum of clinical manifestations that are triggered by the ingestion of gluten. Coeliac disease (CD) or gluten sensitive enteropathy is the most widely recognised, but extra-intestinal manifestations have also been increasingly identified and reported. Such manifestations may exist in the absence of enteropathy. Gluten sensitivity (GS) is another term that has been used to include all GRD, including those where there is serological positivity for GS related antibodies in the absence of an enteropathy. Gluten ataxia (GA) is the commonest extraintestinal neurological manifestation and it has been the subject of many publications. Other movement disorders (MDs) have also been reported in the context of GS. The aim of this review was to assess the current available medical literature concerning MDs and GS with and without enteropathy. A systematic search was performed while using PubMed database. A total of 48 articles met the inclusion criteria and were included in the present review. This review highlights that the phenomenology of gluten related MDs is broader than GA and demonstrates that gluten-free diet (GFD) is beneficial in a great percentage of such cases.

Keywords: movement disorders; coeliac disease; gluten; gluten free diet

---

1. Introduction

The term Gluten related disorders (GRD) covers a broad spectrum of immune-mediated clinical manifestations that are triggered by the same environmental insult; dietary gluten. Coeliac disease (CD) or gluten-sensitive enteropathy is the best-characterized disease within this wide clinical spectrum. Moreover, CD is the most common immune-mediated gastrointestinal (GI) disorder diagnosed both in childhood and adulthood, with an increasing global prevalence [1].

The classical presentation of CD includes GI symptoms (i.e. diarrhoea, abdominal pain, abdominal bloating), malnutrition, anaemia, and weight loss. The treatment is strict adherence to a gluten-free diet (GFD). Rarely patients with CD may no longer respond to GFD and are diagnosed with refractory CD a condition that may require immunosuppressive treatment [2].

Often, patients with gluten sensitivity (GS) can present with subtle or even no GI symptoms and a wide range of extra-intestinal manifestations affecting different organs. Gluten ataxia (GA), defined as sporadic cerebellar ataxia in the presence of circulating antigliadin antibodies and no alternative etiology for the ataxia, is by far the commonest neurological presentation. Nonetheless, several other neurological manifestations have been reported, such as epilepsy [3,4], gluten encephalopathy [5,6], myopathy [7], peripheral neuropathy [8–11], and other movement disorders (MDs). On some occasions, MDs have been recognized as a complication of or co-existing with systemic autoimmune diseases [12,13].

In this paper, we performed a systematically review of the current medical literature on MDs in CD and GS. We have excluded GA as this has been extensively studied and reviewed previously, and as such, it is a well-recognised entity [14,15].

2. Materials and Methods

2.1. Literature and Search Strategy

A systematic computer-based literature search on the topic was conducted on February 12th, 2018 using the Pubmed database. For the search we used two Medical Subject Headings (MeSH) terms in all fields. Term A was "celiac" or "coeliac" or "gluten" and term B was "chorea" or "choreiform" or "choreic" or "choreoathetosis" or "athetosis" or "tremor" or "dystonia" or "hemidystonia" or "torticollis" or "antecollis" or "anterocollis" or "retrocollis" or "laterocollis" or "blepharospasm" or "ballism" or "hemiballism" or "ballismus" or "hemiballismus" or "stiff" or "Parkinson" or "Parkinson's" or "parkinsonism" or "myoclonus" or "myoclonic" or "tic" or "myokymia" or "myorhythmia" or "Huntington" or "Huntington's" or "dyskinesia", and "RLS". Limitations included English language, human species, and full text available. We also perused the reference lists of the papers since the drafting of this paper in order to identify papers not identified through the search strategy.

2.2. Inclusion and Exclusion Criteria

To be included in this review, the articles had to meet the following inclusion criteria:

1. To be original clinical papers.
2. To study human subjects.
3. To involve single cases, case series, or retrospective observational studies with the combination of CD or GS and MDs.

Exclusion criteria included:

1. Reviews, book chapters, letters to editors, and editorials that are not providing new data.
2. Papers referring only to GA.

3. Results

3.1. Search Results

The search strategy that is described above resulted in the identification of 215 articles. After the eligibility assessment, 173 articles were further excluded, as they did not meet our inclusion criteria. Scanning the reference list, six more papers were identified. In total, 48 papers were used for this review. Table 1 summarizes the characteristics of these papers and Figure 1 illustrates the study selection process. Table 2 summarizes the characteristics of the patients and the response to GFD in each movement disorder type.

3.2. Chorea

Chorea is defined as irregular, brief, purposeless movements that flit from one body part to another, and it can be inherited or acquired [16,17]. Vascular, drug-induced, AIDS-related, and metabolic were the most common causes of acquired chorea in the case series published by Piccolo et al. [18] Investigation of chorea should be directed to the most likely causes [19].

The first report suggesting the link between CD and chorea was by Willis and colleagues, who conducted a retrospective observational study to investigate patients with dermatitis herpetiformis (DH), which is another extraintestinal manifestation of CD affecting the skin, for evidence of neurological manifestations [20]. One out of 35 patients with DH suffered chorea. However, of note is that this patient had been on phenytoin over the last 14 years after a single seizure that may have played a role in the development of chorea [21,22]. However, subsequently, case reports and small cases series of patients with chorea and CD or GS, and no other risk factors for developing chorea, have been published [23–26].

Nutrients **2018**, *10*, 1034

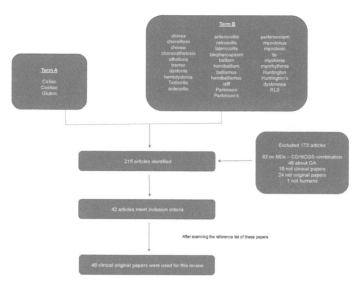

Figure 1. PRISMA chart. To be included in this review, the articles had to meet the following inclusion criteria: (1) To be original clinical papers, (2) to study human subjects, (3) to involve single cases, case series or retrospective observational studies with the combination of Coeliac disease (CD) or gluten sensitivity (GS) and movement disorders (MDs).

Table 1. Characteristics of the papers included in the review.

Number of Papers Related to Each Movement Disorder (%)	
Chorea	5 (11%)
Restless leg syndrome	4 (8%)
Myoclonus	15 (31%)
Palatal tremor	3 (6%)
Dystonia	3 (6%)
Tremor	5 (11%)
Stiff Person Syndrome	2 (5%)
Parkinsonism	3 (6%)
Tics	3 (6%)
Other less commonly reported movement disorders	
Opsoclonus-myoclonus	1 (2%)
Propiospinal myoclonus	1 (2%)
Paroxysmal dyskinesia	1 (2%)
Myorhythmia	1 (2%)
Myokymia	1 (2%)
Demographics	
Female to male ratio	7:2
Mean age (SD), in years	44.6 (22.7)
Types of Publications	
Case reports	30
Case series	8
Retrospective observational studies	9
Prospective pilot study	1
Year of Publication	
Range	1966–2018
Number of Publications per Decade	
Until 1990	5
1991–2000	9
2001–2010	20
2011–2018	14

Table 2. Characteristics of the papers included in the review.

Movement Disorder	Number of Cases of Patients Published until the Date	Male:Female	Mean Age of Onset (SD)/Age of Onset	Response to GFD E, S, N, L	HLA DQ2/DQ8	CD:GS
Chorea	8	1:7	57.4 (12.9)	E 5 (62.5%) S 2 (25%) L 1 (12.5%)	DQ2(+) 2 (25%) DQ2(-) 2 (25%) NA (50%)	5:3
RLS	65	6:59	NA	E 18 (28%) N 16 (25%) L 31 (47%)	NA	65:0
Myoclonus	28	15:13	47.7 (17.3)	S 1 (3%) N 28 (97%)	NA	28:0
Palatal tremor	3	1:2	51.3 (8.1)	E 1 (33%) N 2 (67%)	DQ2(+) 1 (33%) NA: 2 (67%)	1:2
Dystonia	2	1:1	49.50 (2.1)	N 2 (100%)	NA	2:0
Tremor	9	3:6	54.6 (14.9)	E 6 (67%) N 3 (33%)	DQ2(+) 6 (67%) NA: 3 (33%)	9:0
Parkinsonism	3	0:3	54.0 (18.7)	E 1 (33%) N 2 (67%)	NA	3:0
Tics	1	0:1	13	E (100%)	DQ8(+) 1 (100%)	0:1
OM	1	1:0	2	E (100%)	NA	1:0
PSM	1	0:1	23	E (100%)	NA	1:0
Paroxysmal dyskinesia	1	0:1	0.5	E (100%)	NA	1:0
Myorhythmia	1	0:1	68	N (100%)	DQ2 (+) 1 (100%)	1:0
Myokymia	1	0:1	72	N (100%)	NA	1:0

RLS, restless legs syndrome; OM, opsoclonus-myoclonus; PSM, propiospinal myoclonus; NA, not available; GFD, gluten-free diet; E, evident; S, slight; N, none; L, lack of data; CD, coeliac disease; GS, gluten sensitivity.

Demographic data of patients with gluten related chorea were available in seven of the cases. The choreiform movements were described as generalized affecting predominantly the upper limbs. The majority was female (86%) and their mean age of onset was 57.4 ± 12.9 years. Five patients had biopsy proven CD, whereas two patients had only serological evidence of GS. HLA DQ2 was tested in four of the patients, and positive just in two of the cases tested. There was a significant improvement in the choreiform movements after embarking on a GFD in five of the patients and no response in two.

3.3. Restless Legs Syndrome

Restless leg syndrome (RLS) is a circadian disorder appearing typically at the end of the day, being characterised by an intense and irresistible urge to move the lower extremities, either by itself or in response to unpleasant leg sensations. Symptoms typically improve while walking, stretching, or moving the lower limbs [27]. There are five essential diagnostic criteria and all must be met: (1) An urge to move the legs usually but not always accompanied by or felt to be caused by uncomfortable and unpleasant sensations in the legs, (2) Symptoms begin or worsen during periods of rest or inactivity such as lying down or sitting, (3) Symptoms are partially or totally relieved by movement, such as walking or stretching, at least as long as the activity continues, (4) Symptoms only occur or are worse in the evening or night than during the night, and (5) The occurrences of the above features are not solely accounted for as symptoms primary to another medical or behavioral condition [28]. The prevalence of RLS varies among different population surveyed. The data from REST (RLS Epidemiology, Symptoms, and Treatment), which is the largest trial till date with 23.052 patients, revealed that any degree of RLS symptoms was present in 11.9% [29]. The pathogenesis of RLS continues to be only partially understood, but there is substantial evidence for abnormalities in brain iron metabolism and dopaminergic dysfunction probably plays a key role [30]. RLS severity increases with decreased peripheral iron [31]. In fact, its prevalence is significantly greater in individuals with iron-deficiency anaemia [32].

Whether there is a link between RLS and CD or GS remains controversial. The first report suggesting an association between CD and RLS was by Manchanda et al. who presented a consecutive case series of four patients with RLS, low serum ferritin, and biopsy proven CD [33], which was considered to be the underlying cause for low serum ferritin. Subsequently, in two studies RLS was found to be more frequent in patients with CD than in controls [34,35]. On the other hand, however, Cikrikcioglu et al. studied the presence of antibodies relating to GS (tissue transglutaminase antibody IgA and IgG, antiendomyisium antibody IgA and IgG, and/or antigliadin antibody IgA and IgG) in 96 patients with RLS and age, sex, and BMI matching 97 subjects without RLS and could not demonstrate a significant difference between the two groups [36]. Furthermore, contradictory data have hitherto been published related to iron metabolism parameters in coeliac patients with active RLS and coeliac patients without RLS. Weinstock et al., found that concomitant iron deficiency was significantly more common in coeliac patients with RLS than in coeliac patients without RLS, but there were no statistically significant differences in haemoglobin levels between both groups [34]. In contrast, Moccia et al. could not find statistically significant differences in blood levels of iron, ferritin, and MCV between coeliac patients with RLS and coeliac patients without RLS in their study. However, haemoglobin levels were significantly lower in coeliac patients with RLS than in coeliac patients without RLS [35].

There are no data available regarding the age of onset of RLS in patients with CD or GS. The majority of described patients are female (91%). All of the patients had biopsy proven CD. The information about response to GFS is limited; three out of four CD patients with RLS improved on GFD and iron supplementation, whereas one patient improved after being on a GFD without receiving iron supplementation and still having low ferritin levels [33]. Weinstock and colleagues reported that 50% of the CD patients found relief in their RLS symptoms being on GFD, and similarly not all were receiving iron supplementation [34], suggesting that GFD can independently improve the RLS symptoms in people with RLS and CD or GS.

3.4. Myoclonus

Myoclonus is defined as a sudden, brief, shock like involuntary movement caused by active muscle contraction (positive myoclonus), or inhibition of on-going muscle activity (negative myoclonus) [37]. All of the studies that attempt to evaluate the general occurrence of myoclonus have various biases. There is an epidemiological study on myoclonus due to any cause in a defined population where the average annual incidence of pathological and persistent myoclonus for 1976 to 1990 was 13 cases per 100,000 person-years [38]. Progressive myoclonic ataxia (PMA) is a rare syndrome where progressive myoclonus and cerebellar ataxia coexist [39].

The first report suggesting the comorbidity of CD and PMA was by Cook and colleagues in 1966 [40]. Subsequently, several case reports were published [41–47]. Lu and colleagues published a case series of patients with ataxia and myoclonus providing for the first time electrophysiological evidence for the cortical origin of the myoclonus [48]. These findings were further confirmed later in many cases and case series [49–53]. The largest case series was published by Sarrigiannis et al., and included nine patients with CD, myoclonus of cortical origin and ataxia. All of the patients were compliant with a strict GFD, as evident by the elimination of gluten-related antibodies. Nonetheless, there was still evidence of enteropathy in all, and in some it was suggestive of refractory CD type 2. Aggressive immunosuppression improved ataxia and enteropathy in contrast to myoclonus that remained unchanged [54].

The mean age of onset of gluten related PMA is 47.7 ± 17.3 years. The majority of patients are males (55%). All of the patients reported to date had biopsy proven CD. Myoclonus phenomenology was described as often stimulus sensitive, asymmetrical, and irregular, generally focal at onset involving one or more limbs and sometimes the face, with a tendency to become gradually more generalized. However, it tends to still remain asymmetrical. In general, GFD, even in combination with aggressive immunosuppression, shows minimal effect on the myoclonus, but it may improve the enteropathy and the ataxia.

3.5. Palatal Tremor

Palatal tremor is defined as brief, rhythmic involuntary movements of the soft palate. It can be divided into symptomatic palatal tremor (SPT) and essential palatal tremor (EPT). SPT results from an insult in the Mollaret triangle being composed of the inferior olive, red nucleus, and contralateral dentate nucleus. In contrast, in EPT, no lesion is demonstrable. Data regarding the prevalence of SPT or EPT are scarce. SPT rarely can be associated with ataxia and is referred as progressive ataxia palatal tremor syndrome (PAPT) [55].

To date, three case reports of PAPT (one male and two females) in the context of CD have been reported [41,50,56]. The mean age of onset was 51.3 ± 8.1 years. HLA DQ2 was tested just in one of the cases and was positive. Two of the patients had biopsy proven CD, whereas another refused biopsy but it was diagnosed with GS based on the high titer of antigliadin antibodies. In the latter, palatal tremor improved after GFD, whereas no response to GFD was evident on the other two cases.

3.6. Dystonia

Dystonia is defined as a hyperkinetic movement disorder characterized by sustained or intermittent muscle contractions that cause abnormal involuntary repetitive movements, postures, or both [57]. There is significant variability in the reported prevalence of dystonia because to date the epidemiological studies published have adopted different methodologies for case ascertainment. A systematic review and meta-analysis that was published in 2012 reported a prevalence of 16.43 per 100,000, but it is likely to be underestimated, with many cases remaining undiagnosed [58]. The pathophysiology of dystonia is still poorly understood [59].

Two isolated cases of patients (one male and one female) with previous biopsy proven CD diagnosis that presented with dystonia have been reported to date [51,60]. The mean age of onset was 49.5 ± 2.1 years. In both cases, dystonia was focal affecting one limb. There was no response to GFD. In a large study where Bürk et al. screened patients with biopsy proven CD for neurological symptoms or signs, 3 out of 72 patients presented with dystonia [61]. Wittstock and colleagues reported a case of secondary dystonia due to cerebral vasculitis in a patient with biopsy proven CD [62]. This case may only illustrate coincidence of isolated vasculitis and CD. However, dystonia due to vascular lesion in the context of vasculitis and CD were diagnosed simultaneously and the dystonic symptoms improved after being combined with GFD and immunosuppressive therapy. This led the authors to postulate a causative relationship between the dystonia and CD.

3.7. Postural Tremor

Tremor is a rhythmic oscillation of a body part, which is produced by either alternating or synchronous contractions of reciprocally innervated antagonist muscles [63]. Several cases of patients with CD presenting with tremor often in association with or without later development of ataxia have been reported [64–67]. Tremor is focal and generally postural, affecting mainly the limbs, but also head, jaw, and tongue.

The mean age of onset of tremor is 54.6 ± 14.9 years and the male:female ratio was 1:2. All of the patients had biopsy proven CD and 67% had HLA DQ2 positive. There was a significant response to GFD in two-thirds of patients. Of interest is that postural tremor of abrupt onset has also been reported even in childhood in a case of a four year old boy with CD who suffered central pontine myelinolysis without electrolyte abnormalities [68]. The lack of neurophysiological characterisation of the tremor in such reports means that it is not possible to distinguish from myoclonus.

3.8. Stiff-Person Syndrome

Stiff person syndrome (SPS) is characterised by the increased tone of axial and limb muscles, with superimposed muscle spasms leading to lumbar hyperlordosis, impaired gait, falls, and autonomic dysfunction associated with anti-GAD and/or other autoantibodies [69]. This syndrome has a strong concurrence with other autoimmune entities [70–72]. SPS has an estimated prevalence of 1–2 cases per million with an incidence of one case per million per year [73]. In their study, Hadjivassiliou et al. screened patients with neurological disorders of unknown aetiology for GS and showed that such patients had a higher prevalence of circulating antigliadin antibodies [74]. In particular, out of 131 patients with GS and neurological disorders of unknown aetiology, four had the diagnosis of SPS [75]. A higher prevalence of GS in patients with SPS was found than what would be expected in the context of coexistence of two autoimmune diseases [76]. As SPS symptoms follow a relapsing-remitting pattern, the assessment of responsiveness to GFD is challenging. Nevertheless, there is evidence of reduction of the anti-GAD antibody titer after the implementation of GFD suggesting that GFD may be beneficial in treating the condition [77].

3.9. Parkinsonism

Parkinsonism is defined as a hypokinetic syndrome and it is characterised by the presence of resting tremor, rigidity, bradykinesia, and postural instability. The most common primary cause of parkinsonism is idiopathic Parkinson's disease (IPD), with a prevalence of 130 per 100,000 [78], but many secondary or acquired causes of parkinsonism exist [79]. Recently, Di Lazzaro and colleagues reported a case of improvement of parkinsonian symptoms after GFD implementation in a patient with biopsy proven CD [80]. Gonzalez Aleman and colleagues presented the case of a patient with parkinsonism and increased echogenicity in substantia nigra that is associated with biopsy proven CD and clozapine treatment. They postulated that the patient may have had subclinical IPD, which was unveiled after clozapine exposure or that she had a neuroleptic-induced akinetic rigid syndrome. However, they also speculated that CD might have played a role in the pathogenesis, taking into account the young age of the patient [81].

In the study of neurological disorders in a group of unselected patients with biopsy-proven CD conducted by Bürk and colleagues, 2 out of 72 patients fulfilled the diagnostic criteria for PD [61]. However, as these patients had previously followed a GFD and they were considered to be in remission, this finding may have just merely been coincidental. One out of the 10 CD cases reported by Luostarinen and colleagues, which were initially referred to the neurological department because of neurological symptoms and were finally found to have CD, presented with a four-month history of an asymmetrical left sided parkinsonian syndrome. Four years later diagnosis of CD was established, but the patient was never compliant with GFD [65]. In all cases, parkinsonism was described as affecting one side of the body more than the other. The mean age of onset was 54.0 ± 18.7, all the patients were females and had a biopsy proven CD. Only one patient out of three showed a response to GFD. Given that Parakinsonism is a relatively common neurological condition, the co-occurence of CD and Parkinsonism may well be co-incidental.

3.10. Tics

Tics are sudden, rapid, non-rhythmic, intermittent muscle movements (motor tics), or sounds (phonic tics), which can be classified as simple or complex [82,83]. What characterizes tics is an inner urge to make the movement or a local premonitory sensation experienced and temporarily relieved by its performance. Several studies have examined the prevalence of tic disorders. However, wide variation was evident across these studies in terms of specific diagnoses examined and the age of the population under study [84]. Zelnik and colleagues conducted a study to look for a broader spectrum of neurologic disorders in CD. However, an association between CD and Tic disorders was not demonstrated [85]. In the previously mentioned study that was conducted by Bürk and colleagues, two out of 72 suffered with Tics [61].

Gilles de la Tourette syndrome (GTS) is characterised by the presence of multiple motor tics and one vocal or phonic tic persisting for more than a year, from the appearance of the first tic [86]. A case report of a patient with CD, HLA DQ8 positive, and GTS has been reported and it was shown that GFD could be beneficial in managing the tics [87]. Rodrigo et al. carried out a prospective interventional study to analyse and evaluate the efficacy of GFD in a series of childhood and adult patients with GTS. Gluten removal was useful for reducing the intensity and frequency of motor and vocal/phonic tics and OCD symptoms [88].

3.11. Other Movement Disorders

3.11.1. Opsoclonus-Myoclonus

Opsoclonus-myoclonus syndrome is characterised by opsoclonus, myoclonus, and ataxia, associated with behavioural changes [89]. Opsoclonus is encompassed in the group of eye movement abnormalities known as saccadic intrusions, defined as involuntary multidirectional saccades that interrupt steady fixation. [90,91]. Deconinck and colleagues reported the case of a two-year-old male with CD, cerebellar ataxia, palpebral flutter, action myoclonus and opsoclonus. Both GI symptoms, as well as the neurological symptoms, improved after GFD implementation and treatment with steroids and immunoglobulins [92].

3.11.2. Propiospinal Myoclonus

Propiospinal myoclonus (PSM) is an uncommon movement disorder involving axial muscles characterized by painless, usually flexor arrhythmic jerks affecting the trunk, hips, and knees. It is often stimulus sensitive and typically worsens while adopting supine position [93]. The etiology of PSM is most commonly idiopathic [94]. Zhang and colleagues reported a case of a 23-year-old lady who developed PSM in the setting of CD [95]. On examination there were continual relatively rhythmic flexor muscle jerks affecting the neck, shoulders, trunk and hips. The jerks were elicited by patellar tendon tap in the supine position but not while sitting. The myoclonus began minutes to hours after gluten intake. There was complete resolution of the symptoms on GFD.

3.11.3. Paroxysmal Dyskinesia

Paroxysmal dyskinesia is defined as a group of episodic abnormal involuntary movements manifested by recurrent attacks of dystonia, chorea, athetosis, or a combination of these disorders [96]. Most cases are familial and usually autosomal dominant, but some are idiopathic [97]. Hall and colleagues reported the case of a female patient with abnormal movements from the age of six months [98]. The episodes were described as twisting of her upper body to one side, with an outstretched arm as well as a flexed position of the left leg lasting from 5 to 30 min and appearing several times in a day. At the age of eight, she presented with GI and after extensive workup, the diagnosis of biopsy proven CD was established. She was commenced on GFD and the symptoms resolved completely after six months.

3.11.4. Myorhythmia

Myorhythmia is characterised by slow rhythmic movements, usually involving the limb or cranial muscles, and it has been linked with a variety of identifiable etiologies [99]. Dimberg and colleagues reported the case of a 68-year-old lady with refractory CD who presented with myorhythmia [100] of the tongue, cheek, and fingers. Movements were described as continuous, synchronous, semirhythmic contractions occurring at rest as well as with movement. Two months after the onset of myorhythmia, the patient developed an encephalopathy that was confirmed by neuroimaging and neuropathology, that appeared to be inflammatory. An infectious aetiology was excluded by CSF analysis. Screening for autoimmune encephalitis and paraneoplastic syndromes was negative. The patient was HLA-DQ2 and -DQ8 positive.

3.11.5. Myokymia

Myokymia is characterised by spontaneous, fine fascicular contractions of muscle that usually can be seen on the skin as vermicular or continuous rippling movements [101]. A case of a 72-year-old lady with biopsy-confirmed CD, who initially presented with progressive generalized myokymia has been reported [102]. On examination, prominent vermicular, undulating slow movements of her orbicularis oris, mentalis, and right intrinsic hand muscle were noticed. EMG revealed myokymic potentials in several muscles. Subsequently, she developed both, action and stimulus-sensitive myoclonus, as well as ataxia. There was histologic improvement on jejunal biopsy on GFD. In contrast, there was no clinical progression of neurologic symptoms.

4. Conclusions

This paper aimed to systematically review the current literature regarding MDs in CD and GS. To our knowledge, this is the first review on the topic highlighting that the phenomenology of the gluten related movement disorders is broad and that GFD is apparently beneficial in many cases. Our review also indicates the following key points:

1. GS and CD should be considered in the diagnostic workup of MDs of unknown etiology in patients of all ages and both genders, even in the absence of GI symptoms.
2. Neurologic manifestations, including MDs, may precede the diagnosis of GS and CD.
3. Some of the MDs may improve or resolve after dietary gluten removal, so early diagnosis should rapidly lead to the implementation of GFD.
4. Once GFD is implemented, it should generally continue lifelong like in CD. In fact, in some cases, sporadic accidental gluten ingestion continues to trigger the MD.
5. In contrast, other types of MDs, such as ataxia with myoclonus, appear to be linked to refractory CD and when observed, there is prompt need for repeat biopsy of the small intestine and often aggressive immunosuppression.
6. The fact that the majority of the included papers refer to CD rather than the broader spectrum of GS may mean that the relationship of MDs to GS without enteropathy is under-studied.

Author Contributions: This work was carried out in collaboration between the authors. A.V.A. and P.Z. conceived and designed the study; A.V.A. drafted the main part of the manuscript; and the manuscript was edited by P.Z., M.H. and R.A.G. All authors read and approved the final manuscript and take full responsibility for the final content.

Funding: This research received no external funding.

Conflicts of Interest: The authors declare no conflict of interest.

References

1. Kang, J.Y.; Kang, A.H.Y.; Green, A.; Gwee, K.A.; Ho, K.Y. Systematic review: Worldwide variation in the frequency of coeliac disease and changes over time. *Aliment. Pharmacol. Ther.* **2013**, *38*, 226–245. [CrossRef] [PubMed]
2. Daum, S.; Cellier, C.; Mulder, C.J. Refractory coeliac disease. *Best Pract. Res. Clin. Gastroenterol.* **2005**, *19*, 413–424. [CrossRef] [PubMed]
3. Gobbi, G.; Ambrosetto, P.; Zaniboni, M.G.; Lambertini, A.; Ambrosioni, G.; Tassinari, C.A. Celiac disease, posterior cerebral calcifications and epilepsy. *Brain Dev.* **1992**, *14*, 23–29. [CrossRef]
4. Chapman, R.W.; Laidlow, J.M.; Colin-Jones, D.; Eade, O.E.; Smith, C.L. Increased prevalence of epilepsy in coeliac disease. *Br. Med. J.* **1978**, *2*, 250–251. [CrossRef] [PubMed]

5.   Hadjivassiliou, M.; Grünewald, R.A.; Lawden, M.; Davies-Jones, G.A.B.; Powell, T.; Smith, C.M.L. Headache and CNS white matter abnormalities associated with gluten sensitivity. *Neurology* **2001**, *56*, 385–388. [CrossRef] [PubMed]

6.   Kieslich, M.; Errázuriz, G.; Posselt, H.G.; Moeller-Hartmann, W.; Zanella, F.; Boehles, H. Brain white-matter lesions in celiac disease: A prospective study of 75 diet-treated patients. *Pediatrics* **2001**, *108*, E21. [CrossRef] [PubMed]

7.   Hadjivassiliou, M.; Chattopadhyay, A.K.; Grünewald, R.A.; Jarratt, J.A.; Kandler, R.H.; Rao, D.G.; Sanders, D.S.; Wharton, S.B.; Davies-Jones, G.A. Myopathy associated with gluten sensitivity. *Muscle Nerve* **2007**, *35*, 443–450. [CrossRef] [PubMed]

8.   Ludvigsson, J.F.; Olsson, T.; Ekbom, A.; Montgomery, S.M. A population-based study of coeliac disease, neurodegenerative and neuroinflammatory diseases. *Aliment. Pharmacol. Ther.* **2007**, *25*, 1317–1327. [CrossRef] [PubMed]

9.   Chin, R.L.; Sander, H.W.; Brannagan, T.H. Celiac neuropathy. *Neurology* **2003**, *60*, 1581–1585. [CrossRef] [PubMed]

10.   Zis, P.; Rao, D.G.; Sarrigiannis, P.G.; Aeschlimann, P.; Aeschlimann, D.P.; Sanders, D.; Grünewald, R.A.; Hadjivassiliou, M. Transglutaminase 6 antibodies in gluten neuropathy. *Dig. Liver Dis.* **2017**, *49*, 1196–1200. [CrossRef] [PubMed]

11.   Zis, P.; Sarrigiannis, P.G.; Rao, D.G.; Hadjivassiliou, M. Quality of life in patients with gluten neuropathy. *Nutrients* **2018**, *10*, 662. [CrossRef] [PubMed]

12.   Baizabal-carvallo, J.F.; Jankovic, J. Movement disorders in autoimmune diseases. *Mov. Disord.* **2012**, *27*, 935–946. [CrossRef] [PubMed]

13.   Zis, P.; Argiriadou, V.; Temperikidis, P.P.; Zikou, L.; Tzartos, S.J.; Tavernakis, A. Parkinson's disease associated with myasthenia gravis and rheumatoid arthritis. *Neurol. Sci.* **2014**, *35*, 797–799. [CrossRef] [PubMed]

14.   Hadjivassiliou, M.; Sanders, D.D.; Aeschlimann, D.P. Gluten-related disorders: Gluten ataxia. *Dig. Dis.* **2015**, *33*, 264–268. [CrossRef] [PubMed]

15.   Hadjivassiliou, M.; Sanders, D.S.; Woodroofe, N.; Williamson, C.; Grünewald, R.A. Gluten ataxia. *Cerebellum* **2008**, *7*, 494–498. [CrossRef] [PubMed]

16.   Higgins, D.S. Chorea and its disorders. *Neurol. Clin.* **2001**, *19*, 707–722. [CrossRef]

17.   Shannon, K.M. Treatment of chorea. *Contin. Lifelong Learn. Neurol.* **2007**, *13*, 72–93. [CrossRef]

18.   Piccolo, I.; Defanti, C.A.; Soliveri, P. Cause and course in a series of patients with sporadic chorea. *J. Neurol.* **2003**, *250*, 429–435. [CrossRef] [PubMed]

19.   Wild, E.J.; Tabrizi, S.J. The differential diagnosis of chorea. *Pract. Neurol.* **2007**, *7*, 360–373. [CrossRef] [PubMed]

20.   Willis, A.J.; Turner, B.; Lock, R.J.; Johnston, S.L.; Unsworth, D.J.; Fry, L. Dermatitis herpetiformis and neurological dysfunction. *J. Neurol. Neurosurg. Psychiatry* **2002**, *72*, 259–261. [CrossRef]

21.   Shulman, L.; Singer, C.; Weiner, W. Phenytoin-induced focal chorea. *Mov. Disord.* **1996**, *11*, 111–114. [CrossRef] [PubMed]

22.   Haider, Y.; Abbot, R. Phenytoin-induced choreoathetosis. *Postgr. Med. J.* **1990**, *66*, 1089–1990. [CrossRef]

23.   Pereira, A.C.; Edwards, M.J.; Buttery, P.C.; Hawkes, C.H.; Quinn, N.P.; Giovannoni, G.; Hadjivassiliou, M.; Bhatia, K.P. Chorewic syndrome and coeliac disease: A hitherto unrecognised association. *Mov. Disord.* **2004**, *19*, 478–481. [CrossRef] [PubMed]

24.   Andrade, C.; Rocha, H.; Albuquerque, A.; Sá, M.J. Gluten chorea. *Clin. Neurol. Neurosurg.* **2015**, *138*, 8–9. [CrossRef] [PubMed]

25.   Walker, R.H. Further evidence for coeliac disease-associated chorea? *Tremor Other Hyperkinet. Mov.* **2011**, *1*, 1–3. [CrossRef]

26.   Kitiyakara, T.; Jackson, M.; Gorard, D.A. Refractory coeliac disease, small bowel lymphoma and chorea. *J. R. Soc. Med.* **2002**, *95*, 133–134. [CrossRef] [PubMed]

27.   Allen, R.P.; Picchietti, D.; Hening, W.A.; Trenkwalder, C.; Walters, A.S.; Montplaisi, J. The participants in the Restless Legs Syndrome Diagnosis and Epidemiology workshop at the National Institutes of Health in collaboration with members of the International Restless Legs Syndrome Study Group. Restless legs syndrome: Diagnostic criteria, special considerations, and epidemiology. A report from the restless legs syndrome diagnosis and epidemiology workshop at the National Institutes of Health. *Sleep Med.* **2003**, *4*, 101–109. [PubMed]

28. Allen, R.P.; Picchietti, D.L.; Garcia-Borreguero, D.; Ondo, W.G.; Walters, A.S.; Winkelman, J.W.; Zucconi, M.; Ferri, R.; Trenkwalder, C. Restless legs syndrome/Willis-Ekbom disease diagnostic criteria: Updated International Restless Legs Syndrome Study Group (IRLSSG) consensus criteria-history, rationale, description and significance. *Sleep Med.* **2014**, *15*, 860–873. [CrossRef] [PubMed]
29. Hening, W.; Walters, A.S.; Allen, R.P.; Montplaisir, J.; Myers, A.; Ferini-Strambi, L. Impact, diagnosis and treatment of restless legs syndrome (RLS) in a primary care population: The REST (RLS epidemiology, symptoms, and treatment) primary care study. *Sleep Med.* **2004**, *5*, 237–246. [CrossRef] [PubMed]
30. Allen, R. Dopamine and iron in the pathophysiology of restless leg syndrome (RLS). *Sleep Med.* **2004**, *5*, 385–391. [CrossRef] [PubMed]
31. Sun, E.R.; Chen, C.A.; Ho, G.; Earley, C.J.; Allen, R.P. Iron and the restless leg syndrome. *Sleep* **1998**, *21*, 381–387. [CrossRef]
32. Allen, R.P.; Auerbach, S.; Auerbach, M.; Earley, C.J. The prevalence and impact of restless legs syndrome on patients with iron deficiency anemia. *Am. J. Hematol.* **2013**, *88*, 261–264. [CrossRef] [PubMed]
33. Manchanda, S.; Davies, C.R.; Picchietti, D. Celiac disease as a possible cause for low serum ferritin in patients with restless legs syndrome. *Sleep Med.* **2009**, *10*, 763–765. [CrossRef] [PubMed]
34. Weinstock, L.B.; Walters, A.S.; Mullin, G.E.; Duntley, S.P. Celiac disease is associated with restless legs syndrome. *Dig. Dis. Sci.* **2010**, *55*, 1667–1673. [CrossRef] [PubMed]
35. Moccia, M.; Pellecchia, M.T.; Erro, R.; Zingone, F.; Marelli, S.; Barone, D.G.; Ciacci, C.; Strambi, L.F.; Barone, P. Restless legs syndrome is a common feature of adult celiac disease. *Mov. Disord.* **2010**, *25*, 877–881. [CrossRef] [PubMed]
36. Cikrikcioglu, M.A.; Halac, G.; Hursitoglu, M.; Erkal, H.; Cakirca, M.; Kinas, B.E.; Erek, A.; Yetmis, M.; Gundogan, E.; Tukek, T. Prevalence of gluten sensitive enteropathy antibodies in restless legs syndrome. *Acta Neurol. Belg.* **2011**, *111*, 282–286. [PubMed]
37. Marsden, C.; Hallett, M.; Fahn, S. The nosology and pathophysiology of myoclonus. *Mov. Disord.* **1982**, *2*, 196–248.
38. Caviness, J.N.; Alving, L.I.; Maraganore, D.M.; Black, R.A.; McDonnell, S.K.; Rocca, W.A. The incidende and prevalence of myoclonus in Olmsted County, Minnesota. *Mayo Clin. Proc.* **1999**, *74*, 565–569. [CrossRef] [PubMed]
39. Marsden, C.D.; Harding, A.E.; Obeso, J.A.; Lu, C. Progressive Myoclonic Ataxia (The Ramsay Hunt Syndrome). *Arch. Neurol.* **1990**, *47*, 1121–1125. [CrossRef] [PubMed]
40. Cooke, W.; Smith, W. Neurological disorders associated with coeliac disease. *Brain* **1966**, *89*, 683–722. [CrossRef] [PubMed]
41. Finelli, P.F.; McEntee, W.J.; Ambler, M.; Kestenbaum, D. Adult celiac-disease presenting as cerebellar syndrome. *Neurology* **1980**, *30*, 245–249. [CrossRef] [PubMed]
42. Kinney, H.C.; Burger, P.C.; Hurwitz, B.J.; Hijmans, J.C.; Grant, J.P. Degeneration of the central nervous system associated with celiac disease. *J. Neurol. Sci.* **1982**, *53*, 9–22. [CrossRef]
43. Chinnery, P.F.; Reading, P.J.; Milne, D.; Gardner-Medwin, D.; Turnbull, D.M. CSF antigliadin antibodies and the Ramsay Hunt syndrome. *Neurology* **1997**, *49*, 1131–1134. [CrossRef] [PubMed]
44. Hanagasi, H.A.; Gürol, E.; Sahin, H.A.; Emre, M. Atypical neurological involvement associated with celiac disease. *Eur. J. Neurol.* **2001**, *8*, 67–69. [CrossRef] [PubMed]
45. Tüzün, E.; Gürses, C.; Baykan, B.; Büyükbabani, N.; Oztür, A.S.; Gökyigit, A. Lafora body-like inclusions in a case of progressive myoclonic ataxia associated with coeliac disease. *Eur. Neurol.* **2001**, *46*, 157–158. [CrossRef] [PubMed]
46. Sallem, F.S.; Castro, L.M.; Jorge, C.; Marchiori, P.; Barbosa, E. Gluten Sensitivity Presenting as Myoclonic Epilepsy with Cerebellar Syndrome. *Mov. Disord.* **2009**, *24*, 2162–2163. [CrossRef] [PubMed]
47. Siqueira Neto, J.I.; Costa, A.C.; Magalhaes, F.G.; Silva, G.S. Neurological manifestations of celiac disease. *Arq. Neuropsiquiatr.* **2004**, *62*, 969–972. [CrossRef] [PubMed]
48. Lu, C.S.; Thompson, P.D.; Quinn, N.P.; Parkes, J.D.; Marsden, C.D. Ramsay Hunt syndrome and coeliac disease: A new association? *Mov. Disord.* **1986**, *1*, 209–219. [CrossRef] [PubMed]
49. Smith, G.D.; Saldanha, G.; Britton, T.C.; Brown, P. Neurological manifestations of coeliac disease. *J. Neurol. Neurosurg. Psychiatry* **1997**, *63*, 550–551. [CrossRef] [PubMed]
50. Tison, F.; Arne, P.; Henry, P. Myoclonus and adult coeliac disease. *J. Neurol.* **1989**, *236*, 307–308. [CrossRef] [PubMed]

51. Bhatia, K.P.; Brown, P.; Gregory, R.; Lennox, G.G.; Manji, H.; Thompson, P.D.; Ellison, D.W.; Marsden, C.D. Progressive myoclonic ataxia associated with coeliac disease: The myoclonus is of cortical origin, but the pathology is in the cerebellum. *Brain* **1995**, *118*, 1087–1093. [CrossRef] [PubMed]

52. Tijssen, M.A.; Thom, M.; Ellison, D.W.; Wilkins, P.; Barnes, D.; Thompson, P.D.; Brown, P. Cortical myoclonus and cerebellar pathology. *Neurology* **2000**, *54*, 1350–1356. [CrossRef] [PubMed]

53. Javed, S.; Safdar, A.; Forster, A.; Selvan, A.; Chadwick, D.; Nicholson, A.; Jacob, A. refractory coeliac disease associated with late onset epilepsy, ataxia, tremor and progressive myoclonus with giant cortical evoked potentials-A case report and review of literature. *Seizure* **2012**, *21*, 482–485. [CrossRef] [PubMed]

54. Sarrigiannis, P.G.; Hoggard, N.; Aeschlimann, D.; Sanders, D.S.; Grünewald, R.A.; Unwin, Z.C.; Hadjivassiliou, M. Myoclonus ataxia and refractory coeliac disease. *Cerebellum & Ataxias* **2014**, *1*, 11. [CrossRef]

55. Samuel, M.; Torun, N.; Tuite, P.J.; Sharpe, J.A.; Lang, A.E. Progressive ataxia and palatal tremor (PAPT): Clinical and MRI assessment with review of palatal tremors. *Brain* **2004**, *127*, 1252–1268. [CrossRef] [PubMed]

56. Kheder, A.; Currie, S.; Romanowski, C.; Hadjivassiliou, M. Progressive ataxia with palatal tremor due to gluten sensitivity. *Mov. Disord.* **2012**, *27*, 62–63. [CrossRef] [PubMed]

57. Balint, B.; Bhatia, K.P. Dystonia: An update on phenomenology, classification, ptahogenesis and treatment. *Curr. Opin. Neurol.* **2014**, *27*, 468–476. [CrossRef] [PubMed]

58. Steeves, T.D.; Day, L.; Dykeman, J.; Jette, N.; Pringsheim, T. The prevalence of primary dystonia: A systematic review and meta-analysis. *Mov. Disord.* **2012**, *27*, 1789–1796. [CrossRef] [PubMed]

59. Kaji, R.; Bhatia, K.; Graybiel, A.M. Pathogenesis of dystonia: Is it of cerebellar or basal ganglia origin? *J. Neurol. Neurosurg. Psychiatry* **2018**, *89*, 488–492. [CrossRef] [PubMed]

60. Fung, V.S.; Duggins, A.; Morris, J.G.; Lorentz, I.T. Progressive Myoclonic Ataxia Associated With Celiac Disease Presenting as Unilateral Cortical Tremor and Dystonia. *Mov. Disord.* **2000**, *15*, 732–734. [CrossRef]

61. Bürk, K.; Fareki, M.L.; Lamprecht, G.; Roth, G.; Decker, P.; Weller, M.; Rammensee, H.G.; Oertel, W. Neurological symptoms in patients with biopsy proven celiac disease. *Mov. Disord.* **2009**, *24*, 2358–2362. [CrossRef] [PubMed]

62. Wittstock, M.; Grossmann, A.; Kunesch, E. Symptomatic vascular dystonia in Celiac disease. *Mov. Disord.* **2006**, *21*, 427–429. [CrossRef] [PubMed]

63. Deuschl, G.; Bain, P.; Brin, M. Consensus statement of the movement disorder society on tremor. *Mov. Disord.* **1998**, *13*, 2–23. [CrossRef] [PubMed]

64. Hermaszewski, R.A.; Rigby, S.; Dalgleish, A.G. Coeliac disease presenting with cerebellar degeneration. *Postgrad. Med. J.* **1991**, *67*, 1023–1024. [CrossRef] [PubMed]

65. Luostarinen, L.; Himanen, S.L.; Luostarinen, M.; Collin, P.; Pirttilä, T. Neuromuscular and sensory disturbances in patients with well treated coeliac disease. *J. Neurol. Neurosurg. Psychiatry* **2003**, *74*, 490–494. [CrossRef] [PubMed]

66. Habek, M.; Hojsak, I.; Barun, B.; Brinar, V.V. Downbeat nystagmus, ataxia and spastic tetraparesis due to coeliac disease. *Neurol. Sci.* **2011**, *32*, 911–914. [CrossRef] [PubMed]

67. Hernández-Lahoz, C.; Rodrigo-Sáez, L.; Vega-Villar, J.; Mauri-Capdevila, G.; Mier-Juanes, J. Familial gluten ataxia. *Mov. Disord.* **2014**, *29*, 308–310. [CrossRef] [PubMed]

68. Sharma, P.; Sharma, S.; Panwar, N.; Mahto, D.; Kumar, P.; Kumar, A.; Aneja, S. Central pontine myelinolysis presenting with tremor in a child with celiac disease. *J. Child Neurol.* **2014**, *29*, 381–384. [CrossRef] [PubMed]

69. Meinck, H.M.; Thompson, P.D. Stiff man syndrome and related conditions. *Mov. Disord.* **2002**, *17*, 853–866. [CrossRef] [PubMed]

70. O'Sullivan, E.P.; Behan, L.A.; King, T.F.J.; Hardiman, O.; Smith, D. A case of stiff-person syndrome, type 1 diabetes, celiac disease and dermatitis herpetiformis. *Clin. Neurol. Neurosurg.* **2009**, *111*, 384–386. [CrossRef] [PubMed]

71. Bilic, E.; Bilic, E.; Sepec, B.I.; Vranjes, D.; Zagar, M.; Butorac, V.; Cerimagic, D. Stiff-person syndrome in a female patient with type 1 diabetes, dermatitis herpetiformis, celiac disease, microcytic anemia and copper deficiency Just a coincidence or an additional shared pathophysiological mechanism? *Clin. Neurol. Neurosurg.* **2009**, *111*, 644–645. [CrossRef] [PubMed]

72. Soós, Z.; Salamon, M.; Erdei, K.; Kaszás, N.; Folyovich, A.; Szücs, A.; Barcs, G.; Arányi, Z.; Skaliczkis, J.; Vadasdi, K. LADA type diabetes, celiac disease, cerebellar ataxia and stiff person syndrome. A rare association of autoimmune disorders. *Ideggyogy. Sz.* **2014**, *67*, 205–209. [PubMed]

73. Dalakas, M.C. Stiff person syndrome: Advances in pathogenesis and therapeutic interventions. *Curr. Treat. Opt. Neurol.* **2009**, *11*, 102–110. [CrossRef] [PubMed]
74. Hadjivassiliou, M.; Gibson, A.; Davies-Jones, G.A.B.; Lobo, A.J.; Stephenson, T.J.; Milford-Ward, A. Does cryptic gluten sensitivity play a part in neurological illness? *Lancet* **1996**, *347*, 369–371. [CrossRef]
75. Hadjivassiliou, M.; Grünewald, R.A.; Davies-Jones, G.A.B. Gluten sensitivity as a neurological illness. *J. Neurol. Neurosurg. Psychiatry* **2002**, *72*, 560–563. [CrossRef] [PubMed]
76. Hadjivassiliou, M.; Williamson, C.; Grünewald, R.A.; Davies-Jones, G.A.B.; Sanders, D.S.; Sharrack, B.; Woodroofe, N. Glutamic acid Decarboxylase as a Target Antigen in Gluten Sensitivity: The Link to Neurological Manifestation? Available online: https://jnnp.bmj.com/content/76/1/150 (accessed on 7 August 2018).
77. Hadjivassiliou, M.; Aeschlimann, D.; Grünewald, R.A.; Sanders, D.S.; Sharrack, B.; Woodroofe, N. GAD antibody-associated neurological illness and its relationship to gluten sensitivity. *Acta. Neurol. Scand.* **2011**, *123*, 175–180. [CrossRef] [PubMed]
78. Wickremaratchi, M.M.; Perera, D.; O'Loghlen, C.; Sastry, D.; Morgan, E.; Jones, A.; Edwards, P.; Robertson, N.P.; Butler, C.; Morris, H.R.; et al. Prevalence and age of onset of Parkinson's disease in Cardiff: A community based cross sectional study and meta-analysis. *J. Neurol. Neurosurg. Psychiatry* **2009**, *80*, 805–807. [CrossRef] [PubMed]
79. Jankovic, J.; Lang, A.E. *Movement Disorders: Diagnosis and Assessment*, 5th ed.; Butterworth-Heinemann: Philadelphia, PA, USA, 2008.
80. Di Lazzaro, V.; Capone, F.; Cammarota, G.; Di Giud, D.; Ranieri, F. Dramatic improvement of parkinsonian symptoms after gluten-free diet introduction in a patient with silent celiac disease. *J. Neurol.* **2014**, *261*, 443–445. [CrossRef] [PubMed]
81. Gonzalez Aleman, G.; Florenzano, N.; Padilla, E.; Bourdieu, M.; Guerrero, G.; Calvó, M.; Alberio, G.; Strejilevich, S.; de Erausquin, G.A. A 37-year-old woman with celiac disease, recurrent psychosis, and Parkinsonism. *Mov. Disord.* **2006**, *21*, 729–731. [CrossRef] [PubMed]
82. Singer, H.S. Tourette syndrome and other tic disorders. *Hanb. Clin. Neurol.* **2011**, *100*, 641–657. [CrossRef]
83. Cath, D.C.; Hedderly, T.; Ludolph, A.G. European clinical guidelines for Tourette syndrome and other tic disorders. Part I: Assessment. *Eur. Child Adolesc. Psychiatry* **2011**, *20*, 155–171. [CrossRef] [PubMed]
84. Knight, T.; Steeves, T.; Day, L.; Lowerison, M.; Jette, N.; Pringsheim, T. Prevalence of tic disorders: A systematic review and meta-analysis. *Pediatr. Neurol.* **2012**, *47*, 77–90. [CrossRef] [PubMed]
85. Zelnik, N.; Pacht, A.; Obeid, R.; Lerner, A. Range of neurologic disorders in patients with celiac disease. *Pediatrics* **2004**, *113*, 1672–1676. [CrossRef] [PubMed]
86. Jankovic, J. Diagnosis and classification of tics and Tourette syndrome. *Adv. Neurol.* **1992**, *58*, 7–14. [PubMed]
87. Rodrigo, L.; Huerta, M.; Salas-Puig, J. Tourette syndrome and non-celiac gluten sensitivity. Clinical remission with a gluten-free diet: A description case. *J. Sleep Disord. Ther.* **2015**, *4*, 183. [CrossRef]
88. Rodrigo, L.; Nuria, Á.; Fern, E.; Salas-puig, J.; Huerta, M.; Hern, C. Efficacy of a Gluten-Free Diet in the Gilles de la Tourette Syndrome: A Pilot Study. *Nutrients* **2018**, *10*, 573. [CrossRef] [PubMed]
89. Kinsbourne, M. Myoclonic encephalopathy of infants. *J. Neurol. Neurosurg. Psychiatry* **1962**, *25*, 271–276. [CrossRef] [PubMed]
90. Leigh, R.J.; Zee, D.S. *The Neurology of Eye Movements*; Oxford University Press: Philadelphia, PA, USA, 1991.
91. Leigh, R.J.; Averbuch-Heller, L.; Tomsak, R.L. Treatment of abnormal eye movements that impair vision. Strategies based on current concepts of physiology and pharmacology. *Ann. Neurol.* **1994**, *36*, 129–141. [CrossRef] [PubMed]
92. Deconinck, N.; Scaillon, M.; Segers, V.; Groswasser, J.J.; Dan, B. Opsoclonus-Myoclonus Associated with Celiac Disease. *Pediatr. Neurol.* **2006**, *34*, 312–314. [CrossRef] [PubMed]
93. Brown, P.; Thompson, P.D.; Rothwell, J.C.; Day, B.L.; Marsden, C.D. Axial myoclonus of propiospinal origin. *Brain* **1991**, *114*, 197–214. [PubMed]
94. Roze, E.; Bounolleau, P.; Ducreux, D.; Cochen, V.; Leu-Semenescu, S.; Beaugendre, Y. Propiospinal myoclonus revisited: Clinical, neurophysiologic, and neuroradiologic findings. *Neurology* **2009**, *72*, 1301–1309. [CrossRef] [PubMed]
95. Zhang, Y.; Menkes, D.L.; Silvers, D.S. Propriospinal myoclonus associated with gluten sensitivity in a young woman. *J. Neurol. Sci.* **2012**, *315*, 141–142. [CrossRef] [PubMed]

96. Fahn, S. The paroxysmal dyskinesias. In *Movement Disorders*; Oxford University Press: Oxford, UK, 1994; pp. 310–345.

97. Blakeley, J.; Jankovic, J. Secondary Paroxysmal Dyskinesias. *Mov. Disord.* **2002**, *17*, 726–734. [CrossRef] [PubMed]

98. Hall, D.A.; Parsons, J.; Benke, T. Paroxysmal nonkinesigenic dystonia and celiac disease. *Mov. Disord.* **2007**, *22*, 708–710. [CrossRef] [PubMed]

99. Masucci, E.F.; Kurtzke, J.F.; Saini, N. Myorhythmia: A widespread movement disorder. Clinicopathological correlations. *Brain* **1984**, *107*, 53–79. [CrossRef] [PubMed]

100. Dimberg, E.L.; Crowe, S.E.; Trugman, J.M.; Swerdlow, R.H.; Lopes, M.B.; Bourne, T.D.; Burns, T.M. Fatal encephalitis in a patient with refractory celiac disease presenting with myorhythmia and carpal spasm. *Mov. Disord.* **2007**, *22*, 407–411. [CrossRef] [PubMed]

101. Gutmann, L.; Gutmann, L. Myokymia and neuromyotonia 2004. *J. Neurol.* **2004**, *251*, 138–142. [CrossRef] [PubMed]

102. Beydoun, S.R.; Copeland, D.D.; Korula, J. Generalized Myokymia as a Unique Association with Gluten-Sensitive Enteropathy. *Eur. Neurol.* **2000**, *44*, 254–255. [CrossRef] [PubMed]

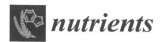

Review

Autoantibodies in the Extraintestinal Manifestations of Celiac Disease

Xuechen B. Yu [1,2,3], **Melanie Uhde** [1,2], **Peter H. Green** [1,2] and **Armin Alaedini** [1,2,3,*]

1 Department of Medicine, Columbia University Medical Center, 1130 Saint Nicholas Ave., New York, NY 10032, USA; xy2314@cumc.columbia.edu (X.B.Y.); melanieuhde86@gmail.com (M.U.); pg11@columbia.edu (P.H.G.)
2 Celiac Disease Center, Columbia University, New York, NY 10032, USA
3 Institute of Human Nutrition, Columbia University, New York, NY 10032, USA
* Correspondence: aa819@columbia.edu

Received: 1 August 2018; Accepted: 17 August 2018; Published: 20 August 2018

Abstract: Increased antibody reactivity towards self-antigens is often indicative of a disruption of homeostatic immune pathways in the body. In celiac disease, an autoimmune enteropathy triggered by the ingestion of gluten from wheat and related cereals in genetically predisposed individuals, autoantibody reactivity to transglutaminase 2 is reflective of the pathogenic role of the enzyme in driving the associated inflammatory immune response. Autoantibody reactivity to transglutaminase 2 closely corresponds with the gluten intake and clinical presentation in affected patients, serving as a highly useful biomarker in the diagnosis of celiac disease. In addition to gastrointestinal symptoms, celiac disease is associated with a number of extraintestinal manifestations, including those affecting skin, bones, and the nervous system. Investigations of these manifestations in celiac disease have identified a number of associated immune abnormalities, including B cell reactivity towards various autoantigens, such as transglutaminase 3, transglutaminase 6, synapsin I, gangliosides, and collagen. Clinical relevance, pathogenic potential, mechanism of development, and diagnostic and prognostic value of the various identified autoantibody reactivities continue to be subjects of investigation and will be reviewed here.

Keywords: celiac disease; gluten; gliadin; autoantibody; B cell; T cell; transglutaminase; synapsin; ganglioside; gluten sensitivity; gastrointestinal symptoms; molecular mimicry; intermolecular help; biomarker

1. Introduction

Celiac disease is a T cell-mediated systemic autoimmune disease triggered by the ingestion of wheat gluten and related proteins in rye and barley in genetically susceptible individuals [1–3]. Gluten is comprised of approximately 70 different proteins (including various gliadins and glutenins), which share a number of immunogenic amino acid sequences found to be pathogenic in the context of celiac disease [4]. Celiac disease has a strong genetic component, with approximately 95% of patients expressing the human leukocyte antigens (HLA)-DQ2 and HLA-DQ8 [5]. The frequency of HLA-DQ2 and -DQ8 and the per capita consumption of wheat are important determinants of celiac disease prevalence [6]. Although formerly considered as a rare condition mainly affecting children, celiac disease is now recognized as one of the most common autoimmune disorders and estimated to affect approximately 1% of the population worldwide [7]. In North America and Europe, celiac disease prevalence has been found to be increasing in recent decades [2,8,9]. The frequency of celiac is also rising in Asia-Pacific regions, where traditional rice-based diets are increasingly replaced by Western-style diets with a larger content of wheat-containing products [10].

The increasing prevalence of celiac disease is also partly attributed to the recent development of highly specific and sensitive serologic tests, which allow for safe and effective screening in individuals suspected of having celiac disease [11]. The gold standard for the diagnosis of celiac disease is based on endoscopic biopsy of the small intestine demonstrating the characteristic histologic features of duodenal lymphocyte infiltration, crypt hyperplasia, and villous atrophy, further supported by positive serologic tests, and the confirmation of remission of symptoms upon the removal of gluten-containing foods from diet [11,12]. Complete elimination of gluten-containing food from diet is currently the only effective and safe treatment for celiac disease [13,14].

The classic gastrointestinal symptoms of celiac disease includes diarrhea, abdominal pain, and malabsorption. However, celiac disease is often also associated with a number of extraintestinal manifestations such as osteoporosis, anemia, and dermatitis herpetiformis, among others [3,14,15]. The clinical picture in some patients can also include other autoimmune diseases, including type 1 diabetes, autoimmune thyroiditis, and autoimmune hepatitis, likely due in part to shared genetic factors [5,16,17].

The production of autoantibodies is an important feature of many autoimmune diseases, indicating a loss of immune tolerance to self-antigens. In celiac disease, a significantly enhanced autoantibody response to the transglutaminase 2 (TG2) enzyme, also known as tissue transglutaminase (tTG), is a hallmark of the pathogenic process and signifies a loss of tolerance to wheat gluten [11,18]. In addition to antibodies against TG2, other autoantibodies have also been reported in patients with celiac disease, particularly in the context of extraintestinal manifestations. In this review, the origin, development, and the potential pathogenic role of autoantibodies associated with extraintestinal manifestations of celiac disease are discussed.

2. Transglutaminases

2.1. Transglutaminase 2

By the 1960s, it was clear that, in addition to antibodies against the immunostimulatory gluten proteins of wheat and related cereals, patients with celiac disease express elevated autoantibody responses to the connective tissue surrounding smooth muscle fibers [19,20]. These antibodies became known as anti-endomysial and anti-reticulin antibodies [21–23]. It was not until 1997, when Dieterich et al. identified TG2 as the major endomysial target autoantigen [24]. Later research has shown that the target of the so-called anti-reticulin antibodies was also TG2 [25].

TG2 is a member of the structurally and functionally related group of transglutaminase proteins that catalyze the modification of proteins by introducing covalent bonds between amine groups (such as a lysine) and γ-carboxamide groups of peptide-bound glutamines [26]. TG2, the first transglutaminase discovered, is unique in some aspects, including that it is a ubiquitously expressed enzyme expressed in various tissues and cell types, and in various locations inside the cell and at the cell surface [26]. Under certain conditions, TG2 may react with H_2O in preference over an amine, converting a specific glutamine to glutamate via deamidation [27]. Intracellular TG2 is involved in signaling events that support cell survival in response to wounding, hypoxia, and oxidative stress [27]. Extracellular TG2 has a role in the regulation of the cytoskeleton by crosslinking extracellular matrix proteins such as fibronectin and integrins, and is believed to function in cell adhesion, matrix assembly, and cell motility [28].

TG2 plays a central role in the initiation of immune reactivity towards dietary gluten in the context of celiac disease [29,30], which also involves the celiac disease susceptibility genes, HLA-DQ2 and -DQ8 [31]. TG2 can effectively deamidate specific glutamine residues of gluten sequences that may have crossed the epithelial barrier and found access to the lamina propria. Antigen presenting cells expressing the HLA-DQ2 and HLA-DQ8 molecules have an increased affinity for these deamidated peptides [32]. Subsequent binding of the generated immunogenic peptides to the HLA molecules results in peptide complexes that can activate host gluten specific CD4$^+$ T cells in the lamina propria.

Activation of these T cells is accompanied by the production of a number of cytokines that can in turn promote inflammation and villous damage in the small intestine through the release of metalloproteinases by fibroblasts and inflammatory cells, as well as providing help to activate gluten-specific B cell responses [30,33].

Gluten-specific CD4$^+$ T cells are speculated to stimulate B cell production of not only anti-gluten antibody, but also anti-TG2 antibody. In the absence of any TG2-specific T cells being identified, the anti-TG2 antibody response is believed to be driven by a process referred to as intermolecular help, similar to the hapten-carrier system. Accordingly, gluten-specific CD4$^+$ T cells are thought to provide help to TG2-specific B cells when TG2–gluten complexes are formed [34]. Such a gluten-specific T cell-driven mechanism would lead to an anti-TG2 immune response without the requirement for TG2-specific T cells. With repeated exposure to TG2–gluten complexes, affinity maturation towards the TG2 antigen can potentially generate specific high-affinity autoantibody reactivity [35–37]. Anti-TG2 autoantibodies are thus gluten-dependent, and the antibody titer decreases rapidly after the elimination of gluten from diet [18,38]. IgA anti-TG2 autoantibodies have high specificity (>90%) and sensitivity (>95%) in celiac disease, currently serving as a particularly useful aid in diagnosis [18,39].

Whether antibodies to TG2 can play a clear role in disease pathogenesis in humans has not been definitively proven. Anti-TG2 antibodies bind to several epitopes of TG2, including the enzymatic core of the protein, and can thus interfere with TG2 bioactivity [40]. As TG2 is involved in epithelial cell differentiation through activation of transforming growth factor β [41], anti-TG2 autoantibodies have been shown to reduce epithelial cell differentiation, increase epithelial cell permeability in an intestinal cell line, and induce monocyte activation upon binding to Toll-like receptor 4 [42–44]. Data from in vitro studies indicate that anti-TG2 antibodies detected along the villous and crypt basement membranes in the jejunum from celiac disease patients may take part in the intestinal damage, particularly the remodeling of the small bowel mucosal architecture and the development of villous atrophy as well as crypt hyperplasia [43,45–47].

Because TG2 is the most widely expressed member of the transglutaminase family of proteins in the body, being present in almost all cell types, and participates in various biological reactions, the autoantibodies have the potential to negatively affect the activity of the enzyme and its biological role in tissues outside of the gastrointestinal tract as well [48]. The presence of IgA deposits colocalizing with TG2 in the liver, lymph nodes, muscle, thyroid, bone, and brain indicates that the circulating autoantibodies originating from the small intestine can access the autoantigen throughout the body and may potentially exert certain pathogenic effects [42,49–51]. Although the significance of anti-TG2 antibody binding to thyroid tissue or bone is not clear, both thyroid dysfunction and reduced bone density are common in celiac disease, raising the possibility that the antibodies may affect target organ function [49,50,52]. Anti-TG2 autoantibodies found within the muscular layer of brain vessels have also been speculated to cause disruption of the blood–brain barrier, which may further expose the central nervous system to other autoantibodies and potential toxins [51]. In mice, the injection of anti-TG2 antibodies in the lateral ventricle of the brain has been shown to cause deficits in motor coordination [53]. The data suggest that once exposed to the central nervous system, anti-TG2 antibodies may play a role in inducing neurologic deficits. Anti-TG2 antibodies isolated from celiac disease patients also have the potential to cross-react with other members of the transglutaminase family of enzymes due to some level of sequence homology, suggesting that such autoantibodies may additionally affect the activity of other transglutaminases [53]. Taken together, the data are suggestive of a pathogenic role for anti-TG2 autoantibodies in some of the extraintestinal manifestations of celiac disease.

2.2. Transglutaminase 3

The skin manifestation of celiac disease, known as dermatitis herpetiformis, was first described by Louis Adolphus Duhring in 1884 as an itchy, blistering, skin disease [54]. Dermatitis herpetiformis is characterized by the deposition of pathognomonic granular IgA in the dermal papillae, sometimes without significant gastrointestinal symptoms, and shares the same HLA associations with celiac disease [5]. In 2002, epidermal transglutaminase (eTG), also known as transglutaminase 3 (TG3), was identified as the main autoantigen target in skin IgA deposits in dermatitis herpetiformis [55]. In addition to increased anti-TG2 antibodies, dermatitis herpetiformis patients also present with elevated levels of antibody directed at TG3 [55,56].

TG3 is mainly expressed in the cornified layer of the epidermis and has been shown to play an important role in epidermal keratinization and in the formation of cornified envelope, which is essential for the maintenance for skin homeostasis [57]. Serum levels of anti-TG2 and anti-TG3 antibodies appear to correlate in celiac disease patients without skin manifestation, but not in patients with dermatitis herpetiformis, suggesting there is antibody reactivity to specific non-cross-reactive epitopes of TG3 in dermatitis herpetiformis [55,58]. IgA autoantibodies against TG3 have been reported to be detected in as much as 95% of dermatitis herpetiformis patients, substantially more than those against TG2 (79% of patients) [59]. In addition, detection of IgA antibody to TG3 has been found to efficiently distinguish untreated dermatitis herpetiformis from other dermatological itchy diseases and to be highly sensitive to a gluten-free diet [60]. IgA anti-TG3 antibody has been proposed as a useful diagnostic marker for dermatitis herpetiformis in both pediatric and adult patients [59–61].

The production of anti-TG3 antibodies may begin as a result of cross-reactivity of anti-TG2 IgA antibodies with TG3, which is released from epidermal keratinocytes and can diffuse through the basement membrane in regions of trauma [62]. Prolonged gluten immune stimulation may allow for epitope spreading and further maturation of these antibodies, resulting in the development of high affinity anti-TG3 antibodies [55,62,63]. Disappearance of anti-TG3 IgA antibody in response to dietary exclusion of gluten is slow and may take longer than for antibody response to TG2, suggesting that mechanisms other than homology between TG2 and TG3 might trigger the production of anti-TG3 antibodies [64–66].

Deposition of IgA antibodies in dermatitis herpetiformis is believed to play a role in the infiltration of neutrophils into the papillary dermis and in the formation of basement membrane zone vesicles in the lamina lucida [55]. TG3 in the papillary dermis has been found to overlap with the deposits of IgA antibodies in dermatitis herpetiformis patients, implying that TG3 is bound by the IgA autoantibodies [55,63]. It is hypothesized that active TG3 may cross-link anti-TG3 antibodies to certain dermal structural elements, leading to the dermal deposition of anti-TG3 IgA, which can in turn invoke skin pathology such as the associated blisters and papules [55]. However, anti-TG3 IgA deposits have also been found in uninvolved skin in affected patients, in areas away from lesions, suggesting that factors beyond these immune complexes may be necessary for lesion formation [62,63].

2.3. Transglutaminase 6

In addition to the well-characterized gastrointestinal and skin manifestations, a number of studies have reported on various other symptoms associated with celiac disease. Neurologic deficits, including peripheral neuropathy and cerebellar ataxia, are among the most common extraintestinal symptoms reported in conjunction with celiac disease [67,68]. Furthermore, elevated levels of anti-gliadin antibody have been associated with idiopathic neuropathy and idiopathic ataxia, even in the apparent absence of the characteristic mucosal pathology [69–72]. The terms "gluten ataxia" and "gluten neuropathy" have been used to describe these conditions, although the significance of the anti-gliadin antibodies in the absence of biopsy-proven intestinal damage has been debated [70,72,73].

Among these, idiopathic or sporadic ataxia associated with anti-gliadin antibodies has been the best studied in terms of understanding its frequency in different populations of ataxia patients and its potential etiology and pathogenic mechanism. A recent meta-analysis of several studies further validates the presence of significantly increased levels of antibody to gliadin among patients with non-hereditary ataxia [74]. There have been suggestions that gluten ataxia would fit better within the spectrum of non-celiac wheat/gluten sensitivity (NCWS) rather than celiac disease, based on serologic, histologic, and genetic markers [75,76]. In 2008, a novel neuronal transglutaminase, TG6, was reported as a target autoantigen in patients with gluten ataxia [77]. Antibodies to TG6 were later also detected in patients with gluten neuropathy [78]. However, the specificity of anti-TG6 antibodies in gluten ataxia and gluten neuropathy needs further investigation, as other studies have found such antibodies in patients with other conditions and in those without neurologic symptoms as well [77–81].

TG6 is predominantly expressed in a subset of neurons and plays a role in neurogenesis, particularly in the context of nervous system development and motor function [82]. TG6 is encoded on the same chromosome (20q11–12) as TG2 in humans [83]. Similarly to TG2, when TG6 is incubated with gluten peptides, it can both deamidate and transamidate glutamine residues, and there is a large degree of overlap in glutamine donor substrates of TG6 and TG2 [82]. TG6 can also form the previously mentioned hapten-carrier complexes with gluten, but to a lesser extent when compared with TG2 [84]. Therefore, it is conceivable that, in the event of blood–brain or blood–nerve barrier disruption, TG6 may become exposed to gluten-derived antigens. As such, gluten-specific $CD4^+$ T cells may be able to provide help to TG6-specific B cells, leading to the production of anti-TG6 autoantibodies in a similar fashion to anti-TG2 antibodies.

The relationship between gluten intake and the development of anti-TG6 antibodies has been examined. Lindfors et al. did not observe a decrease in anti-TG6 IgA antibodies in celiac disease patients on a gluten-free diet, suggesting a lack of gluten-dependency of TG6 autoantibodies [81]. However, a more recent study on a pediatric cohort of celiac disease patients found anti-TG6 antibody reactivity to correlate with the duration of gluten exposure, and to decline in response to the introduction of a gluten-free diet [79].

Similar to what has been described for anti-TG2 autoantibodies, anti-TG6 antibodies have the potential to disrupt TG6's biological functions. In mice, the injection of celiac disease patient-derived TG2 antibody that can cross-react with TG6 into mouse brain has been shown to cause deficits in motor coordination [53]. Recently, missense mutations in the of transglutaminase 6 gene have been identified in families of Chinese patients with spinocerebellar ataxia type 35 (SCA35) [85]. However, a causative link between neurological manifestations and autoantibodies to TG6 remains unclear [86]. Future studies on anti-TG6 antibodies can help in further clarifying their diagnostic and pathogenic potential in the context of neurologic and other manifestations in celiac disease and gluten sensitivity.

3. Gangliosides

Gangliosides are sialic acid-containing glycosphingolipids present in high concentrations in the nervous system, as well as on gut epithelial cells [87,88]. Antibodies to gangliosides, especially GM1, GD1a, GD1b, and GQ1b, are associated with and serve as diagnostic markers for a number of immune-mediated peripheral neuropathies, such as multifocal motor neuropathy and Guillain-Barré syndrome [89–91]. The antibodies are directed at carbohydrate epitopes of the ganglioside molecule [89]. The presence of anti-ganglioside antibodies in celiac disease patients with peripheral neuropathy was first reported by our team in 2002 [92]. A number of subsequent studies have confirmed the presence of various anti-ganglioside antibodies in conjunction with neurologic symptoms in celiac disease patients and those with immune reactivity to gluten [93–99]. At least one study has found that anti-ganglioside antibody reactivity responds to the exclusion of gluten from diet in a significant subset of patients with celiac disease [96].

Generation of anti-ganglioside antibodies is speculated to be linked to the intestinal immune response to ingested gluten. In acute immune-mediated neuropathies, the presence of anti-ganglioside antibodies has been demonstrated to result from molecular mimicry between gangliosides and bacterial or viral oligosaccharides [100,101]. While some gliadins may be glycosylated, epitopes that resemble gangliosides have not been found [102], making molecular mimicry less likely. However, it should be noted that while most gluten proteins appear to bear few or no carbohydrates, glycosylation of gluten can take place during or after the processing of flour and especially in food preparation under elevated temperatures [103]. A role for such Maillard reaction modifications of gluten in triggering an immune response that may target other autoantigens cannot be ruled out.

An alternative mechanism by which the antibody response to GM1 and other gangliosides could be generated may be through intermolecular help in a way similar to anti-TG2 autoantibodies in celiac disease [30]. In fact, it has been shown that gliadin can bind to the ganglioside-rich intestinal brush border membrane in an enzyme-independent way and can form stable complexes with GM1 ganglioside that are resistant to denaturing conditions [102]. The binding appears to take place at least partially through the ganglioside's pentasaccharide chain [102]. The reported dependence of anti-ganglioside antibodies on gluten intake would support such a mechanism of intermolecular help [96].

4. Synapsin I

The development of IgG and IgA antibody reactivity to gluten is a hallmark of celiac disease [11,14]. Whether anti-gluten antibodies can cross-react with autoantigens has been the subject of speculation and investigation for some time, especially in the context of extraintestinal manifestation of celiac disease. In a study by our group, we demonstrated that affinity-purified anti-gliadin antibodies from both immunized animals and celiac disease patients, particularly those with neurologic symptoms, can cross-react strongly with synapsin I (SYN1), a neuron-specific cytosolic phosphoprotein present in most nerve terminals [104]. The anti-gliadin antibodies bound to both isomers of SYN1, a and b, which have similar amino acid sequences.

SYN1 is primarily associated with synaptic vesicle membranes at the cytoplasmic surface [105]. It is a major substrate for protein kinases and its state of phosphorylation can affect synaptic function [105]. The similarity in certain repeat amino acid sequences found in both gliadin proteins and SYN1, with high frequencies of proline and glutamine residues and the presence of PQP and PQQP motifs, is believed to contribute to the cross-reactivity between anti-gliadin antibodies and SYN1 [104]. While SYN1 is known to carry O-linked N-acetylglucosamine and fucosyl groups [106,107], the removal of these carbohydrates do not inhibit the binding of anti-gliadin antibodies to the protein, ruling out a major role for them as target epitopes.

Whether SYN1-cross-reactive anti-gliadin antibodies can exert a pathogenic effect in humans is unknown. Synapsins are multifunctional proteins, containing different domains with distinct activities [108]. In addition to binding synaptic vesicles and various cytoskeletal proteins [109–111], synapsins may have enzymatic functions as well [112,113]. Disruption of SYN1 activity via the use of anti-SYN1 antibodies to the aplysia sea slug homologue of synapsin has been shown to reduce post-tetanic potentiation, and to increase the rate and extent of synaptic depression [114]. However, sufficient data to clearly link anti-SYN1 antibodies to neurologic manifestations in the context of autoimmunity does not exist yet. The data from celiac disease patients demonstrate that only certain subsets of anti-gliadin antibodies cross-react with SYN1 [104]. Because of the large number and heterogeneous nature of gluten proteins and associated epitopes [115], the anti-gliadin immune response involves a diverse repertoire of antigenic determinants. Therefore, varying degrees of cross-reactivity to SYN1 would be expected in different individuals with an elevated immune response to gluten. Such differences in the degree of cross-reactivity may explain and reveal clues about the association of such antibodies with specific extraintestinal complications, including neurologic manifestations. Ultimately, the type and specificity of the immune response, local integrity of the blood–nerve and blood–brain barriers, and other pro-inflammatory factors are likely contribute to and influence the potential pathogenic role of SYN1-cross-reactive anti-gliadin antibodies [116]. It is worth noting that the pathogenic effect of anti-synapsin immune reactivity might not be limited to the nervous system, as the presence of low levels of SYN1 has been demonstrated in non-neuronal cells as well, including liver epithelial cells [117] and pancreatic β cells [118]. It is expected that these tissues would be more accessible to antibodies and T cells than the nervous system.

5. Other Autoantigens in Celiac Disease

A number of studies have reported on antibodies to cytoskeletal actin in the context of celiac disease [119–121]. Although these antibodies are not specific to celiac disease and have also been associated with chronic hepatitis [122,123], IgA anti-actin antibodies do appear to correlate with the degree of villous atrophy [121,124]. These findings suggest that anti-actin antibodies are linked with mucosal injury and may result from the release of actin from injured or dying cells, thus triggering an autoantibody response. In addition, their appearance in celiac disease is dependent on gluten intake [125]. It is not clear whether they are associated with or play any role in the extraintestinal manifestations of celiac disease. IgA autoantibodies to collagen types I, III, V, and VI have also been found in association with celiac disease. No specific clinical manifestation is reported to be associated with these antibodies yet, but the prevalence of connective tissue diseases in patients with celiac disease may be related to an anti-collagen immune reactivity. Antibody reactivity to single- and double-stranded DNA, ATP synthase β chain, cardiolipin, and enolase α has also been found in some celiac disease patients [120,126], but their clinical relevance remains to be assessed.

As celiac disease is associated with several other autoimmune disorders, including type 1 diabetes and autoimmune thyroiditis, autoantibodies specifically linked to these disorders can be found in patients with celiac disease [127]. A list of such antibodies and associated conditions is included in Table 1. The link between celiac disease and associated autoimmune disorders is believed to be primarily due to common genetic background, particularly in the HLA region of chromosome 6 [127–130]. Whether gluten intake can contribute to the development of these organ-specific autoantibodies is not entirely clear yet. However, there are reports showing that diabetes- and thyroid disease-related antibodies in children with celiac disease may disappear in response to the exclusion of gluten-containing foods from diet [131].

6. Autoantibodies in Non-Celiac Wheat Sensitivity

Some individuals experience a range of symptoms in response to the ingestion of gluten-containing foods, i.e., wheat, rye, and barley, without the characteristic serologic or histologic markers of celiac disease and wheat allergy [132–135]. The condition is variably referred to as non-celiac gluten sensitivity or non-celiac wheat sensitivity (NCWS). NCWS is associated with gastrointestinal symptoms, commonly including bloating, abdominal pain, and diarrhea, as well as extra-intestinal symptoms, among which fatigue, headache, anxiety, and cognitive difficulties are predominant [133]. Accurate figures for the prevalence of NCWS are not known, but current estimates put the number at similar to or greater than for celiac disease [136,137]. The identity of the exact component(s) of wheat and related cereals responsible for triggering the associated symptoms remains uncertain. While recent controlled trials have indicated a prominent role for gluten [134,138], non-gluten proteins and fermentable short chain carbohydrates have also been suggested by some studies to drive aberrant immune responses or to be associated with symptoms [139,140].

Recent research indicates that NCWS is associated with increased innate and adaptive systemic immune activation in response to microbial translocation [141]. Affected individuals also have elevated levels of intestinal fatty acid-binding protein that correlates with the markers of immune activation, suggesting a compromised intestinal epithelial barrier integrity [141]. By definition, NCWS patients do not have elevated levels of antibody to TG2, the celiac disease-specific autoantibody. Whether there is any autoimmune component to NCWS is not clear. However, one study has found that compared with irritable bowel syndrome (IBS) patients, an increased proportion of individuals with NCWS develops an autoimmune disease [142]. In addition, the study reported an increased frequency of anti-nuclear antibodies (ANA) in NCWS patients, as detected by indirect immunofluorescence using HEp-2 cells [142]. Anti-nuclear antibodies bind to proteins in the cell nucleus and are found to be elevated in some systemic autoimmune disorders, including systemic lupus erythematosus. The specific target antigen(s) and pathogenic relevance of these antibodies, or their association with specific extraintestinal manifestations, in the context of NCWS remains to be determined.

Table 1. Autoantibody reactivities associated with other autoimmune diseases found in patients with celiac disease.

Autoantibody Target	Associated Autoimmune Disease	Reference
Islet cells; Glutamic acid decarboxylase	Type 1 diabetes mellitus	[16,131,143]
Thyroperoxidase; Thyroglobulin, Thyroid stimulating hormone receptor; Thyroid microsomal antigen	Autoimmune thyroid disease	[16,131,144,145]
Liver-kidney microsomal antigen	Autoimmune liver disease	[16,146,147]
Double-stranded DNA; Nuclear antigen	Systemic lupus Erythematosus	[16,37,148]
Sjögren syndrome-related antigen A (Ro), Sjögren syndrome-related antigen B (La); Nuclear antigen	Sjögren syndrome	[16,149]
Cardiolipin; Phophatidylserine/prothrombin	Anti-phospholipid syndrome	[126,150–153]

7. Conclusions

Celiac disease is a systemic autoimmune condition with intestinal and extraintestinal manifestations. Autoantibody reactivity against a number of autoantigens has been described in the context of the various manifestations of the disease. The clinical relevance and pathogenic role of such antibodies continue to be the subject of investigation and debate. Questions regarding the mechanisms by which such autoantibodies are generated and how they may access target tissues, such as the nervous system, also remain incompletely resolved. Identification of autoantibody biomarkers closely associated with specific extraintestinal manifestations of celiac disease can be particularly useful for the development of predictive and diagnostic tests, in addition to providing novel clues regarding disease mechanism and therapeutic approaches. Although a number of advances in the identification and understanding of autoantibody reactivity in celiac disease have been made in the past 20 years, further research and confirmatory studies with larger cohorts of patients and controls, as well as more in-depth preclinical mechanistic studies will be needed to clarify remaining questions.

Author Contributions: Conceptualization: X.B.Y. and A.A.; First draft of the manuscript: X.B.Y. and A.A.; Critical revision of the manuscript for important intellectual content: M.U., P.H.G. and A.A.

Funding: This research received no external funding.

Conflicts of Interest: The authors declare no conflict of interest.

References

1. Ludvigsson, J.F.; Leffler, D.A.; Julio, B.; Biagi, F.; Fasano, A.; Green, P.H.; Hadjivassiliou, M.; Kaukinen, K.; Kelly, C.; Leonard, J.N.; et al. The Oslo definitions for coeliac disease and related terms. *Gut* **2013**, *62*, 43–52. [CrossRef] [PubMed]
2. Rubio-Tapia, A.; Ludvigsson, J.F.; Brantner, T.; Murray, J.A.; Everhart, J.E. The prevalence of celiac disease in the United States. *Am. J. Gastroenterol.* **2012**, *107*, 1538–1544. [CrossRef] [PubMed]
3. Re, V.D.; Magris, R.; Cannizzaro, R. New insights into the pathogenesis of celiac disease. *Front. Med.* **2017**, *4*, 1–11.
4. Dupont, F.M.; Vensel, W.H.; Tanaka, C.K.; Hurkman, W.J.; Altenbach, S.B. Deciphering the complexities of the wheat flour proteome using quantitative two-dimensional electrophoresis, three proteases and tandem mass spectrometry. *Proteome Sci.* **2011**, *9*, 10. [CrossRef] [PubMed]
5. Spurkland, A.; Ingvarsson, G.; Falk, E.S.; Sollid, L.M.; Thorsby, E. Dermatitis herpetiformis and celiac disease are both primarily associated with the HLA-DQ(α1*0501, β1*02) or the HLA-DQ (α1*03, β1*0302) heterodimers. *Tissue Antigens* **1997**, *49*, 29–34. [CrossRef] [PubMed]
6. Cummins, A.G.; Roberts-Thomson, I.C. Prevalence of celiac disease in the Asia-Pacific region. *J. Gastroenterol. Hepatol.* **2009**, *24*, 1347–1351. [CrossRef] [PubMed]
7. Biagi, F.; Klersy, C.; Balducci, D.; Corazza, G.R. Are we not over-estimating the prevalence of celiac disease in the general population? *Ann. Med.* **2010**, *42*, 557–561. [CrossRef] [PubMed]
8. Green, P.H.; Cellier, C. Celiac disease. *N. Engl. J. Med.* **2007**, *357*, 1731–1743. [CrossRef] [PubMed]

9. Lebwohl, B.; Ludvigsson, J.F.; Green, P.H. Celiac disease and non-celiac gluten sensitivity. *BMJ* **2015**, *351*, h4347. [CrossRef] [PubMed]
10. Wang, X.; Liu, W.; Xu, C. Celiac disease in children with diarrhea in 4 cities in China. *J. Pediatr. Gastroenterol. Nutr.* **2011**, *53*, 368–370. [PubMed]
11. Byrne, G.; Feighery, C.F. Celiac Disease: Diagnosis. In *Celiac Disease Methods and Protocols*; Ryan, A.W., Ed.; Humana Press: New York, NY, USA, 2015.
12. Troncone, R.; Jabri, B. Coeliac disease and gluten sensitivity. *J. Int. Med.* **2011**, *269*, 582–590. [CrossRef] [PubMed]
13. Fasano, A.; Catassi, C. Current approaches to diagnosis and treatment of celia disease: An evolving spectrum. *Gastroenterology* **2001**, *120*, 631–651. [CrossRef]
14. Gujral, N.; Freeman, H.J.; Thomson, A.B. Celiac disease: Prevalence, diagnosis, pathogenesis and treatment. *World J. Gastroenterol.* **2012**, *18*, 6036–6059. [PubMed]
15. Najmeh, A.; Farshad, A.S. Extra intestinal manifestations of celiac disease and associated disorders. *Int. J. Celiac Dis.* **2017**, *5*, 1–9.
16. Caglar, E.; Ugurlu, S.; Ozenoglu, A.; Can, G.; Kadioglu, P.; Dobrucali, A. Autoantibody frequency in celiac disease. *Clinics* **2009**, *64*, 1195–1200. [CrossRef] [PubMed]
17. Lauret, E.; Rodrigo, L. Celiac disease and autoimmune-associated conditions. *BioMed. Res. Int.* **2013**, *2013*, 127589. [CrossRef] [PubMed]
18. Rauhavirta, T.; Hietikko, M.; Salmi, T.; Lindfors, K. Transglutaminase 2 and transglutaminase 2 autoantibodies in celiac disease: A review. *Clin. Rev. Allergy Immunol.* **2016**, 1–16. [CrossRef]
19. Rubin, W.; Fauci, A.S.; Marvin, S.F.; Sleisenger, M.H.; Jefries, G.H. Immunofluorescent Studies in Adult Celiac Disease. *J. Clin. Investig.* **1965**, *44*, 475–485. [CrossRef] [PubMed]
20. Malik, G.B.; Watson, W.C.; Murray, D.; Cruickshank, B. Immunofluorescent Antibody Studies in Idiopathic Steatorrhoea. *Lancet* **1964**, *13*, 1127–1129. [CrossRef]
21. Seah, P.P.; Fry, L. Tissue antibodies in dermatitis herpetiformis and adult coeliac disease. *Lancet* **1971**, 834–836. [CrossRef]
22. Alp, M.H.; Wright, R. Autoantibodies to reticulin in patients with idiopathic steatorrhoea, coeliac disease, and Crohn's disease, and their relation to immunoglobulins and dietary antibodies. *Lancet* **1971**, *2*, 682–685. [CrossRef]
23. Chorzelski, T.P.; Beutner, E.H.; Sulej, J.; Tchorzewska, H.; Jablonska, S.; Skumar, V.; Kapuscinska, A. IgA anti-endomysium antibody. A new immunological marker of dermatitis herpetiformis and coeliac disease. *Br. J. Dermatol.* **1984**, *3*, 395–402. [CrossRef]
24. Dieterich, W.; Ehnis, T.; Bauer, M.; Donner, P.; Volta, U.; Riecken, E.O.; Schuppan, D. Identification of tissue transglutaminase as the autoantigen of celiac disease. *Nat. Med.* **1997**, *3*, 797–801. [CrossRef] [PubMed]
25. Korponay-Szabo, I.R.; Laurila, K.; Szondy, Z.; Halttunen, T.; Szalai, Z.; Dahlbom, I.; Rantala, I.; Kovacs, J.; Fesus, L.; Maki, M. Missing endomysial and reticulin binding of coeliac antibodies in transglutaminase 2 knockout tissues. *Gut* **2003**, *52*, 199–204. [CrossRef] [PubMed]
26. Eckert, R.L.; Kaartinen, M.T.; Nurminskaya, M.; Belkin, A.M.; Colak, G.; Johnson, G.V.; Mehta, K. Transglutaminase regulation of cell function. *Physiol. Rev.* **2014**, *94*, 383–417. [PubMed]
27. Lerner, A.; Neidhofer, S.; Matthias, T. Transglutaminase 2 and anti-transglutaminase 2 autoantibodies in celiac disease and beyond: TG2 double-edged sword: Gut and extraintestinal involvement. *Immunome. Res.* **2015**, *11*, 1–5. [CrossRef]
28. Klock, C.; DiRaimondo, T.R.; Khosla, C. Role of transglutaminase 2 in celiac disease pathogenesis. *Semin. Immunopathol.* **2012**, *34*, 513–522. [CrossRef] [PubMed]
29. Sollid, L.M.; Jabri, B. Celiac disease and transglutaminase 2: A model for posttranslational modification of antigens and HLA association in the pathogenesis of autoimmune disorders. *Immunology* **2011**, *23*.
30. Alaedini, A.; Green, P.H. Narrative review: Celiac disease: Understanding a complex autoimmune disorder. *Ann. Intern. Med.* **2005**, *142*, 289–298. [PubMed]
31. Taylor, A.K.; Lebwohl, B.; Snyder, C.L.; Green, P.H.R. Celiac disease. In *GeneReviews*; Adam, M., Ardinger, H., Pagon, R., Eds.; University of Washington: Seattle, WA, USA, 2008.
32. Stamnaes, J.; Fleckenstein, B.; Sollid, L.M. The propensity for deamidation and transamidation of peptides by transglutaminase 2 is dependent on substrate affinity and reaction conditions. *Biochim. Biophys. Acta* **2008**, *1784*, 1804–1811. [CrossRef] [PubMed]

33. Jabri, B.; Kasarda, D.D.; Green, P.H. Innate and adaptive immunity: The yin and yang of celiac disease. *Immunol. Rev.* **2005**, *206*, 219–231. [CrossRef] [PubMed]

34. Fleckenstein, B.; Qiao, S.W.; Larsen, M.R.; Jung, G.; Roepstorff, P.; Sollid, L.M. Molecular characterization of covalent complexes between tissue transglutaminase and gliadin peptides. *J. Biol. Chem.* **2004**, *279*, 17607–17616. [CrossRef] [PubMed]

35. Korponay-Szabo, I.R.; Vescei, Z.; Kiraly, R. Homology of Deamidated Peptides with Tissue Transglutaminase. Proceedings of the 9th International Conference of TG Protein Crosslinking 2007. Available online: https://www.researchgate.net/publication/298270098_Homology_of_deamidated_gliadin_peptides_and_tissue_transglutaminase (accessed on 19 August 2018).

36. Pinkas, D.M.; Strop, P.; Brunger, A.T.; Khosla, C. Transglutaminase 2 undergoes a large conformational change upon activation. *PLoS Biol.* **2007**, *5*, e327. [CrossRef] [PubMed]

37. Alaedini, A.; Green, P.H.R. Autoantibodies in celiac disease. *Autoimmunity* **2008**, *41*, 19–26. [CrossRef] [PubMed]

38. Sulkanen, S.; Halttunen, T.; Laurila, K.; Kolho, K.L.; Korponay-Szabo, I.R.; Sarnesto, A.; Savilahti, E.; Collin, P.; Maki, M. Tissue transglutaminase autoantibody enzyme-linked immunosorbent assay in detecting celiac disease. *Gastroenterology* **1998**, *115*, 1322–1328. [CrossRef]

39. Briani, C.; Samaroo, D.; Alaedini, A. Celiac disease: From gluten to autoimmunity. *Autoimmun. Rev.* **2008**, *7*, 644–650. [CrossRef] [PubMed]

40. Hnida, K.; Stamnaes, J.; du Pré, M.F.; Mysling, S.; Jorgensen, T.J.D.; Sollid, L.M.; Iversen, R. Epitope-dependent functional effects of celiac disease autoantibodies on transglutaminase 2. *J. Biol. Chem.* **2016**, *291*, 25542–25552. [CrossRef] [PubMed]

41. Nunes, I.; Gleizes, P.E.; Metz, C.N.; Rifkin, D.B. Latent transforming growth factor-beta binding protein domains involved in activation and transglutaminase-dependent cross-linking of latent transforming growth factor-beta. *J. Cell Biol.* **1997**, *136*, 1151–1163. [CrossRef] [PubMed]

42. Korponay-Szabo, I.R.; Halttunen, T.; Szalai, Z.; Laurila, K.; Kiraly, R.; Kovacs, J.B.; Fesus, L.; Maki, M. In vivo targeting of intestinal and extraintestinal transglutaminase 2 by coeliac autoantibodies. *Gut* **2004**, *53*, 641–648. [CrossRef] [PubMed]

43. Zanoni, G.; Navone, R.; Lunardi, C. In celiac disease, a subset of autoantibodies against transglutaminase binds toll-like receptor 4 and induces activation of monocytes. *PLoS Med.* **2006**, *3*, e358. [CrossRef] [PubMed]

44. Halttunen, T.; Maki, M. Serum immunoglobulin A from patients with celiac disease inhibits human T84 intestinal crypt epithelial cell differentiation. *Gastroenterology* **1999**, *116*, 566–572. [CrossRef]

45. Barone, M.V.; Caputo, I.; Ribecco, M.T.; Maglio, M.; Marzari, R.; Sblattero, D.; Trocone, R.; Auricchio, S.; Esposito, C. Humoral immune response to tissue transglutaminase is related to epithelial cell proliferation in celiac disease. *Gastroenterology* **2007**, *132*, 1245–1253. [CrossRef] [PubMed]

46. Myrsky, E.; Syrjanen, M.; Korponay-Szabo, I.R.; Maki, M.; Kaukinen, K.; Lindfors, K. Altered small-bowel mucosal vascular network in untreated coeliac disease. *Scand. J. Gastroenterol.* **2009**, *44*, 162–167. [CrossRef] [PubMed]

47. Caja, S.; Maki, M.; Kaukinen, K.; Lindfors, K. Antibodies in celiac disease: Implications beyond diagnostics. *Cell. Mol. Radioimmunol.* **2011**, *8*, 103–109. [CrossRef] [PubMed]

48. Gundemir, S.; Colak, G.; Tucholski, J.; Johnson, G.V. Transglutaminase 2: A molecular Swiss army knife. *Biochim. Biophys. Acta* **2012**, *1823*, 406–419. [CrossRef] [PubMed]

49. Naiyer, A.J.; Shah, J.; Hernandez, L.; Kim, S.Y.; Ciaccio, E.J.; Cheng, J.; Manavalan, S.; Bhagat, G.; Green, P.H. Tissue transglutaminase antibodies in individuals with celiac disease bind to thyroid follicles and extracellular matrix and may contribute to thyroid dysfunction. *Thyroid* **2008**, *18*, 1171–1178. [CrossRef] [PubMed]

50. Sugai, E.; Chernavsky, A.; Pedreira, S.; Smecuol, E.; Vazquez, H.; Niveloni, S.; Mazure, R.; Mauriro, E.; Rabinovich, G.A.; Bai, J.C. Bone-specific antibodies in sera from patients with celiac disease: Characterization and implications in osteoporosis. *J. Clin. Immunol.* **2002**, *22*, 353–362. [CrossRef] [PubMed]

51. Hadjivassiliou, M.; Maki, M.; Sanders, D.S.; Willamson, C.A.; Grunewald, R.A.; Woodroofe, N.M.; Korponay-Szabo, I.R. Autoantibody targeting of brain and intestinal transglutaminase in gluten ataxia. *Neurology* **2006**, *66*, 373–377. [CrossRef] [PubMed]

52. Alaedini, A. Celiac disease and bone health. In *Nutrition and Bone Health*; Holick, M., Nieves, J., Eds.; Springer: New York, NY, USA, 2015; pp. 33–40.

53. Boscolo, S.; Lorenzon, A.; Sblattero, D.; Florian, F.; Stebel, M.; Marzari, R.; Not, T.; Aeschlimann, D.; Ventura, A.; Hadjivassiliou, M.; et al. Anti transglutaminase antibodies cause ataxia in mice. *PLoS ONE* **2010**, *5*, 1–9. [CrossRef] [PubMed]

54. Duhring, L.A. Dermatitis Herpetiformis. *JAMA* **1884**, *3*, 225–229. [CrossRef]

55. Sardy, M.; Karpati, S.; Merkl, B.; Paulsson, M.; Smyth, N. Epidermal transglutaminase (TGase 3) is the autoantigen of dermatitis herpetiformis. *J. Exp. Med.* **2002**, *195*, 747–757. [CrossRef] [PubMed]

56. Hull, C.M.; Liddle, M.; Hansen, N.; Meyer, L.J.; Schmidt, L.; Taylor, T.; Jaskowski, T.D.; Hill, H.R.; Zone, J.J. Elevation of IgA anti-epidermal transglutaminase antibodies in dermatitis herpetiformis. *J. Biol. Chem.* **2008**, *159*, 120–124. [CrossRef] [PubMed]

57. Mack, J.A.; Anand, S.; Maytin, E.V. Proliferation and cornification during development of the mammalian epidermis. *Birth Defects Res.* **2006**, *75*, 314–329. [CrossRef] [PubMed]

58. Kim, I.G.; McBridge, O.W.; Wang, M.; Kim, S.Y.; Idler, W.W.; Steinert, P.M. Structure and organization of the human transglutaminase 1 gene. *J. Biol. Chem.* **1992**, *267*, 7710–7717. [PubMed]

59. Rose, C.; Armbruster, F.P.; Ruppert, J.; Igl, B.-W.; Zillikens, D.; Shimanovich, I. Autoantibodies against epidermal transglutaminase are a sensitive diagnostic marker in patients with dermatitis herpetiformis on a normal or gluten-free diet. *J. Am. Acad. Dermatol.* **2009**, *61*, 39–43. [CrossRef] [PubMed]

60. Borroni, G.; Biagi, F.; Ciocca, O.; Vassallo, C.; Carugno, A.; Cananzi, R.; Campanella, J.; Bianchi, P.I.; Brazzelli, V.; Corazza, G.R. IgA anti-epidermal transglutaminase autoantibodies: A sensible and sensitive marker for diagnosis of dermatitis herpetiformis in adult patients. *J. Eur. Acad. Dermatol. Venereol.* **2013**, *27*, 836–841. [CrossRef] [PubMed]

61. Jaskowski, T.D.; Hamblin, T.; Wilson, A.R.; Hill, H.R.; Brook, L.S. IgA anti-epidermal transglutaminase antibodies in dermatitis herpetiformis and pediatric celiac disease. *J. Investig. Dermatol.* **2009**, *129*, 2728–2730. [CrossRef] [PubMed]

62. Nakajima, K. Recent advances in dermatitis herpetiformis. *Clin. Dev. Immunol.* **2012**, *2012*, 4. [CrossRef] [PubMed]

63. Donaldson, M.R.; Zone, J.J.; Schmidt, L.A.; Taylor, T.B.; Neuhausen, S.L.; Hull, C.M.; Meyer, L.J. Epidermal transglutaminase deposits in perilesional and uninvolved skin in patients with dermatitis herpetiformis. *J. Investig. Dermatol.* **2007**, *127*, 1268–1271. [CrossRef] [PubMed]

64. Paolella, G.; Caputo, I.; Marabotti, A.; Lepretti, M.; Salzano, A.M.; Scaloni, A.; Vitale, M.; Zambrano, N.; Sblattero, D.; Esposito, C. Celiac anti-type 2 transglutaminase antibodies induce phosphoproteome modification in intestinal epithelial caco-2 cells. *PLoS ONE* **2013**, *8*, e84403. [CrossRef] [PubMed]

65. Reunala, R.; Salmi, T.T.; Hervonen, K.; Laurila, K.; Kautiainen, H.; Collin, P.; Kaukinen, K. IgA antiepidermal transglutaminase antibodies in dermatitis herpetiformis: A significant but not complete response to a gluten-free diet treatment. *Br. J. Dermatol.* **2015**, *172*, 1139–1141. [CrossRef] [PubMed]

66. Hietikko, M.; Hervonen, K.; Salmi, T.; Ilus, T.; Zone, J.J.; Kaukinen, K.; Reunala, T.; Lindfors, K. Disappearance of epidermal transglutaminase and IgA deposits from the papillary dermis of patients with dermatitis herpetiformis after a long-term gluten-free diet. *Br. J. Dermatol.* **2018**, *178*, e198–e201. [CrossRef] [PubMed]

67. Bushara, K.O. Neurologic presentation of celiac disease. *Gastroenterology* **2005**, *128*, S92–S97. [CrossRef] [PubMed]

68. Green, P.H.; Alaedini, A.; Sander, H.W.; Brannagan, T.H., III; Latov, N.; Chin, R.L. Mechanisms underlying celiac disease and its neurologic manifestations. *Cell. Mol. Life Sci.* **2005**, *62*, 791–799. [CrossRef] [PubMed]

69. Bushara, K.O.; Goebel, S.U.; Shill, H.; Goldfarb, L.G.; Hallett, M. Gluten sensitivity in sporadic and hereditary cerebellar ataxia. *Ann. Neurol.* **2001**, *49*, 540–543. [CrossRef] [PubMed]

70. Hadjivassiliou, M.; Grunewald, R.A.; Chattopadhyay, A.K.; Davies-Jones, G.A.; Gibson, A.; Jarratt, J.A.; Kandler, R.H.; Lobo, A.; Powell, T.; Smith, C.M. Clinical, radiological, neurophysiological, and neuropathological characteristics of gluten ataxia. *Lancet* **1998**, *352*, 1582–1585. [CrossRef]

71. Burk, K.; Bosch, S.; Muller, C.A.; Melms, A.; Zuhlke, C.; Stern, M.; Besenthal, I.; Skalej, M.; Ruck, P.; Ferber, S.; et al. Sporadic cerebellar ataxia associated with gluten sensitivity. *Brain* **2001**, *124*, 1013–1019. [CrossRef] [PubMed]

72. Hadjivassiliou, M.; Grunewald, R.A.; Kandler, R.H.; Chattopadhyay, A.K.; Jarratt, J.A.; Sanders, D.S.; Sharrack, B.; Wharton, S.B.; Davies-Jones, G.A. Neuropathy associated with gluten sensitivity. *J. Neurol. Neurosurg. Psychiatry* **2006**, *77*, 1262–1266. [CrossRef] [PubMed]

73. Wills, A.J.; Unsworth, D.J. Gluten ataxia 'in perspective'. *Brain* **2003**, *126*, E4. [CrossRef] [PubMed]

74. Lin, C.Y.; Wang, M.J.; Tse, W.; Pinotti, R.; Alaedini, A.; Green, P.H.R.; Kuo, S.H. Serum antigliadin antibodies in cerebellar ataxias: A systematic review and meta-analysis. *J. Neurol. Neurosurg. Psychiatry* **2018**. [CrossRef] [PubMed]

75. Lundin, K.E.; Alaedini, A. Non-celiac gluten sensitivity. *Gastrointest. Endosc. Clin. N. Am.* **2012**, *22*, 723–734. [CrossRef] [PubMed]

76. Rodrigo, L.; Hernandez-Lahoz, C.; Lauret, E.; Rodriguez-Pelaez, M.; Soucek, M.; Ciccocioppo, R.; Kruzliak, P. Gluten ataxia is better classified as non-celiac gluten sensitivity than as celiac disease: A comparative clinical study. *Immunol. Res.* **2016**, *64*, 558–564. [CrossRef] [PubMed]

77. Hadjivassiliou, M.; Aeschlimann, P.; Strigun, A.; Sanders, D.D.; Woodroofe, N.; Aeschlimann, D. Autoantibodies in gluten ataxia recognize a novel neuronal transglutaminase. *Br. J. Dermatol.* **2008**, *64*, 332–343.

78. Zis, P.; Rao, D.G.; Sarrigiannis, P.G.; Aeschlimann, P.; Aeschlimann, D.P.; Sanders, D.; Grunewald, R.A.; Hadjivassiliou, M. Transglutaminase 6 antibodies in gluten neuropathy. *Br. J. Dermatol.* **2017**, *49*, 1196–1200. [CrossRef] [PubMed]

79. De Leo, L.; Aeschlimann, D.; Hadjivassiliou, M.; Aeschlimann, P.; Salce, N.; Vatta, S.; Ziberna, F.; Cozzi, G.; Martelossi, S.; Ventura, A.; et al. Anti-transglutaminase 6 antibody development in children with celiac disease correlates with duration of gluten exposure. *JPGN* **2018**, *66*, 64–68. [CrossRef] [PubMed]

80. Sato, K.; Nanri, K. Gluten Ataxia: Anti-Transglutaminase-6 Antibody as a New Biomarker. *Brain Nerve* **2017**, *69*, 933–940. [PubMed]

81. Lindfors, K.; Koskinen, O.; Laurila, K.; Collin, P.; Saavalainen, P.; Haimila, K.; Partanen, J.; Maki, M.; Kaukinen, K. IgA-class autoantibodies against neuronal transglutaminase, TG6 in celiac disease: No evidence for gluten dependency. *Clin. Chim. Acta* **2011**, *412*, 1187–1190. [CrossRef] [PubMed]

82. Thomas, H.; Beck, K.; Adamczyk, M.; Aeschlimann, P.; Langley, M.; Oita, R.C.; Thiebach, L.; Hils, M.; Aeschlimann, D. Transglutaminase 6: A protein associated with central nervous system development and motor function. *Amino Acids* **2013**, 161–177. [CrossRef] [PubMed]

83. Grenard, P.; Bates, M.K.; Aeschlimann, D. Evolution of transglutaminase genes: Identification of transglutaminase gene cluster on human chromosome 15q15. Structure of the gene encoding transglutaminase X and a novel gene family member, transglutaminase Z. *J. Biol. Chem.* **2001**, *276*, 33066–33078. [CrossRef] [PubMed]

84. Stamnaes, J.; Dorum, S.; Fleckenstein, B.; Aeschlimann, D.; Sollid, L.M. Gluten T cell epitope targeting by TG3 and TG6; implications for dermatitis herpetiformis and gluten ataxia. *Amino Acids* **2010**, *39*, 1183–1191. [CrossRef] [PubMed]

85. Wang, J.L.; Yang, X.; Xia, K.; Hu, Z.M.; Weng, L.; Jin, X.; Jiang, H.; Zhang, P.; Shen, L.; Guo, J.F.; et al. TGM6 identified as a novel causative gene of spinocerebellar ataxias using exome sequencing. *Brain* **2010**, *133*, 3510–3518. [CrossRef] [PubMed]

86. Mulder, C.J.J.; Rouvroye, M.D.; van Dam, A.-M. Transglutaminase 6 antibodies are not yet mainstream in neuro-coeliac disease. *Dig. Liver Dis.* **2018**, *50*, 96–97. [CrossRef] [PubMed]

87. Sato, E.; Uezato, T.; Fujita, M.; Nishimura, K. Developmental profiles of glycolipids in mouse small intestine. *J. Biochem. (Tokyo)* **1982**, *91*, 2013–2019. [CrossRef]

88. Hansson, H.A.; Holmgren, J.; Svennerholm, L. Ultrastructural localization of cell membrane GM1 ganglioside by cholera toxin. *Proc. Natl. Acad. Sci. USA* **1977**, *74*, 3782–3786. [CrossRef] [PubMed]

89. O'Leary, C.P.; Willison, H.J. The role of antiglycolipid antibodies in peripheral neuropathies. *Curr. Opin. Neurol.* **2000**, *13*, 583–588. [CrossRef] [PubMed]

90. Alaedini, A.; Briani, C.; Wirguin, I.; Siciliano, G.; D'Avino, C.; Latov, N. Detection of anti-ganglioside antibodies in Guillain-Barre syndrome and its variants by the agglutination assay. *J. Neurol. Sci.* **2002**, *196*, 41–44. [CrossRef]

91. Alaedini, A.; Latov, N. A surface plasmon resonance biosensor assay for measurement of anti-GM(1) antibodies in neuropathy. *Neurology* **2001**, *56*, 855–860. [CrossRef] [PubMed]

92. Alaedini, A.; Green, P.H.; Sander, H.W.; Hays, A.P.; Gamboa, E.T.; Fasano, A.; Sonnenberg, M.; Lewis, L.D.; Latov, N. Ganglioside reactive antibodies in the neuropathy associated with celiac disease. *J. Neuroimmunol.* **2002**, *127*, 145–148. [CrossRef]

93. Tursi, A.; Giorgetti, G.M.; Iani, C.; Arciprete, F.; Brandimarte, G.; Capria, A.; Fontana, L. Peripheral neurological disturbances, autonomic dysfunction, and antineuronal antibodies in adult celiac disease before and after a gluten-free diet. *Dig. Dis. Sci.* **2006**, *51*, 1869–1874. [CrossRef] [PubMed]

94. Shill, H.A.; Alaedini, A.; Bushara, K.O.; Latov, N.; Hallett, M. Anti-ganglioside antibodies in idiopathic and hereditary cerebellar degeneration. *Neurology* **2003**, *60*, 1672–1673. [CrossRef] [PubMed]

95. Volta, U.; Granito, A.; De Giorgio, R. Antibodies to gangliosides in coeliac disease with neurological manifestations. *Aliment. Pharmacol. Ther.* **2005**, *21*, 291–292; author reply 292–293. [CrossRef] [PubMed]

96. Volta, U.; De Giorgio, R.; Granito, A.; Stanghellini, V.; Barbara, G.; Avoni, P.; Liguori, R.; Petrolini, N.; Fiorini, E.; Montagna, P.; et al. Anti-ganglioside antibodies in coeliac disease with neurological disorders. *Dig. Liver. Dis.* **2006**. [CrossRef] [PubMed]

97. Przybylska-Felus, M.; Zwolinska-Wcislo, M.; Piatek-Guziewicz, A.; Furgala, A.; Salapa, K.; Mach, T. Concentrations of antiganglioside M1 antibodies, neuron-specific enolase, and interleukin 10 as potential markers of autonomic nervous system impairment in celiac disease. *Pol. Arch. Med. Wewn.* **2016**, *126*, 763–771. [PubMed]

98. Briani, C.; Zara, G.; Alaedini, A.; Grassivaro, F.; Ruggero, S.; Toffanin, E.; Albergoni, M.P.; Luca, M.; Giometto, B.; Ermani, M.; et al. Neurological complications of celiac disease and autoimmune mechanisms: A prospective study. *J. Neuroimmunol.* **2008**, *195*, 171–175. [CrossRef] [PubMed]

99. Chin, R.L.; Sander, H.W.; Brannagan, T.H.; Green, P.H.; Hays, A.P.; Alaedini, A.; Latov, N. Celiac neuropathy. *Neurology* **2003**, *60*, 1581–1585. [CrossRef] [PubMed]

100. Yuki, N.; Susuki, K.; Koga, M.; Nishimoto, Y.; Odaka, M.; Hirata, K.; Taguchi, K.; Miyatake, T.; Furukawa, K.; Kobata, T.; et al. Carbohydrate mimicry between human ganglioside GM1 and Campylobacter jejuni lipooligosaccharide causes Guillain-Barre syndrome. *Proc. Natl. Acad. Sci. USA* **2004**, *101*, 11404–11409. [CrossRef] [PubMed]

101. Mori, M.; Kuwabara, S.; Miyake, M.; Dezawa, M.; Adachi-Usami, E.; Kuroki, H.; Noda, M.; Hattori, T. Haemophilus influenzae has a GM1 ganglioside-like structure and elicits Guillain-Barre syndrome. *Neurology* **1999**, *52*, 1282–1284. [CrossRef] [PubMed]

102. Alaedini, A.; Latov, N. Transglutaminase-independent binding of gliadin to intestinal brush border membrane and GM1 ganglioside. *J. Neuroimmunol.* **2006**, *177*, 167–172. [CrossRef] [PubMed]

103. Thorpe, S.R.; Baynes, J.W. Maillard reaction products in tissue proteins: New products and new perspectives. *Amino Acids* **2003**, *25*, 275–281. [CrossRef] [PubMed]

104. Alaedini, A.; Okamoto, H.; Briani, C.; Wollenberg, K.; Shill, H.A.; Bushara, K.O.; Sander, H.W.; Green, P.H.R.; Hallett, M.; Latov, N. Immune Cross-Reactivity in Celiac Disease: Anti-Gliadin Antibodies Bind to Neuronal Synapsin I. *J. Immunol.* **2007**, 6590–6595. [CrossRef]

105. Huttner, W.B.; Schiebler, W.; Greengard, P.; Camilli, P.D. Synapsin I (protein I), a nerve terminal-specific phosphoprotein. III. its association with synaptic vesicles studied in a highly purified synaptic vesicle preparation. *J. Cell Biol.* **1983**, *96*, 1374–1388. [CrossRef] [PubMed]

106. Murrey, H.E.; Gama, C.I.; Kalovidouris, S.A.; Luo, W.I.; Driggers, E.M.; Porton, B.; Hsieh-Wilson, L.C. Protein fucosylation regulates synapsin Ia/Ib expression and neuronal morphology in primary hippocampal neurons. *Proc. Natl. Acad. Sci. USA* **2006**, *103*, 21–26. [CrossRef] [PubMed]

107. Luthi, T.; Haltiwanger, R.S.; Greengard, P.; Bahler, M. Synapsins contain O-linked N-acetylglucosamine. *J. Neurochem.* **1991**, *56*, 1493–1498. [CrossRef] [PubMed]

108. Hilfiker, S.; Benfenati, F.; Doussau, F.; Nairn, A.C.; Czernik, A.J.; Augustine, G.J.; Greengard, P. Structural domains involved in the regulation of transmitter release by synapsins. *J. Neurosci.* **2005**, *25*, 2658–2669. [CrossRef] [PubMed]

109. Baines, A.J.; Bennett, V. Synapsin I is a spectrin-binding protein immunologically related to erythrocyte protein 4.1. *Nature* **1985**, *315*, 410–413. [CrossRef] [PubMed]

110. Schiebler, W.; Jahn, R.; Doucet, J.P.; Rothlein, J.; Greengard, P. Characterization of synapsin I binding to small synaptic vesicles. *J. Biol. Chem.* **1986**, *261*, 8383–8390. [PubMed]

111. Bahler, M.; Greengard, P. Synapsin I bundles F-actin in a phosphorylation-dependent manner. *Nature* **1987**, *326*, 704–707. [CrossRef] [PubMed]

112. Esser, L.; Wang, C.R.; Hosaka, M.; Smagula, C.S.; Sudhof, T.C.; Deisenhofer, J. Synapsin I is structurally similar to ATP-utilizing enzymes. *EMBO J.* **1998**, *17*, 977–984. [CrossRef] [PubMed]

113. Hosaka, M.; Sudhof, T.C. Synapsins I and II are ATP-binding proteins with differential Ca^{2+} regulation. *J. Biol. Chem.* **1998**, *273*, 1425–1429. [CrossRef] [PubMed]

114. Humeau, Y.; Doussau, F.; Vitiello, F.; Greengard, P.; Benfenati, F.; Poulain, B. Synapsin controls both reserve and releasable synaptic vesicle pools during neuronal activity and short-term plasticity in Aplysia. *J. Neurosci.* **2001**, *21*, 4195–4206. [CrossRef] [PubMed]

115. Mamone, G.; Addeo, F.; Chianese, L.; Di Luccia, A.; De Martino, A.; Nappo, A.; Formisano, A.; De Vivo, P.; Ferranti, P. Characterization of wheat gliadin proteins by combined two-dimensional gel electrophoresis and tandem mass spectrometry. *Proteomics* **2005**, *5*, 2859–2865. [CrossRef] [PubMed]

116. Vojdani, A.; O'Bryan, T.; Kellermann, G.H. The immunology of gluten sensitivity beyond the intestinal tract. *Int. J. Inflam.* **2008**, *6*, 49–57. [CrossRef]

117. Bustos, R.; Kolen, E.R.; Braiterman, L.; Baines, A.J.; Gorelick, F.S.; Hubbard, A.L. Synapsin I is expressed in epithelial cells: Localization to a unique trans-Golgi compartment. *J. Cell Sci.* **2001**, *114*, 3695–3704. [PubMed]

118. Krueger, K.A.; Ings, E.I.; Brun, A.M.; Landt, M.; Easom, R.A. Site-specific phosphorylation of synapsin I by Ca^{2+}/calmodulin-dependent protein kinase II in pancreatic betaTC3 cells: Synapsin I is not associated with insulin secretory granules. *Diabetes* **1999**, *48*, 499–506. [CrossRef] [PubMed]

119. Clemente, M.G.; Musu, M.P.; Frau, F.; Brusco, G.; Sole, G.; Corazza, G.R.; De Virgiliis, S. Immune reaction against the cytoskeleton in coeliac disease. *Gut* **2000**, *47*, 520–526. [CrossRef] [PubMed]

120. Stulik, J.; Hernychova, L.; Porkertova, S.; Pozler, O.; Tuckova, L.; Sanchez, D.; Bures, J. Identification of new celiac disease autoantigens using proteomic analysis. *Proteomics* **2003**, *3*, 951–956. [CrossRef] [PubMed]

121. Pedreira, S.; Sugai, E.; Moreno, M.L.; Vazquez, H.; Niveloni, S.; Smecuol, E.; Mazure, R.; Kogan, Z.; Maurino, E.; Bai, J.C. Significance of smooth muscle/anti-actin autoantibodies in celiac disease. *Acta Gastroenterol. Latinoam.* **2005**, *35*, 83–93. [PubMed]

122. Lidman, K.; Biberfeld, G.; Fagraeus, A.; Norberg, R.; Torstensson, R.; Utter, G.; Carlsson, L.; Luca, J.; Lindberg, U. Anti-actin specificity of human smooth muscle antibodies in chronic active hepatitis. *Clin. Exp. Immunol.* **1976**, *24*, 266–272. [PubMed]

123. Krupickova, S.; Tuckova, L.; Flegelova, Z.; Michalak, M.; Walters, J.R.; Whelan, A.; Harries, J.; Vencovsky, J.; Tlaskalova-Hogenova, H. Identification of common epitopes on gliadin, enterocytes, and calreticulin recognised by antigliadin antibodies of patients with coeliac disease. *Gut* **1999**, *44*, 168–173. [CrossRef] [PubMed]

124. Carroccio, A.; Fabiani, E.; Iannitto, E.; Giannitrapani, L.; Gravina, F.; Montalto, G.; Catassi, C. Tissue transglutaminase autoantibodies in patients with non-Hodgkin's lymphoma. Case reports. *Digestion* **2000**, *62*, 271–275. [CrossRef] [PubMed]

125. Bailey, D.S.; Freedman, A.R.; Price, S.C.; Chescoe, D.; Ciclitira, P.J. Early biochemical responses of the small intestine of coeliac patients to wheat gluten. *Gut* **1989**, *30*, 78–85. [CrossRef] [PubMed]

126. Lerner, A.; Blank, M.; Lahat, N.; Shoenfeld, Y. Increased prevalence of autoantibodies in celiac disease. *Dig. Dis. Sci.* **1998**, *43*, 723–726. [CrossRef] [PubMed]

127. Collin, P.; Kaukinen, K.; Valimaki, M.; Salmi, J. Endocrinological disorders and celiac disease. *Endocr. Rev.* **2002**, *23*, 464–483. [CrossRef] [PubMed]

128. Dalton, T.A.; Bennett, J.C. Autoimmune disease and the major histocompatibility complex: Therapeutic implications. *Am. J. Med.* **1992**, *92*, 183–188. [CrossRef]

129. Atkinson, M.A.; Eisenbarth, G.S. Type 1 diabetes: New perspectives on disease pathogenesis and treatment. *Lancet* **2001**, *358*, 221–229. [CrossRef]

130. Buzzetti, R.; Quattrocchi, C.C.; Nistico, L. Dissecting the genetics of type 1 diabetes: Relevance for familial clustering and differences in incidence. *Diabetes Metab. Rev.* **1998**, *14*, 111–128. [CrossRef]

131. Ventura, A.; Neri, E.; Ughi, C.; Leopaldi, A.; Citta, A.; Not, T. Gluten-dependent diabetes-related and thyroid-related autoantibodies in patients with celiac disease. *J. Pediatr.* **2000**, *137*, 263–265. [CrossRef] [PubMed]

132. Carroccio, A.; Mansueto, P.; Iacono, G.; Soresi, M.; D'Alcamo, A.; Cavataio, F.; Brusca, I.; Florena, A.M.; Ambrosiano, G.; Seidita, A.; et al. Non-celiac wheat sensitivity diagnosed by double-blind placebo-controlled challenge: Exploring a new clinical entity. *Am. J. Gastroenterol.* **2012**, *107*, 1898–1906. [CrossRef] [PubMed]

133. Volta, U.; Bardella, M.T.; Calabro, A.; Troncone, R.; Corazza, G.R. An Italian prospective multicenter survey on patients suspected of having non-celiac gluten sensitivity. *BMC Med.* **2014**, *12*, 85. [CrossRef] [PubMed]

134. Biesiekierski, J.R.; Newnham, E.D.; Irving, P.M.; Barrett, J.S.; Haines, M.; Doecke, J.D.; Shepherd, S.J.; Muir, J.G.; Gibson, P.R. Gluten causes gastrointestinal symptoms in subjects without celiac disease: A double-blind randomized placebo-controlled trial. *Am. J. Gastroenterol.* **2011**, *106*, 508–514. [CrossRef] [PubMed]

135. Peters, S.L.; Biesiekierski, J.R.; Yelland, G.W.; Muir, J.G.; Gibson, P.R. Randomised clinical trial: Gluten may cause depression in subjects with non-coeliac gluten sensitivity—An exploratory clinical study. *Aliment. Pharmacol. Ther.* **2014**, *39*, 1104–1112. [CrossRef] [PubMed]

136. Fasano, A.; Sapone, A.; Zevallos, V.; Schuppan, D. Nonceliac gluten sensitivity. *Gastroenterology* **2015**, *148*, 1195–1204. [CrossRef] [PubMed]

137. Green, P.H.; Lebwohl, B.; Greywoode, R. Celiac disease. *J. Allergy Clin. Immunol.* **2015**, *135*, 1099–1106. [CrossRef] [PubMed]

138. Di Sabatino, A.; Volta, U.; Salvatore, C.; Biancheri, P.; Caio, G.; De Giorgio, R.; Di Stefano, M.; Corazza, G.R. Small Amounts of Gluten in Subjects With Suspected Nonceliac Gluten Sensitivity: A Randomized, Double-Blind, Placebo-Controlled, Cross-Over Trial. *Clin. Gastroenterol. Hepatol.* **2015**, *13*, 1604–1612. [CrossRef] [PubMed]

139. Junker, Y.; Zeissig, S.; Kim, S.J.; Barisani, D.; Wieser, H.; Leffler, D.A.; Zevallos, V.; Libermann, T.A.; Dillon, S.; Freitag, T.L.; et al. Wheat amylase trypsin inhibitors drive intestinal inflammation via activation of toll-like receptor 4. *J. Exp. Med.* **2012**, *209*, 2395–2408. [CrossRef] [PubMed]

140. Biesiekierski, J.R.; Peters, S.L.; Newnham, E.D.; Rosella, O.; Muir, J.G.; Gibson, P.R. No effects of gluten in patients with self-reported non-celiac gluten sensitivity after dietary reduction of fermentable, poorly absorbed, short-chain carbohydrates. *Gastroenterology* **2013**, *145*, 320–328. [CrossRef] [PubMed]

141. Uhde, M.; Ajamian, M.; Caio, G.; De Giorgio, R.; Indart, A.; Green, P.H.; Verna, E.C.; Volta, U.; Alaedini, A. Intestinal cell damage and systemic immune activation in individuals reporting sensitivity to wheat in the absence of coeliac disease. *Gut* **2016**, *65*, 1930–1937. [CrossRef] [PubMed]

142. Carroccio, A.; D'Alcamo, A.; Cavataio, F.; Soresi, M.; Seidita, A.; Sciume, C.; Geraci, G.; Iacono, G.; Mansueto, P. High Proportions of People With Nonceliac Wheat Sensitivity Have Autoimmune Disease or Antinuclear Antibodies. *Gastroenterology* **2015**, *149*, 596–603.e1. [CrossRef] [PubMed]

143. Galli-Tsinopoulou, A.; Nousia-Arvanitakis, S.; Dracoulacos, D.; Xefteri, M.; Karamouzis, M. Autoantibodies predicting diabetes mellitus type I in celiac disease. *Horm. Res.* **1999**, *52*, 119–124. [CrossRef] [PubMed]

144. Ansaldi, N.; Palmas, T.; Corrias, A.; Barbato, M.; D'Altiglia, M.R.; Campanozzi, A.; Baldassarre, M.; Rea, F.; Pluvio, R.; Bonamico, M.; et al. Autoimmune thyroid disease and celiac disease in children. *J. Pediatr. Gastroenterol. Nutr.* **2003**, *37*, 63–66. [CrossRef] [PubMed]

145. Altintas, A.; Pasa, S.; Cil, T.; Bayan, K.; Gokalp, D.; Ayyildiz, O. Thyroid and celiac diseases autoantibodies in patients with adult chronic idiopathic thrombocytopenic purpura. *Platelets* **2008**, *19*, 252–257. [CrossRef] [PubMed]

146. Garg, A.; Reddy, C.; Duseja, A.; Chawla, Y.; Dhiman, R.K. Association between celiac disease and chronic hepatitis C virus infection. *J. Clin. Exp. Hepatol.* **2011**, *1*, 41–44. [CrossRef]

147. Caprai, S.; Vajro, P.; Ventura, A.; Sciveres, M.; Maggiore, G. Autoimmune liver disease associated with celiac disease in childhood: A multicenter study. *Clin. Gastroenterol. Hepatol.* **2008**, *6*, 803–806. [CrossRef] [PubMed]

148. Shaoul, R.; Lerner, A. Associated autoantibodies in celiac disease. *Autoimmun. Rev.* **2007**, *6*, 559–565. [CrossRef] [PubMed]

149. Erbasan, F.; Coban, D.T.; Karasu, U.; Cekin, Y.; Yesil, B.; Cekin, A.H.; Suren, D.; Terzioglu, M.E. Primary Sjögren's syndrome in patients with celiac disease. *Turk. J. Med. Sci.* **2017**, *47*, 430–434. [CrossRef] [PubMed]

150. Kechida, M.; Villalba, N.L. Coeliac disease associated with sarcoidosis and antiphospholipid syndrome: A case report. *Egypt. Rheumatol.* **2017**, *39*, 191–193. [CrossRef]

151. Lerner, A.; Agmon-Levin, N.; Shapira, Y.; Gilburd, B.; Reuter, S.; Lavi, I.; Shoenfeld, Y. The thrombophilic network of autoantibodies in celiac disease. *BMC Med.* **2013**, *11*, 1–7. [CrossRef] [PubMed]

152. Laine, O.; Pitkanen, K.; Lindfors, K.; Huhtala, H.; Niemela, O.; Collin, P.; Kurppa, K.; Kaukinen, K. Elevated serum antiphospholipid antibodies in adults with celiac disease. *Dig. Liver Dis.* **2018**, *50*, 457–461. [CrossRef] [PubMed]

153. Karoui, S.; Sellami, M.K.; Laatar, A.B.; Zitouni, M.; Matri, S.; Laadhar, L.; Fekih, M.; Boubaker, J.; Makni, S.; Filali, A. Prevalence of anticardiolipin and anti-β2-glycoprotein I antibodies in celiac disease. *Dig. Dis. Sci.* **2007**, *52*, 1096–1100. [CrossRef] [PubMed]

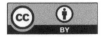

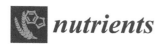

Article

There Is No Association between Coeliac Disease and Autoimmune Pancreatitis

Giulia De Marchi [1], Giovanna Zanoni [2], Maria Cristina Conti Bellocchi [1], Elena Betti [3], Monica Brentegani [2], Paola Capelli [4], Valeria Zuliani [1], Luca Frulloni [1], Catherine Klersy [5] and Rachele Ciccocioppo [1,*]

[1] Gastroenterology Unit, Department of Medicine, AOUI Policlinico G.B. Rossi, University of Verona; Piazzale L.A. Scuro, 10, 37134 Verona, Italy; giuli.dema@yahoo.it (G.D.M.); mcristina.contibellocchi@gmail.com (M.C.C.B.); valeria.zuliani@univr.it (V.Z.); luca.frulloni@univr.it (L.F.)
[2] Immunology Unit, Department of Pathology and Diagnostics, AOUI Policlinico G.B. Rossi, Piazzale L.A. Scuro, 10, 37134 Verona, Italy; giovanna.zanoni@aovr.veneto.it (G.Z.); monica.brentegani@aovr.veneto.it (M.B.)
[3] Clinica Medica I, Department of Internal Medicine, IRCCS Policlinico San Matteo Foundation, Piazzale Golgi, 19, 27100 Pavia, Italy; elena.betti19@gmail.com
[4] Pathology Unit, Department of Pathology and Diagnostics, AOUI Policlinico G.B. Rossi, Piazzale L.A. Scuro, 10, 37134 Verona, Italy; paola.capelli@aovr.veneto.it
[5] Clinical Epidemiology & Biometry Unit, IRCCS Fondazione Policlinico San Matteo; Viale Golgi 19, 27100 Pavia, Italy; klersy@smatteo.pv.it
* Correspondence: rachele.ciccocioppo@univr.it; Tel.: +39-045-812-4578

Received: 1 August 2018; Accepted: 22 August 2018; Published: 24 August 2018

Abstract: Autoimmune pancreatitis (AIP) is a rare disorder whose association with coeliac disease (CD) has never been investigated, although CD patients display a high prevalence of both endocrine and exocrine pancreatic affections. Therefore, we sought to evaluate the frequency of CD in patients with AIP and in further medical pancreatic disorders. The screening for CD was carried out through the detection of tissue transglutaminase (tTG) autoantibodies in sera of patients retrospectively enrolled and divided in four groups: AIP, chronic pancreatitis, chronic asymptomatic pancreatic hyperenzymemia (CAPH), and control subjects with functional dyspepsia. The search for anti-endomysium autoantibodies was performed in those cases with borderline or positive anti-tTG values. Duodenal biopsy was offered to all cases showing positive results. One patient out of 72 (1.4%) with AIP had already been diagnosed with CD and was following a gluten-free diet, while one case out of 71 (1.4%) with chronic pancreatitis and one out of 92 (1.1%) control subjects were diagnosed with de novo CD. No cases of CD were detected in the CAPH group. By contrast, a high prevalence of cases with ulcerative colitis was found in the AIP group (13.8%). Despite a mutual association between CD and several autoimmune disorders, our data do not support the serologic screening for CD in AIP. Further studies will clarify the usefulness of CD serologic screening in other pancreatic disorders.

Keywords: autoimmune pancreatitis; coeliac disease; pancreatic disorders; screening

1. Introduction

Coeliac disease (CD) is an autoimmune condition affecting the small bowel mucosa of a proportion of subjects carrying the human leukocyte antigen (HLA)-DQ2 or -DQ8 haplotypes upon gluten ingestion [1]. Its prevalence, as assessed by serologic tests, is 0.4% in South America, 0.5% in Africa and North America, 0.6% in Asia, and 0.8% in Europe and Oceania, with higher values in female versus male individuals (0.6% vs. 0.4%; $p < 0.001$) [2]. The intestinal lesions encompass a variable degree of villous atrophy and crypt hyperplasia, with a heavy lymphocytic infiltrate of both the epithelial and lamina propria layers (Figure 1) [3]. The clinical picture is multifaceted, ranging from an overt malabsorption syndrome to apparently asymptomatic forms, with anaemia, isolated fatigue, cryptic hypertransaminasaemia, infertility, peripheral and central neurologic disorders, osteopenia, short stature, and dental enamel defects, being the main findings [1,4]. A gluten-free diet leads to an almost complete recovery of both mucosal lesions and clinical features in the vast majority of cases [1]. Remarkably, owing the same genetic and/or environmental predisposing factors, CD patients are at risk of developing further systemic or organ-specific immune-mediated disorders, with type 1 diabetes being the most prevalent and widely studied association, thus justifying the mutual serologic screening [5]. By contrast, no information about the possible association between CD and autoimmune pancreatitis (AIP), the immune-mediated condition affecting the exocrine component of the pancreas, is available so far.

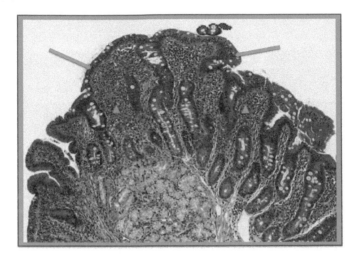

Figure 1. Histological features of duodenal mucosa of active coeliac disease showing subtotal villous atrophy with crypt hyperplasia and heavy lymphocytic inflammatory infiltrate in both the epithelial (arrows) and lamina propria (head arrows) compartments (hematoxylin-eosin, original magnification × 100).

AIP is a rare (estimated prevalence of 0.82:100,000 [6]), chronic fibro-inflammatory condition affecting the whole or a part of the gland, characterized by specific histological, radiological and serological aspects that disappear following a course of steroid therapy [7]. Two different types of AIP (type 1 and type 2) can be distinguished histologically. The first is the so called lymphoplasmacytic sclerosing pancreatitis displaying a dense periductal infiltration of plasma cells, mainly immunoglobulin (Ig)G4 positive, and lymphocytes, peculiar storiform fibrosis, and oblitering venulitis (Figure 2). The second, also called idiopathic duct-centric pancreatitis, is characterized by the presence of intraluminal and intraepithelial neutrophils in medium-sized and small ducts as well as in acini, often leading to destruction and obliteration of the duct lumen. However, the diagnosis of type 1 or type 2 AIP can be made even in the absence of histology by applying a combination of two or more of the following International Consensus Diagnostic Criteria [8]: (1) characteristic imaging features of both the parenchyma and main duct, i.e., a diffuse enlargement with delayed enhancement of the parenchyma with a long or multiple duct strictures without marked upstream dilatation in the typical form, while a segmental/focal enlargement with delayed enhancement of the parenchyma with segmental short duct narrowing in the atypical one; (2) increased level of IgG4; (3) other organ involvement, i.e., biliary duct, retroperitoneum, kidneys, salivary/lachrymal gland, as assessed histologically or radiologically; (4) response to steroid therapy. In those cases where distinctive criteria cannot be identified, the diagnosis of AIP not otherwise specified is given.

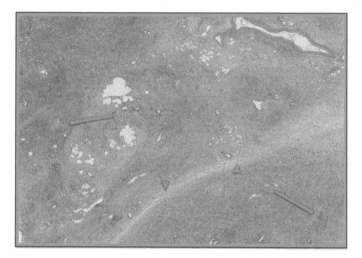

Figure 2. Histological features of autoimmune pancreatitis showing a dense periductal infiltration of plasma cells and lymphocytes leading to obliteration of the affected veins (**arrows**), and peculiar storiform fibrosis (**head arrows**) (hematoxylin-eosin, original magnification × 100).

At variance with AIP, some evidence is available in the literature about the association between CD and non-immune-mediated disorders of the exocrine pancreas. Indeed, CD patients have been found to be at increased risk of developing both acute and chronic pancreatitis in comparison to the general population [9,10]. In addition, patients with villous atrophy, including CD, may carry an exocrine pancreatic insufficiency [11]. Finally, asymptomatic pancreatic hyperamylasemia, which usually precedes the diagnosis of CD and often disappears following a gluten-free diet, has been also described [12]. Similarly, macroamylasemia, a benign condition caused by circulating complexes of pancreatic or salivary amylases bound to plasma proteins that cannot be cleared by the renal glomeruli, has also been described in adulthood CD, but it possibly decreases or resolves after a strict gluten-free diet [13].

The aim of this study, therefore, was to establish the prevalence of CD in patients suffering from AIP by using the sera collected in the Biobank of a Tertiary Italian referral centre for pancreatic diseases. This gave us the unique opportunity to include also patients with non-immune-mediated pancreatic disorders, i.e., chronic pancreatitis and chronic asymptomatic pancreatic hyperenzymemia (CAPH), as control diseased groups, other than control subjects.

2. Patients and Methods

2.1. Study Population

Four groups of adult patients not taking steroids or immunosuppressive therapy at the time of blood sample harvest were enrolled in this study, as detailed below:

Group 1 (AIP). The sera of 72 out of 259 patients diagnosed with AIP (type 1 n = 43, type 2 n = 16, not otherwise specified n = 13) according to the International Consensus Diagnostic Criteria [8] were collected at the Pancreas Institute of the Policlinico G.B. Rossi (AOUI and University of Verona, Italy), from January 2003 through December 2017. Specifically, 40 out of 43 with type 1 AIP (93%), 2 out of 16 with type 2 AIP (12.5%), and 0 out of 13 with not otherwise specified AIP (0%) displayed IgG4 positivity.

Group 2 (chronic pancreatitis). A cohort of 71 out of 492 patients diagnosed with chronic pancreatitis from January 2012 to December 2017 was included in the study. The diagnostic criteria, as adapted following our experience, included at least one of the following criteria: (1) presence of pancreatic-type pain, history of acute/recurrent pancreatitis, presence of steatorrhea or diabetes, weight loss; (2) imaging findings of pancreatic parenchyma atrophy, main pancreatic duct dilation >6 mm and/or presence of irregularities, secondary ducts dilation, presence of pancreatic calcifications; (3) laboratory findings of decreased level of faecal elastase-1 (<100 μg/g of stool), glycated haemoglobin >6.5%; (4) histological features of chronic pancreatitis (loss of acinar cells, presence of interlobular fibrosis, infiltration of inflammatory cells and relative conservation of intralobular ducts and islets) in surgical specimens [14].

Group 3 (CAPH). This group comprised 32 out of 160 patients who were found with CAPH from January 2012 to December 2017. The diagnosis was made when the serum levels of lipases and/or pancreatic amylases were found above the upper normal limits (>10%) for at least three consecutive times lasting for more than six months in the absence of pancreatic-type pain [15]. Moreover, in all cases no lesions of the parenchyma and/or the ductal system were evident at the magnetic resonance of the abdomen with cholangiopancreatography sequences.

Group 4 (control subjects). The serum samples of a cohort of 92 patients suffering from functional dyspepsia, as assessed following the Rome III criteria [16], were collected from June 2012 to December 2016. The presence of relevant co-morbidities, such as primary immunodeficiencies, cancer, active infections or organ failure, was considered an exclusion criterion.

The demographic and clinical features of the study groups are listed in Table 1.

Table 1. Demographic and clinical features of the study population.

	Autoimmune Pancreatitis	Chronic Pancreatitis	Chronic Pancreatic Hyperenzymemia	Control Subjects
Number of cases	72	71	32	92
Male/female ratio	55/17	57/14	18/14	48/44
Mean age in years (SD)	56.5 (16.9)	55.1 (13.2)	52.7 (14.6)	45.7 (18.3)
Body mass index: kg/m^2 (mean ± SD)	25.1 ± 4.1	23.2 ± 5.7	24.9 ± 4.4	22.7 ± 5.2
Time from diagnosis in months (mean ± SD)	25.4 ± 29.3	81 ± 37.5	n.a.	n.a.
Concomitant autoimmune disorders: IBD	13 (10 UC)	1 (Crohn)	0	1 (UC)
Thyroiditis	5	1	1	2
Psoriasis	3	0	0	1
Asthma	1	2	0	2
Coeliac disease	1 *	0	0	0
Rheumatic diseases	2	1	0	3
Thrombocytopenia	1	0	0	0

Abbreviation: SD: Standard Deviation; IBD: inflammatory bowel disease; n.a.: not applicable; UC: ulcerative colitis.
* case already diagnosed with coeliac disease.

The Biobank of the Pancreas Institute, Policlinico G.B. Rossi, AOUI and University of Verona, Italy had been previously approved by the local Ethics Committee (Protocol number 5604, 2 February 2012). This study was approved by the local Ethics Committee (Protocol number 49061, 7 July 2018) and each enrolled patient gave written informed consent.

2.2. Screening for Coeliac Disease

Detection of tissue transglutaminase (tTG) IgA antibody was performed by using a commercial Elisa test (Eu-tTG®IgA kit, Eurospital, Trieste, Italy; cut-off levels: negative < 9 U/mL, borderline 9–15 U/mL, positive > 15 U/mL). Patients with borderline or positive tTG IgA results underwent investigation for IgA anti-endomysium antibodies (EMA-IgA), which was performed by indirect immunofluorescent technique (Eurospital), according to the manufacturer's instructions. Sera with low tTG IgA levels (<1 U/mL) were also evaluated by tTG IgG antibody determination (Eu-tTG®IgG kit, Eurospital, Trieste, Italy; cut-off levels: negative < 20 U/mL, positive ≥ 20 U/mL).

Duodenal mucosal sampling was offered to all cases with positive tTG-IgA and/or EMA-IgA. Four biopsies from the second part of the duodenum and two from the bulb were taken during upper endoscopy for the histological examination according to the Corazza–Villanacci classification [3].

2.3. Statistical Analysis

Continuous variables were expressed as the mean and standard deviation (SD). Discrete data were tabulated as numbers and percentages. The prevalence of CD was computed, together with its 95% exact binomial confidence intervals (95% CI) overall, for pancreatic disorders as a whole and by diagnostic group. Stata 15 (StataCorp, College Station, TX, USA) was used for computation.

3. Results

A total of 267 serum samples harvested from 178 males and 89 females (mean age: 51.8 years, range: 18–85) were included in this study, with 175 being from patients with pancreatic disorders and 92 from control subjects with functional dyspepsia. Worth of note, a large prevalence of males was found in both AIP and chronic pancreatitis groups, accordingly with literature data [7,17], whereas a similar proportion of both genders was observed in the other two groups. As shown in Table 1, one case out of 72 patients of group 1 (1.4%), who was diagnosed with type 1 AIP, had already received the diagnosis of CD two years earlier because of unexplained hypertransaminasemia and weight loss. Since then, he was following a strict gluten-free diet with full recovery of laboratory and clinical features. Therefore, his CD serology resulted negative, and a normal mucosal architecture was found at histology (see Table 2). The radiological findings that led to the diagnosis of AIP type 1, together with a high level of IgG4, are shown in Figure 3. The serologic screening did not detect any further case of CD among patients affected by AIP. However, in two cases a search for tTG-IgG was carried out because of a very low level of tTG-IgA (less than 1.0 U/mL), giving negative results (4.34 and 6.25 U/mL). Remarkably, a consistent number of patients with AIP (13 out 72, 20.8%, of whom three had type 1 and 10 had type 2 AIP) was also affected by inflammatory bowel disease, mostly ulcerative colitis (10 out of 13 cases, while two had indeterminate colitis and one had Crohn's disease). Specifically, one case was diagnosed with ulcerative colitis and AIP simultaneously, whereas the diagnosis of ulcerative colitis preceded that of AIP by a median interval of 28 months (range, 3 to 67 months) in the remaining patients. The vast majority of ulcerative colitis patients (eight out of 10) were not taking systemic corticosteroids at the time of diagnosis of AIP, although they had previously undergone this therapy; only a small proportion of them (three out of 10) was under biological agents (anti-tumour necrosis factor monoclonal antibody). Also, one patient amongst the 71 with chronic pancreatitis (1.4%) showed a positive value of both tTG-IgA antibodies, although at low titre (15,875 U/mL), and EMA-IgA at 1:5 dilution. The histologic examination of the duodenal biopsies showed the characteristic lesions, thus confirming the diagnosis of CD (see Table 2), and the patient was willing to start a gluten-free diet. When collecting his clinical history, aphthous stomatitis appeared evident. One further case was found within the group of patients with functional dyspepsia (1.1%), displaying positivity for both tTG-IgA (value 123 U/mL) and EMA-IgA at 1:16 dilution, thus leading to a definitive diagnosis of CD upon the demonstration of the characteristic lesions at histologic examination of the duodenal biopsies (see Table 2). Interestingly, she complained of infertility. An additional two cases in this group showed borderline values of tTG-IgA (12.44 and 13.47 U/mL) but was negative for the EMA test; hence, they did not undergo endoscopy, whereas in four cases a search for tTG-IgG was carried out because of a very low level of tTG-IgA (less than 1.0 U/mL), giving negative results (5.42, 5.73, 5.8, 8.15 U/mL). By contrast, no cases of positive CD serology were detected among the 32 patients with CAPH (mean value of tTG-IgA: 2.93 U/mL, range 1.276–7.537 U/mL). Therefore, as shown in

Table 2, a total of three cases were identified to suffer from CD (two active and one treated) in the study population; that prevalence was similar in patients with pancreatic disorders and control subjects (overall prevalence 1.1%). Confidence intervals were consistent and ranged from 0% to about 10% in the single diagnostic groups and up to 4% in aggregated diagnoses.

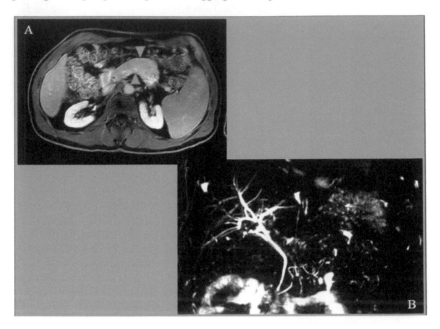

Figure 3. Abdominal magnetic resonance scan showing a diffuse enlargement of the body of the pancreas, with a "sausage-like" aspect (**A**), and multiple long stenosis of the main pancreatic duct at the cholangiopancreatography sequences (**B**).

Table 2. Cases with positive results at the serological screening with their histological findings.

	N	tTG IgA	tTg IgG	EMA	Histology [§]	Prevalence (95% CI)
Group 1	72	0	0	0	Grade A lesions *	1.4% (0.0–7.5)
Group 2	71	1	0	1	Grade B1 lesions	2.4% (0.0–7.6)
Group 3	32	0	0	0	Not performed	0% (0.0–10.9)
Group 4	92	1 + 2 borderline	0	1	Grade B2 lesions	1.1% (0.0–5.9)
Pancreatic disorders	175	1	0	1	–	1.1% (0.1–4.1)
Total	267	2	0	2	3	1.1% (0.2–3.2)

Abbreviations. EMA: anti-endomysium autoantibody; IgA: class A immunoglobulin; IgG: class G immunoglobulin; N: number of cases; tTG: tissue transglutaminase. [§] Following the Corazza–Villanacci classification [3]. * case already diagnosed with coeliac disease.

4. Discussion

Limited information is available about the occurrence of exocrine pancreatic disorders during the course of CD [18], while strong evidence demonstrates an association between CD and type 1 diabetes [5,19]. In fact, approximately 90% of patients with type 1 diabetes carry either HLA-DQ2 or -DQ8 haplotypes as compared to 30% of the general population [20], with those diabetic cases homozygous for DR3-DQ2 having a 33% risk for the presence of tTG autoantibodies [21]. This is why the heterodimers encoded by these HLA haplotypes efficiently bind negatively charged peptides derived from gliadin upon tTG deamidation, thus eliciting a T- and B-cell mediated immune response [22]. This, in turn, leads to an upregulation of key pro-inflammatory molecules, such as interferon-γ [23] and interleukin (IL)-21 [24], responsible for tissue damage. It has also been suggested that dietary gluten could be involved in the pathogenesis of type 1 diabetes [25]. Conversely, a gluten-free diet largely prevented diabetes onset in non-obese diabetic mice, possibly through a modification of the gut microbiota [26].

However, autoimmune attack against the pancreas may involve not only the endocrine component, but also the exocrine one, giving rise to AIP. This is the pancreatic manifestation of the IgG4-related disease, whose genetic susceptibility and pathogenic mechanisms are still poorly understood [7]. Nonetheless, almost all of the candidate genes are directly or indirectly implicated in the regulation of the immune response [7]. A further aspect supporting an autoimmune background is the large proportion of AIP patients displaying autoantibodies, mostly against enzymes, such as lactoferrin, carbonic anhydrases, pancreatic secretory trypsin inhibitor, and trypsinogens [27,28]. Even CD is characterized by the presence of autoantibodies against a ubiquitous enzyme, tTG2, which, besides being the main autoantigen and target of the anti-endomysium autoantibodies [29], catalyses a specific and ordered deamidation of gliadin peptides, giving rise to immunodominant epitopes [22]. In addition, tTG2 seems to play a crucial role in the development of secondary autoimmunity through a post-translational modification of additional proteins, leading to the generation of neoantigens [30]. Also of note, transgenic HLA-DQ8 mice, grown in germ-free conditions and fed a gluten-free diet, developed acute pancreatitis after intra-peritoneal injection of cerulein, a cholecystokinin analogue that causes hyperstimulation of the exocrine component [31]. Whether or not gliadin was then introduced in the diet of these mice, an increased level of IgG1 (homologous of human IgG4) was observed, together with a histological pattern resembling that of human AIP [31]. Moreover, an increased level of serum IgG4 was documented in patients suffering from both CD and pancreatic exocrine insufficiency [32], while an increased number of IgG4+ cells was occasionally found at the mucosal levels of CD patients [33]. Finally, it is conceivable that the mucosal dysbiosis found in CD patients [34] might also contribute to an autoimmune attack in close organs, like the pancreas.

Despite these hypotheses, only one case suffering from both CD and AIP has been reported so far [35], thus we sought to investigate a putative association between these two immune-mediated conditions, taking advantage of the sera collected at the Biobank of a Tertiary Referral centre for pancreatic diseases. We found one patient among the 72 AIP patients who had already received the diagnosis of CD two years earlier. Therefore, the same prevalence of CD in AIP as that of the general population [2] was evident (1.4%). This also suggests that a gluten-free diet does not protect against the development of AIP. One possible explanation may lie in the different genetic predisposition since, at least in the Japanese population, an association of the DRB1*0405-DQB1*0401 haplotype with AIP was found [36], whereas CD is associated with the HLA-DQ2 and -DQ8 ones [1,5]. Moreover, unlike classic autoimmune diseases in which T-cells with regulatory effect are defective in number and/or function, they are likely activated in AIP. Indeed, an increased rate of transcription factor Forkhead box P3+CD4+CD25+ T-cells in both pancreatic tissue [37] and peripheral blood [38] was found in AIP patients, together with upregulation of two cytokines with modulatory functions, i.e., IL-10 and transforming growth factor-β [7]. These seem to be key molecules since the former contributes to IgG4 class switching [39], while the latter is involved in the development of fibrosis [40].

At variance with CD, a strong association between AIP and IBD (18.0% of cases), mostly ulcerative colitis (13.9%), has been found in our cohort of Caucasian patients, thus confirming previous reports [41,42]. However, the prevalence was higher than that found in either an American [41] or an Asiatic [42] study, where a frequency of 5.6% and 5.8%, respectively, was found. Likewise, both have a retrospective design and a similar sample size (71 and 104 AIP cases, respectively) [41,42]. However, the tools applied for the diagnosis of AIP were different, since the HISORt criteria for AIP [43] were used in the former, whereas the Asian Diagnostic Criteria for AIP [44] were used in the latter, thus possibly affecting the final results. The discrepancy may also be partly related to ethnic differences and to the relatively small number of patients recruited. Interestingly, the course of ulcerative colitis was worst in those suffering from both diseases since, during the follow-up period of 10 years, 33.3% of patients underwent a colectomy versus none of those suffering from ulcerative colitis alone [42]. Finally, although Berkson's bias (patients with two uncommon diseases are more likely to be referred to a tertiary medical centre than patients with just one such disease) [45] could have inflated the magnitude of this association, our data strongly suggest that the AIP and ulcerative colitis are related to some degree whose extent deserves further investigation.

As far as the non-immune-mediated pancreatic disorders are concerned, it is widely acknowledged that both functional and anatomical changes of the gland may be caused by or coexist with CD [18]. A Swedish register study, indeed, found an increased risk of both acute and chronic pancreatitis in patients with adulthood CD during the observational period of 1964 to 2003 [9]. Furthermore, it was estimated that over 20% of patients with CD have defective exocrine pancreatic function [10]. This seems to be related to an impaired secretion of cholecystokinin pancreozymin secondary to enteropathy and/or malnutrition, since normalization of both intestinal mucosa and nutritional status restores the secretion of digestive hormones and enzymes [46]. Nevertheless, no information on the prevalence of CD in non-immune-mediated pancreatic disorders is available so far. We found one case in the chronic pancreatitis group (1.4%) and one in the control subject group (1.1%), again overlapping with the prevalence in the general population [2]. Thus, despite a relationship between CD and pancreatic disorders having been demonstrated, the opposite does not seem true. Accordingly, we did not find any positivity at the serologic screening for CD in the CAPH group, even though an abnormal elevation of serum amylase and/or lipase was found in CD patients but disappeared upon a course of gluten-free diet [12].

Obviously, our study has strengths and weaknesses. A point of strength is that this is the first study investigating the prevalence of CD in patients suffering from pancreatic disorders, whereas the studies published so far did the opposite. Moreover, if we consider that AIP is a rare and difficult-to-diagnose condition, the large sample size available, together with the appropriateness of the diagnosis, put us in a privileged situation where the putative higher prevalence of CD in this clinical setting might have been demonstrated, if there was any. The limitations include the retrospective design and the small sample size (and thus the relatively large confidence intervals) of the CAPH and chronic pancreatitis groups in comparison with the overall institutional cohorts due to the low level of willingness to give serum samples for future unknown studies, whereas the lack of sex and age matching among AIP and chronic pancreatitis patients with CAPH and control cases was largely expected [7,47]. In addition, serum IgG or IgG4 levels were not available in non-AIP groups because they are not routinely measured. Despite these limitations, our cohort of 72 patients with AIP represents one of the largest single-centre experiments to date.

5. Conclusions

In summary, our findings suggest that there is a low probability of there being an association of CD with AIP, thus serological screening for CD is not recommended in patients with AIP. By contrast, a strong association between AIP and ulcerative colitis appears evident. AIP is a relatively "new" diagnostic entity, thus further prospective and multicentre studies are needed to confirm the conclusions of this study.

Author Contributions: Conceptualization, R.C.; data curation, G.D.M. and E.B.; formal analysis, C.K., V.Z. and L.F.; funding acquisition, R.C.; investigation, R.C.; methodology, G.Z. and M.B.; project administration, M.C.C.B.; resources, P.C.; supervision, L.F.; validation, R.C.; writing—original draft, G.D.M.; writing—review & editing, C.K. and R.C.

Funding: This research was partially funded by a grant from the Fondazione Celiachia (Italy), project number: N. 016_FC_2015 to R.C. This source of funding did not influence the study design, collection, analysis and interpretation of data, writing of the manuscript, or decision to submit the article for publication.

Conflicts of Interest: The authors have no conflicts of interest to declare.

Abbreviations

AIP	autoimmune pancreatitis
CD	coeliac disease
CAPH	chronic asymptomatic pancreatic hyperenzymemia
CI	confidence interval
EMA	anti-endomysium antibodies
HLA	human leukocyte antigen
Ig	immunoglobulin
SD	standard deviation
tTG	tissue transglutaminase

References

1. Lebwohl, B.; Sanders, D.S.; Green, P.H.R. Coeliac disease. *Lancet* **2018**, *391*, 70–81. [CrossRef]
2. Singh, P.; Arora, A.; Strand, T.A.; Leffler, D.A.; Catassi, C.; Green, P.H.; Kelly, C.P.; Ahuja, V.; Makharia, G.K. Global prevalence of celiac disease: Systematic review and meta-analysis. *Clin. Gastroenterol. Hepatol.* **2018**, *16*, 823–836. [CrossRef] [PubMed]
3. Corazza, G.R.; Villanacci, V.; Zambelli, C.; Milione, M.; Luinetti, O.; Vindigni, C.; Chioda, C.; Albarello, L.; Bartolini, D.; Donato, F. Comparison of the interobserver reproducibility with different histologic criteria used in celiac disease. *Clin. Gastroenterol. Hepatol.* **2007**, *5*, 838–843. [CrossRef] [PubMed]
4. Leffler, D.A.; Green, P.H.R.; Fasano, A. Extraintestinal manifestations of coeliac disease. *Nat. Rev. Gastroenterol Hepatol.* **2015**, *12*, 561–571. [CrossRef] [PubMed]
5. Lundin, K.E.A.; Wijmenga, C. Coeliac disease and autoimmune disease—Genetic overlap and screening. *Nat. Rev. Gastroenterol. Hepatol.* **2015**, *12*, 507–515. [CrossRef] [PubMed]
6. Uchida, K.; Masamune, A.; Shimosegawa, T.; Okazaki, K. Prevalence of IgG4-related disease in Japan based on nationwide survey in 2009. *Int. J. Rheumatol.* **2012**, *2012*, 358371. [CrossRef] [PubMed]
7. Hart, P.A.; Zen, Y.; Chari, S.T. Recent advances in autoimmune pancreatitis. *Gastroenterology* **2015**, *149*, 39–51. [CrossRef] [PubMed]
8. Shimosegawa, T.; Chari, S.T.; Frulloni, L.; Kamisawa, T.; Kawa, S.; Mino-Kenudson, M.; Kim, M.H.; Kloppel, G.; Lerch, M.M.; Lohr, M.; et al. International consensus diagnostic criteria for autoimmune pancreatitis: Guidelines of the International Association of Pancreatology. *Pancreas* **2011**, *40*, 352–358. [CrossRef] [PubMed]
9. Ludvigsson, J.F.; Montgomery, S.M.; Ekbom, A. Risk of pancreatitis in 14,000 individuals with celiac disease. *Clin. Gastroenterol. Hepatol.* **2007**, *5*, 1347–1353. [CrossRef] [PubMed]
10. Sadr-Azodi, O.; Sanders, D.S.; Murray, J.A.; Ludvigsson, J.F. Patients with celiac disease have an increased risk for pancreatitis. *Clin. Gastroenterol. Hepatol.* **2012**, *10*, 1136–1142. [CrossRef] [PubMed]
11. Walkowiak, J.; Herzig, K.H. Fecal elastase-1 is decreased in villous atrophy regardless of the underlying disease. *Eur. J. Clin. Investig.* **2001**, *31*, 425–430. [CrossRef]
12. Carroccio, A.; Di Prima, L.; Scalici, C.; Soresi, M.; Cefalù, A.B.; Noto, D.; Averna, M.R.; Montalto, G.; Iacono, G. Unexplained elevated serum pancreatic enzymes: A reason to suspect celiac disease. *Clin. Gastroenterol. Hepatol.* **2006**, *4*, 455–459. [CrossRef] [PubMed]
13. Rajvanshi, P.; Chowdhury, J.R.; Gupta, S. Celiac sprue and macroamylasaemia: Potential clinical and pathophysiological implications. Case study. *J. Clin. Gastroenterol.* **1995**, *20*, 304–306. [CrossRef] [PubMed]
14. Duggan, S.N.; Ni Chonchubhair, H.M.; Lawal, O.; O'Connor, D.B.; Conlon, K.C. Chronic pancreatitis: A diagnostic dilemma. *World J. Gastroenterol.* **2016**, *22*, 2304–2313. [CrossRef] [PubMed]
15. Amodio, A.; Manfredi, R.; Katsotourchi, A.M.; Gabbrielli, A.; Benini, L.; Mucelli, R.P.; Vantini, I.; Frulloni, L. Prospective evaluation of subjects with chronic asymptomatic pancreatic hyperenzymemia. *Am. J. Gastroenterol.* **2012**, *107*, 1089–1095. [CrossRef] [PubMed]
16. Longstreth, G.F.; Thompson, W.G.; Chey, W.D.; Houghton, L.A.; Mearin, F.; Spiller, R.C. Functional bowel disorders. *Gastroenterology* **2006**, *130*, 1480–1491. [CrossRef] [PubMed]
17. Yadav, D.; Lowenfels, A.B. The epidemiology of pancreatitis and pancreatic cancer. *Gastroenterology* **2013**, *144*, 1252–1261. [CrossRef] [PubMed]

18. Pezzilli, R. Exocrine pancreas involvement in celiac disease: A review. *Recent. Pat. Inflamm. Allergy Drug Discov.* **2014**, *8*, 167–172. [CrossRef] [PubMed]

19. Weiss, B.; Pinhas-Hamiel, O. Celiac disease and diabetes: When to test and treat. *J. Pediatr. Gastroenterol. Nutr.* **2017**, *64*, 175–179. [CrossRef] [PubMed]

20. Smyth, D.J.; Plagnol, V.; Walker, N.M.; Cooper, J.D.; Downes, K.; Yang, J.H.; Howson, J.M.; Stevens, H.; McManus, R.; Wijmenga, C.; et al. Shared and distinct genetic variants in type 1 diabetes and celiac disease. *N. Engl. J. Med.* **2008**, *359*, 2767–2777. [CrossRef] [PubMed]

21. Bao, F.; Yu, L.; Babu, S.; Wang, T.; Hoffenberg, E.J.; Rewers, M.; Eisenbarth, G.S. One third of HLA DQ2 homozygous patients with type 1 diabetes express celiac disease associated transglutaminase autoantibodies. *J. Autoimmun.* **1999**, *13*, 143–148. [CrossRef] [PubMed]

22. Stamnaes, J.; Sollid, L.M. Celiac disease: Autoimmunity in response to food antigen. *Semin. Immunol.* **2015**, *27*, 343–352. [CrossRef] [PubMed]

23. Nilsen, E.M.; Lundin, K.E.; Krajci, P.; Scott, H.; Sollid, L.M.; Brandtzaeg, P. Gluten specific, HLA-DQ restricted T cells from coeliac mucosa produce cytokines with Th1 or Th0 profile dominated by interferon gamma. *Gut* **1995**, *37*, 766–776. [CrossRef] [PubMed]

24. Fina, D.; Sarra, M.; Caruso, R.; Del Vecchio Blanco, G.; Pallone, F.; MacDonald, T.T.; Monteleone, G. Interleukin-21 contributes to the mucosal T helper cell type 1 response in coeliac disease. *Gut* **2008**, *57*, 887–892. [CrossRef] [PubMed]

25. Troncone, R.; Discepolo, V. Celiac disease and autoimmunity. *J. Pediatr. Gastroenterol. Nutr.* **2014**, *59*, S9–S11. [CrossRef] [PubMed]

26. Marietta, E.V.; Gomez, A.M.; Yeoman, C.; Tilahun, A.Y.; Clark, C.R.; Luckey, D.H.; Murray, J.A.; White, B.A.; Kudva, Y.C.; Rajagopalan, G. Low incidence of spontaneous type 1 diabetes in non-obese diabetic mice raised on gluten-free diets is associated with changes in the intestinal microbiome. *PLoS ONE* **2013**, *8*, e78687. [CrossRef] [PubMed]

27. Okazaki, K.; Uchida, K.; Ohana, M.; Nakase, H.; Uose, S.; Inai, M.; Matsushima, Y.; Katamura, K.; Ohmori, K.; Chiba, T. Autoimmune-related pancreatitis is associated with autoantibodies and a Th1/Th2-type cellular immune response. *Gastroenterology* **2000**, *118*, 573–581. [CrossRef]

28. Lohr, J.M.; Faissner, R.; Koczan, D.; Bewerunge, P.; Bassi, C.; Brors, B.; Eils, R.; Frulloni, L.; Funk, A.; Halangk, W.; et al. Autoantibodies against the exocrine pancreas in autoimmune pancreatitis: Gene and protein expression profiling and immunoassays identify pancreatic enzymes as a major target of the inflammatory process. *Am. J. Gastroenterol.* **2010**, *105*, 2060–2071. [CrossRef] [PubMed]

29. Brusco, G.; Muzi, P.; Ciccocioppo, R.; Biagi, F.; Cifone, M.G.; Corazza, G.R. Transglutaminase and coeliac disease: Endomysial reactivity and small bowel expression. *Clin. Exp. Immunol.* **1999**, *118*, 371–375. [CrossRef] [PubMed]

30. Martucci, S.; Corazza, G.R. Spreading and focusing of gluten epitopes in celiac disease. *Gastroenterology* **2002**, *122*, 2072–2075. [CrossRef] [PubMed]

31. Moon, S.H.; Kim, J.; Kim, M.Y.; Park, D.H.; Song, T.J.; Kim, S.A.; Lee, S.S.; Seo, D.W.; Lee, S.K.; Kim, M.H. Sensitization to and challenge with gliadin induce pancreatitis and extrapancreatic inflammation in HLA-DQ8 Mice: An animal model of type 1 autoimmune pancreatitis. *Gut Liver.* **2016**, *10*, 842–850. [CrossRef] [PubMed]

32. Leeds, J.S.; Sanders, D.S. Risk of pancreatitis in patients with celiac disease: Is autoimmune pancreatitis a biologically plausible mechanism? *Clin. Gastroenterol. Hepatol.* **2008**, *6*, 951. [CrossRef] [PubMed]

33. Cebe, K.M.; Swanson, P.E.; Upton, M.P.; Westerhoff, M. Increased IgG4+ cells in duodenal biopsies are not specific for autoimmune pancreatitis. *Am. J. Clin. Pathol.* **2013**, *139*, 323–329. [CrossRef] [PubMed]

34. D'Argenio, V.; Casaburi, G.; Precone, V.; Pagliuca, C.; Colicchio, R.; Sarnataro, D.; Discepolo, V.; Kim, S.M.; Russo, I.; Del Vecchio Blanco, G.; et al. Metagenomics reveals dysbiosis and a potentially pathogenic N. flavescens strain in duodenum of adult celiac patients. *Am. J. Gastroenterol.* **2016**, *11*, 879–890. [CrossRef] [PubMed]

35. Masoodi, I.; Wani, H.; Alsayari, K.; Sulaiman, T.; Hassan, N.S.; Nazmi Alqutub, A.; Al Omair, A.; H Al-Lehibi, A. Celiac disease and autoimmune pancreatitis: An uncommon association. A case report. *Eur. J. Gastroenterol. Hepatol.* **2011**, *23*, 1270–1272. [CrossRef] [PubMed]

36. Kawa, S.; Ota, M.; Yoshizawa, K.; Horiuchi, A.; Hamano, H.; Ochi, Y.; Nakayama, K.; Tokutake, Y.; Katsuyama, Y.; Saito, S.; et al. HLA DRB10405-DQB10401 haplotype is associated with autoimmune pancreatitis in the Japanese population. *Gastroenterology* **2002**, *122*, 1264–1269. [CrossRef] [PubMed]

37. Zen, Y.; Fujii, T.; Harada, K.; Kawano, M.; Yamada, K.; Takahira, M.; Nakanuma, Y. Th2 and regulatory immune reactions are increased in immunoglobin G4-related sclerosing pancreatitis and cholangitis. *Hepatology* **2007**, *45*, 1538–1546. [CrossRef] [PubMed]

38. Miyoshi, H.; Uchida, K.; Taniguchi, T.; Yazumi, S.; Matsushita, M.; Takaoka, M.; Okazaki, K. Circulating naive and CD4+CD25high regulatory T cells in patients with autoimmune pancreatitis. *Pancreas* **2008**, *36*, 133–140. [CrossRef] [PubMed]

39. Jeannin, P.; Lecoanet, S.; Delneste, Y.; Gauchat, J.F.; Bonnefoy, J.Y. IgE versus IgG4 production can be differentially regulated by IL-10. *J. Immunol.* **1998**, *160*, 3555–3561. [PubMed]

40. Yamamoto, M.; Shimizu, Y.; Takahashi, H.; Yajima, H.; Yokoyama, Y.; Ishigami, K.; Tabeya, T.; Suzuki, C.; Matsui, M.; Naishiro, Y.; et al. CCAAT/enhancer binding protein alpha (C/EBPalpha)(+) M2 macrophages contribute to fibrosis in IgG4-related disease? *Mod. Rheumatol.* **2015**, *25*, 484–486. [CrossRef] [PubMed]

41. Ravi, K.; Chari, S.T.; Vege, S.S.; Sandborn, W.J.; Smyrk, T.C.; Loftus, E.V., Jr. Inflammatory bowel disease in the setting of autoimmune pancreatitis. *Inflamm. Bowel Dis.* **2009**, *15*, 1326–1330. [CrossRef] [PubMed]

42. Park, S.H.; Kim, D.; Ye, B.D.; Yang, S.-K.; Kim, J.-H.; Yang, D.-H.; Jung, K.W.; Kim, K.-J.; Byeon, J.-S.; Myung, S.-J.; et al. The characteristics of ulcerative colitis associated with autoimmune pancreatitis. *J. Clin. Gastroenterol.* **2013**, *47*, 520–525. [CrossRef] [PubMed]

43. Chari, S.T. Diagnosis of autoimmune pancreatitis using its five cardinal features: Introducing the Mayo Clinic's HISORt criteria. *J. Gastroenterol.* **2007**, *42*, 39–41. [CrossRef] [PubMed]

44. Otsuki, M.; Chung, J.B.; Okazaki, K.; Kim, M.H.; Kamisawa, T.; Kawa, S.; Park, S.W.; Shimosegawa, T.; Lee, K.; Ito, T.; et al. Asian diagnostic criteria for autoimmune pancreatitis: Consensus of the Japan-Korea Symposium on Autoimmune Pancreatitis. *J. Gastroenterol.* **2008**, *43*, 403–408. [CrossRef] [PubMed]

45. Berkson, J. Limitations of the application of fourfold tables to hospital data. *Biometr. Bull.* **1946**, *2*, 47–53. [CrossRef] [PubMed]

46. Nousia-Arvanitakis, S.; Fotoulaki, M.; Tendzidou, K.; Vassilaki, C.; Agguridaki, C.; Karamouzis, M. Subclinical exocrine pancreatic dysfunction resulting from decreased cholecystokinin secretion in the presence of intestinal villous atrophy. *J. Pediatr. Gastroenterol. Nutr.* **2006**, *43*, 307–312. [CrossRef] [PubMed]

47. Hart, P.A.; Kamisawa, T.; Brugge, W.R.; Chung, J.B.; Culver, E.L.; Czakó, L.; Frulloni, L.; Go, V.L.; Gress, T.M.; Kim, M.H.; et al. Long-term outcomes of autoimmune pancreatitis: A multicentre, international analysis. *Gut* **2013**, *62*, 1771–1776. [CrossRef] [PubMed]

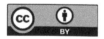

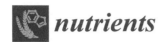

Article

The Significance of Low Titre Antigliadin Antibodies in the Diagnosis of Gluten Ataxia

Marios Hadjivassiliou [1,*], Richard A Grünewald [1], David S Sanders [2], Panagiotis Zis [1],
Iain Croall [1], Priya D Shanmugarajah [1], Ptolemaios G Sarrigiannis [1], Nick Trott [3], Graeme Wild [4]
and Nigel Hoggard [2]

[1] Academic Departments of Neurosciences and Neuroradiology, Sheffield Teaching Hospitals NHS Trust,
Sheffield S10 2JF, UK; r.a.grunewald@sheffield.ac.uk (R.A.G.); takiszis@gmail.com (P.Z.);
i.croall@sheffield.ac.uk (I.C.); p.d.shanmugarajah@sheffield.ac.uk (P.D.S.);
p.sarrigiannis@sheffield.ac.uk (P.G.S.); n.hoggard@sheffield.ac.uk (N.H.)

[2] Departments of Gastroenterology, Sheffield Teaching Hospitals NHS Trust, Sheffield S10 2JF, UK;
David.Sanders@sth.nhs.uk (D.S.S.)

[3] Departments of Dietetics, Sheffield Teaching Hospitals NHS Trust, Sheffield S10 2JF, UK;
Nick.Trott@sth.nhs.uk (N.T.)

[4] Departments of Immunology, Sheffield Teaching Hospitals NHS Trust, Sheffield S10 2JF, UK;
Graeme.Wild@sth.nhs.uk (G.W)

* Correspondence: m.hadjivassiliou@sheffield.ac.uk; Tel.: +44-114-2712502

Received: 6 September 2018; Accepted: 4 October 2018; Published: 5 October 2018

Abstract: Background: Patients with gluten ataxia (GA) without enteropathy have lower levels of antigliadin antibodies (AGA) compared to patients with coeliac disease (CD). Magnetic Resonance Spectroscopy (NAA/Cr area ratio) of the cerebellum improves in patients with GA following a strict gluten-free diet (GFD). This is associated with clinical improvement. We present our experience of the effect of a GFD in patients with ataxia and low levels of AGA antibodies measured by a commercial assay. Methods: Consecutive patients with ataxia and serum AGA levels below the positive cut-off for CD but above a re-defined cut-off in the context of GA underwent MR spectroscopy at baseline and after a GFD. Results: Twenty-one consecutive patients with GA were included. Ten were on a strict GFD with elimination of AGA, 5 were on a GFD but continued to have AGA, and 6 patients did not go on a GFD. The NAA/Cr area ratio from the cerebellar vermis increased in all patients on a strict GFD, increased in only 1 out of 5 (20%) patients on a GFD with persisting circulating AGA, and decreased in all patients not on a GFD. Conclusion: Patients with ataxia and low titres of AGA benefit from a strict GFD. The results suggest an urgent need to redefine the serological cut-off for circulating AGA in diagnosing GA.

Keywords: Gluten ataxia; antigliadin antibodies; coeliac disease; MR spectroscopy; gluten sensitive enteropathy; antigliadin antibody titre

1. Introduction

Gluten ataxia (GA) is defined as otherwise idiopathic sporadic ataxia with serological evidence of gluten sensitivity in the absence of an alternative cause [1]. The presence or absence of an enteropathy is not a prerequisite for its diagnosis [2]. Indeed, up to 50% of patients with GA do not have an enteropathy, yet they still benefit from a gluten-free diet (GFD) [2]. For this reason, IgG and IgA native antigliadin antibodies (AGA) are currently the most sensitive marker for GA when compared to endomysium (EMA) and transglutaminase 2 antibodies (TG2), both of which are specific for the presence of enteropathy (Coeliac Disease-CD) [2]. Despite this, the majority of immunology laboratories in the UK and other countries have abandoned the use of native AGA assays in the diagnosis of CD because of poor specificity. Estimation of specificity, however, is based on the presence of a gold standard, in this case the presence of enteropathy (CD). It is now widely accepted that sensitivity to gluten can be present without enteropathy [3]. The only current serological biomarker helpful in diagnosing gluten sensitivity without enteropathy is AGA [4].

Patients with CD often have high titres of circulating AGA, whereas patients with GA and no enteropathy tend to have low titres. The serological cut-off for significant titre in commercially available AGA assays is calculated to maximize diagnostic specificity using data from patients with CD. This would not necessarily be applicable to those patients with gluten sensitivity who do not have enteropathy and those patients with extraintestinal manifestations.

Having previously demonstrated the beneficial effect of a GFD in patients with GA using MR spectroscopy of the cerebellum, in this report we present our experience of the effect of a GFD in patients with ataxia and AGA levels that are below what is considered positive, as defined by the manufacturer, but above a newly defined cut-off AGA level based on our extensive experience in managing patients with GA and the re-evaluation of over 500 patients with GA.

2. Methods

This report is based on prospective observational case series of patients regularly attending the gluten sensitivity/neurology clinic run by one of the authors (M.H.). The South Yorkshire Research Ethics Committee has confirmed that no ethical approval is indicated given that a gluten-free diet is a recognized treatment for suspected patients with GA and that all investigations/interventions were clinically indicated and did not form part of a research study.

2.1. AGA Serological Testing

In January 2015, the immunology lab at Sheffield Teaching Hospitals NHS Trust changed the ELISA AGA (IgG and IgA) assay to Phadia 2500 [5]. The decision was based on the benefits of an automated high throughput process. After consultation with the clinicians using the AGA assay, a decision was made to provide numerical values for the AGA results instead of just positive/negative results.

The manufacturers provided the following information regarding positivity (for both IgA and IgG) of their assay: 0–7 U/mL negative, 7–10 U/mL borderline, >10 U/mL positive.

2.2. Patient Selection and Follow-up

The Sheffield Ataxia Centre cares for over 1800 patients with progressive ataxia, including over 500 patients with GA. All patients with ataxia undergo extensive investigations to try and identify a cause [6]. Such investigations include serological testing for AGA, EMA and TG2. Our previous report on the effect of a GFD on MR spectroscopy in 117 patients with GA was based on those patients with AGA serological positivity (with or without serological positivity for TG2 and EMA antibodies and/or enteropathy) using previous commercial AGA assays by our immunology lab, or those patients who had a value of over 7 U/mL using the new assay [7]. Fifty percent of our cohort of patients with GA have an enteropathy (CD). As expected in patients with enteropathy, EMA and TTG antibodies are also positive. All patients diagnosed with GA at our centre are routinely advised to adopt a strict GFD and are referred to an experienced dietitian for GFD advice. Strict adherence to a GFD is assumed when there is elimination of all gluten related antibodies. If patients have persistently positive antibodies, they are reviewed by an experienced dietitian (NT) for further advice. Patients who still have persistently positive AGA are assumed not to be strict with a GFD.

In the current report we have included only those consecutive patients with serological results for IgG and/or IgA AGA over 3 U/mL but less than 7 U/mL. The lower cut-off value of 3 U/mL was derived based on our experience in the diagnosis and management of over 500 patients with GA who regularly attend the Sheffield Ataxia Centre and either did not adopt a GFD or were on a partial (non-strict) GFD. All of these patients were repeatedly tested using the new assay, irrespective of their GFD status. The new serological cut-off was also based on AGA estimation in those GA patients already on a strict GFD who had persistently absent circulating AGA, using previous assays and with evidence of improvement of their ataxia clinically and on MR spectroscopy. All of these patients with GA who remained neurologically stable had values below 3 U/mL on the new assay. Patients on partial or no GFD had levels above 3 U/mL but often less than 7 U/mL. We therefore used the cut-off of 3 U/mL, below which we assumed strict adherence to a GFD.

Consecutive patients included in this report attend the Sheffield Ataxia Centre on a 6 monthly basis. All patients had undergone more than one clinical MR spectroscopy scan for the purpose of diagnosis and monitoring of their ataxia since 2015, the year of the introduction of the new AGA assay. Only a third of the patients reported here underwent gastroscopy and duodenal biopsy to establish the presence of enteropathy (triad of villus atrophy, crypt hyperplasia and increased intraepithelial lymphocytes). This was based on patient choice after informing them of their serological results, including the negative serology for TG2 and EMA antibodies. None of these patients had enteropathy as predicted by the negative EMA and TG2 antibodies, but presence or not of enteropathy was not an exclusion criterion. Patients were reviewed by an experienced dietitian (NT) who provided detailed advice on a GFD with further monitoring by telephone or face-to-face consultations. The patients underwent repeat clinical evaluation and further serological testing at approximately 6 monthly intervals. Strict adherence to a GFD was indicated by serological elimination of circulating AGA (<3 U/mL). For the purpose of this report, the patients were divided into 3 groups: those with strict adherence to GFD with AGA levels of <3 U/mL, those with partial adherence to a GFD as evident from the presence of AGA (above 3 U/mL but less that 7 U/mL), and a third group consisting of patients that declined GFD (AGA level above 3 U/mL and less than 7 U/mL).

We also reviewed the AGA results in patients with classical CD presenting to gastroenterology clinics and patients with idiopathic sporadic ataxia. Data on the prevalence of AGA (range between 3–7 U/mL) was also available from healthy volunteers as part of another ongoing study.

2.3. MR Spectroscopy

In addition to volumetric 3T MR imaging, all patients underwent single-voxel H^1 MR spectroscopy of the cerebellum. This imaging protocol is in clinical use as part of the investigation of all patients with cerebellar ataxia attending the Sheffield Ataxia Centre. The brain imaging protocol for structural, volumetric, and spectroscopy studies has been previously described [7]. The main measurement is the NAA/Cr area ratio within the cerebellar vermis. N-acetyl aspartate (NAA) reflects the health of neurons and is a reliable marker of monitoring neuronal energy impairment and dysfunction. Creatine (Cr) is a stable metabolite with little variation between different pathologies. As such, it is typically used as an internal standard in MR spectroscopy from which metabolite ratios can be calculated.

A baseline MR spectroscopy scan was done on all patients and a repeat scan was done after the introduction of the GFD. In common with other immune-mediated ataxias, the cerebellar vermis is primarily involved in GA; therefore, MR spectroscopy results reported here are measurements from the cerebellar vermis.

2.4. Statistical Analysis

Change in mean values between the groups was compared with Student's two-tailed *t*-test for unpaired samples. A value of $p < 0.05$ was considered significant.

3. Results

A total of 21 consecutive patients with GA were included at the time of writing this report. Detailed clinical characteristics of patients with GA have been described previously. The patients included in this report did not differ in any way from those patients with GA described previously [1,8].

All patients had two MR spectroscopy scans at baseline and the second after a mean interval of 19 months (range 5 months to 36 months). Of the 21 patients, 10 were on a strict GFD with elimination of all antibodies (IgG and/or IgA AGA <3 U/mL), 5 were on a GFD but still had serological evidence of circulating AGA, indicating ongoing exposure to gluten (IgG and/or IgA >3 U/mL), and 6 patients were not on the diet (IgG and/or IgA AGA >3 U/ml and <7 U/mL). There were no significant differences in the duration of ataxia between the 3 groups. The patients on partial GFD were significantly younger that the other 2 groups. There were, however, no significant differences in age between the strict GFD and no GFD groups. Those patients that declined a GFD also had a repeat scan for monitoring purposes. The NAA/Cr area ratio taken from the cerebellar vermis increased in all 10 patients on a strict diet, but in only 1 out of 5 (20%) patients on a partial GFD with persistent circulating AGA. In the remaining 4, the NAA/Cr area ratio decreased. In all of the 6 patients not on a diet, there was a decrease in NAA/Cr area ratio on repeat scanning. These results are illustrated in Figures 1 and 2. A Chi squared contingency table looking at numbers improved on MR spectroscopy on a strict diet compared with no diet was significant $p < 0.0001$. A comparison of the change in MR spectroscopy values from baseline between the 3 groups showed the following: no diet mean change −0.098, Standard error of the Mean (SEM) 0.06, partial diet mean change −0.028, SEM 0.087 and strict diet mean change +0.092, SEM 0.06. Comparison between the strict diet and no diet groups was significant ($p < 0.0001$), as was the comparison between partial diet and no diet ($p = 0.0028$).

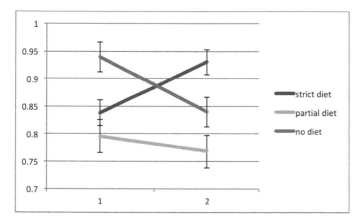

Figure 1. NAA/Cr area ratio in patients with gluten ataxia without enteropathy following the introduction of a gluten-free diet (GFD) in the 2 sub-groups (number of patients on gluten free diet 10, partial diet 5). The third subgroup consisted of 6 patients who declined a GFD. All patients had antigliadin antibodies (AGA) IgG and/or IgA of >3 U/mL and <7 U/mL at baseline. Both the partial diet and no diet groups still had AGA values >3 U/mL at the time of the second scan. All 10 patients on a strict GFD showed improvement of the NAA/Cr area ratio (vertical axis) of the vermis 4 of the 5 patients on partial GFD and all 6 patients not on GFD showed deterioration of the NAA/Cr ratio. A Chi squared contingency table looking at numbers improved on magnetic resonance spectroscopy on a strict diet compared with no diet was significant $p < 0.0001$.

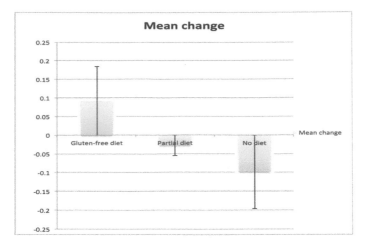

Figure 2. Mean change of the area ratio of NAA/Cr from baseline in the 3 groups.

Using the same serological cut-off for AGA titres of >3 U/mL, the prevalence of AGA positivity amongst 68 patients with classical CD presenting to the gastroenterologists was 100%. The mean baseline value for AGA titre in this classical CD group was 46.5 U/mL. This compares to a mean AGA titre of 4.1 U/mL in the 21 patients reported here. The prevalence amongst 28 healthy controls was 7%, and the prevalence amongst 197 patients with otherwise idiopathic sporadic ataxia was 39%. This group of 197 did not include patients with ataxia who had AGA levels over 7 U/mL or those who also had enteropathy. Table 1 summarises the clinical and serological characteristics of the GA groups.

Table 1. Summary of clinical characteristics and the change in magnetic resonance spectroscopy and antigliadin antibody titre at baseline and at the time of the second scan in the 3 groups. The differences in numbers improved and in the changes in MR spectroscopy between the strict GFD and the not on GFD groups were significant $p < 0.0001$. There were no significant clinical differences between the strict GFD and the partial or not on diet groups. The patients on partial GFD were significantly younger than the other 2 groups. GA = gluten ataxia; NAA/Cr = N Acetyl Aspartate to Creatine ratio; GFD = Gluten Free Diet; AGA = Antigliadin antibodies; SD standard deviation.

Dietary Status in GA Groups	Numb per Group	Mean Age	Mean Duration of Ataxia in Years	Mean MR Spectroscopy Change from Baseline (NAA/Cr Area Ratio)	Numb Improv-ed	Mean AGA Antibody Titre at Baseline (SD)	Mean AGA Antibody Titre at the Time of 2nd Scan (SD)
strict GFD	10	65	6.4	+0.092	10	3.6 (0.46)	1.8 (0.74)
partial GFD	5	50	6.6	−0.028	1	4.5 (1.3)	3.8 (1)
not on diet	6	77	7.3	−0.098	0	4.2 (1.3)	4.2 (1.8)

4. Discussion

We have previously demonstrated clinical and MR spectroscopic improvement in patients with GA after a year of strict adherence to a gluten-free diet [7,9]. The current study demonstrates that in patients with GA with low titres of AGA, NAA/Cr area ratio within the cerebellar vermis improves with strict adherence to a gluten-free diet, worsens with on-going exposure to gluten, and also largely worsens with partial adherence to a gluten-free diet, as indicated by persistently positive circulating AGA. The improvement in MR spectroscopy was accompanied by clinical improvement or stabilisation of the ataxia in the strict GFD group.

The advantage of MR spectroscopy as a monitoring tool is that it can be easily performed as part of routine MR imaging, it is reproducible in an individual on a particular scanner, and relies on objective measurements such as the NAA/Cr area ratio [7,10]. It therefore overcomes the disadvantages of the clinical scales (interrater variability, fluctuation of ataxia symptoms and signs due to fatigue, insensitive scales in disabled patients and ceiling effect). Other groups have also demonstrated good correlation between MR spectroscopy and the clinical status as assessed by ataxia rating scales [11]. This report also demonstrates the importance of strict adherence to the GFD. Amongst those patients on the diet, but not strict, only 20% improved on MR spectroscopy as opposed to 100% in those on a strict GFD. Strict diet with serological evidence of elimination of all antibodies appears to have the potential to stabilise and partially reverse immune mediated damage to the cerebellum.

This report also demonstrates that for extraintestinal manifestations of gluten sensitivity, and in particular for those patients without enteropathy, the level of circulating AGA that is still significant is lower than that seen in the context of enteropathy. This means that the serological cut-off titre for diagnosing GA requires adjustment. This has major implications for the diagnosis of GA. Our data from 197 patients with idiopathic sporadic ataxia collected since 2015 (the year of the introduction of the new assay), excluding those with positive AGA (using the manufacturer's serum cut-off level for positivity) and those with CD, showed that 39% had AGA levels between 3 and 7 U/mL. As we have shown here, these patients also benefited from a strict GFD. Up until now, such patients would have remained undiagnosed and therefore followed a progressive course as a result of ongoing exposure to gluten. Indeed, some of these patients had been under regular follow-up in our ataxia clinic but were negative for AGA on previous assays used by our immunology lab.

We have found MR spectroscopy a reliable and useful tool in the monitoring of patients with GA and other ataxias. Improvement of NAA/Cr in patients adherent to a GFD bolsters the diagnosis of GA and, in our experience, is accompanied by clinical improvement [9]. Such improvement also acts as a motivation for patients to continue with the GFD. The commonest cause for the lack of improvement tends to be poor adherence to the GFD.

Both this report and previous publications from our group have highlighted the importance of using the correct serological markers for the diagnosis of GA. The presence of enteropathy (associated with the presence of positive TG2 and endomysium antibodies) does not influence the response to the GFD, and thus any patient with positive antigliadin antibodies and no other cause of ataxia should be offered a strict gluten-free diet, even in the absence of enteropathy.

In conclusion, using MR spectroscopy data we have demonstrated that patients with ataxia and low titre of AGA improve on a strict GFD. We are therefore proposing a new AGA titre cut-off level that should be used in the diagnosis of GA.

Author Contributions: M.H. runs the Gluten Sensitivity/Neurology Clinic and with P.D.S. runs dedicated ataxia clinics from where all patients were identified. D.S.S. runs the coeliac clinic and was responsible for all the gastroscopies and duodenal biopsies as well as serological testing of patients with CD. P.Z. performed the serological testing of healthy cotrols. N.H. and I.C. were responsible for MR spectroscopy. N.T. provided all the dietetic input. G.W. was responsible for the AGA assay and the provision of numerical data for the AGA results. R.A.G., P.G.S and P.Z. provided all the statistical advice. M.H. produced the first draft with contributions from all authors. The final version was approved by all the authors.

Funding: This research received no external funding.

Acknowledgments: This is a summary of independent research supported by BRC and carried out at the National Institute for Health Research (NIHR) Sheffield Clinical Research Facility. The views expressed are those of the authors and not necessarily those of the BRC, NHS, the NIHR, or the Department of Health.

Conflicts of Interest: The authors declare no conflicts of interest.

References

1. Hadjivassiliou, M.; Grünewald, R.A.; Chattopadhyay, A.K.; Davies-Jones, G.A.B.; Gibson, A.; Jarratt, J.A.; Kandler, R.H.; Lobo, A.; Powell, T.; Smith, C.M.L. Clinical, radiological, neurophysiological and neuropathological characteristics of gluten ataxia. *Lancet* **1998**, *352*, 1582–1585. [CrossRef]

2. Hadjivassiliou, M.; Rao, D.G.; Grunewald, R.A.; Aeschlimann, D.P.; Sarrigiannis, P.G.; Hoggard, N.; Aeschlimann, P.; Mooney, P.D.; Sanders, D.S. Neurological dysfunction in Coeliac Disease and Non-Coeliac Gluten Sensitivity. *Am. J. Gastroenterol.* **2016**, *111*, 561–567. [CrossRef] [PubMed]
3. Aziz, I.; Hadjivassiliou, M.; Sanders, D.S. Does gluten sensitivity in the absence of coeliac disease exist? *BMJ* **2012**, *345*, e7907. [CrossRef] [PubMed]
4. Aziz, I.; Hadjivassiliou, M.; Sanders, D.S. The spectrum of non-coeliac gluten sensitivity. *Nat. Rev. Gastroenterol. Hepatol.* **2015**, *12*, 516–526. [CrossRef] [PubMed]
5. Available online: www.phadia.com/da/Products/Phadia-Laboratory-Systems/Phadia-2500/ (accessed on 4 September 2018).
6. Hadjivassiliou, M.; Martindale, J.; Shanmugarajah, P.; Grunewald, R.A.; Sarrigiannis, P.G.; Beauchamp, N.; Garrard, K.; Warburton, R.; Sanders, D.S.; Friend, D.; et al. Causes of progressive cerebellar ataxia: Prospective evaluation of 1500 patients. *J. Neurol. Neurosurg. Psychiatry* **2016**, *88*, 301–309. [CrossRef] [PubMed]
7. Hadjivassiliou, M.; Grunewald, R.A.; Sanders, D.S.; Shanmugarajah, P.; Hoggard, N. Effect of gluten-free diet on MR spectroscopy in gluten ataxia. *Neurology* **2017**, *89*, 1–5. [CrossRef] [PubMed]
8. Hadjivassiliou, M. Advances in Therapies of Cerebellar Disorders: Immune mediated Ataxias. *CNS Neurol. Disord. Drug Targets* **2018**. [CrossRef] [PubMed]
9. Hadjivassiliou, M.; Davies-Jones, G.A.B.; Sanders, D.S.; Grünewald, R.A. Dietary treatment of gluten ataxia. *J. Neurol. Neurosurg. Psychiatry* **2003**, *74*, 1221–1224. [CrossRef] [PubMed]
10. Currie, S.; Hadjivassiliou, M.; Craven, I.J.; Wilkinson, I.D.; Griffiths, P.D.; Hoggard, N. Magnetic resonance spectroscopy of the brain. *Postgrad. Med. J..* [CrossRef] [PubMed]
11. Oz, G.; Hutter, D.; Tkac, I.; Clark, H.B.; Gross, M.D.; Jiang, H.; Eberly, L.E.; Bushara, K.O.; Gomez, C.M. Neurochemical alterations in spinocerebellar ataxia type 1 and their correlations with clinical status. *Mov. Disord.* **2010**, *25*, 1253–1261. [CrossRef] [PubMed]

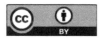

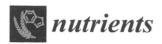

Review

Headache Associated with Coeliac Disease: A Systematic Review and Meta-Analysis

Panagiotis Zis [1,*], Thomas Julian [2] and Marios Hadjivassiliou [1]

[1]   Academic Department of Neurosciences, Sheffield Teaching Hospitals NHS Foundation Trust, Sheffield S10 2JF, UK; m.hadjivassiliou@sheffield.ac.uk

[2]   Medical School, University of Sheffield, Sheffield S10 2TN, UK; thjulian07@gmail.com

*   Correspondence: takiszis@gmail.com

Received: 18 September 2018; Accepted: 29 September 2018; Published: 6 October 2018

Abstract: Objective: The aim of this systematic review was to explore the relationship between coeliac disease (CD) and headache. The objectives were to establish the prevalence of each entity amongst the other, to explore the role of gluten free diet (GFD), and to describe the imaging findings in those affected by headaches associated with CD. Methodology: A systematic computer-based literature search was conducted on the PubMed database. Information regarding study type, population size, the age group included, prevalence of CD amongst those with headache and vice versa, imaging results, the nature of headache, and response to GFD. Results: In total, 40 articles published between 1987 and 2017 qualified for inclusion in this review. The mean pooled prevalence of headache amongst those with CD was 26% (95% CI 19.5–33.9%) in adult populations and 18.3% (95% CI 10.4–30.2%) in paediatric populations. The headaches are most often migraine-like. In children with idiopathic headache, the prevalence of CD is 2.4% (95% CI 1.5–3.7%), whereas data for adult populations is presently unavailable. Brain imaging can be normal, although, cerebral calcifications on CT, white matter abnormalities on MRI and deranged regional cerebral blood flow on SPECT can be present. GFD appears to be an effective management for headache in the context of CD, leading to total resolution of headaches in up to 75% of patients. Conclusions: There is an increased prevalence of CD amongst idiopathic headache and vice versa. Therefore, patients with headache of unknown origin should be screened for CD, as such patients may symptomatically benefit from a GFD.

Keywords: gluten sensitivity; coeliac disease; gluten free diet; migraine; headache

1. Introduction

Gluten-related disorders (GRDs) represent a diverse spectrum of clinical entities for which the ingestion of gluten is a common trigger.

Coeliac disease (CD) is the best-recognised GRD and it is characterized by a small bowel enteropathy occurring in genetically susceptible individuals whilst exposed to the protein gliadin [1]. Non-coeliac gluten sensitivity (NCGS) is a term that is used by gastroenterologists to describe patients with primarily gastrointestinal (GI) symptoms that are related to the ingestion of wheat, barley, and rye, who do not have enteropathy, but do symptomatically benefit from a gluten free diet (GFD) [2] However, in the context of neurological manifestations, patients might have serological evidence of gluten sensitivity (GS); usually anti-gliadin IgG and/or IgA (AGA), with or without transglutaminase (TG) or endomysial antibodies (EMA), but no histological changes on biopsy of the bowel to suggest CD [3]. Such patients might still benefit neurologically from a strict GFD.

Although the gastrointestinal manifestations of GRDs are the most prevalent, a range of debilitating neurological manifestations are increasingly being recognised in clinical practice, often preceding or in the absence of GI symptoms. The most well-known neurological GRDs are cerebellar ataxia [4] and peripheral neuropathy [5], however clear links between GS/CD and epilepsy [3], various movement disorders [6], and headaches [7] have also been described.

The aim of this paper is to systematically review the current literature in order to establish the relationship between headache and CD.

2. Methods

2.1. Literature Search Strategy

This study is reported in accordance with the Preferred Reporting Items for Systematic Reviews and Meta-Analysis (PRISMA) guidelines [8]. A systematic search was performed on the 29 August 2018 using the PubMed database. For the search, two medical subject headings (MeSH terms) were used and they were restricted to title/abstract fields. Term A was "coeliac" or "celiac" or "gluten". Term B was "headache" or "migraine". English language was applied as a filter. The reference lists of included articles were examined in order to identify further relevant articles.

2.2. Inclusion and Exclusion Criteria

Articles to be included in the review were required to meet the following criteria:

1. The study subjects were diagnosed with idiopathic headache and gluten sensitivity or coeliac disease.
2. The study subjects were human.
3. The study contained original data.
4. The study was available as a full-text, English language article, or contained utilisable information in an English language abstract.
5. For randomised control trials, a JADAD score [9] of above 3 to ensure good quality and to reduce any potential bias.

Details of the inclusion process are detailed in the PRISMA chart, Figure 1.

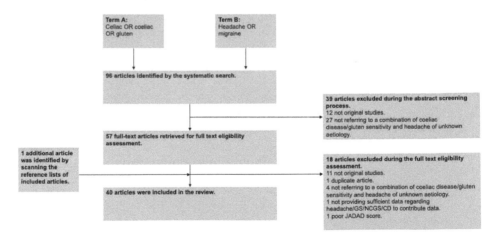

Figure 1. Preferred Reporting Items for Systematic Reviews and Meta-Analysis (PRISMA) chart.

2.3. Statistical Analyses

A database was developed using IBM SPSS Statistics (version 23.0 for Mac, IBM. New York, United States). Data were extracted from each study and included: study type; population size; the age group included; prevalence of GRD/headache; imaging results; the nature of headache; and, response to GFD. Frequencies and descriptive statistics were examined for each variable. The outcomes of interest were the proportion of patients with CD or GS suffering from headache and the proportion of patients suffering from idiopathic headache that had CD or GS.

Meta-analysis of the pooled proportions was conducted in R language [10] while using the default settings of the "meta" package using the "metaprop" function. The meta-analysis of odds ratios was conducted using the RevMan program [11], as suggested by the Cochrane Collaboration Group. Heterogeneity between studies was assessed using the I2 statistic. Data were analysed using a random effects model.

A value of $p < 0.05$ was considered to be statistically significant.

2.4. Compliance with Ethical Guidelines

This article is based upon previously published studies. The article is in compliance with the journal's ethical guidelines.

3. Results

3.1. Selected Studies

The search strategy identified 96 articles. A total of 57 articles were excluded during the eligibility assessment. After perusing the reference lists of included studies, one additional article meeting our inclusion criteria was identified, which had not already been discovered in the aforementioned search strategy. Therefore, in total 40 articles published between 1987 and 2017 qualified for inclusion in this review, studying a total of 42,388 individuals with either headache or GRD (mean number of patients per citation 1059.7 ± 4626.5). The characteristics of the included papers are summarised in Table 1. Figure 1 illustrates the study selection process.

Table 1. Descriptive of studies included in the review.

Parameter	Value
Number of papers	40
Population (%)	
Adult	18 (45.0)
Children	18 (45.0)
Mixed	4 (10.0)
Type of study	
Case report	9 (22.5)
Cohort/Case series	16 (40.0)
Case-controlled study	11 (27.5)
Population-based	2 (5.0)
Survey	2 (5.0)
Gluten-related disorder	
Coeliac disease	36 (90.0)
Mixed group: CD/GS	1 (2.5)
Mixed group: NCGS/GS	3 (7.5)
Type of headache reported	
Migraine	16 (40.0)
All types	6 (15.0)
Not specified	14 (35.0)
Idiopathic intracranial hypertension–related	2 (5.0)
Encephalopathy syndrome	2 (5.0)
Imaging *	
MRI	8 (20.0)
CT	7 (17.5)
SPECT	2 (5.0)
No imaging data	24 (60.0)

Table 1. *Cont.*

Parameter	Value
Year of publication (%)	
Until 2000	5 (12.5)
2000–2009	15 (37.5)
2010–2018	20 (50.0)

* Some citations had data on more than one imaging types.

3.2. Prevalence of Headache in Patients with CD

Only one population based epidemiological study, inclusive of all ages, has been conducted to date [12]. In this population-based retrospective cohort study that was conducted in Sweden, Lebwohl et al. reported that among 28,638 patients with CD and 143,126 controls, headache-related visits occurred in 4.7% and 2.9% of each group, respectively, suggesting a hazard ratio of 1.7 (95% CI 1.6–1.8; $p < 0.0001$). However, in this study, there was no information provided regarding the criteria for headache diagnosis used and if diagnosed, its exact type.

Information about prevalence of headache in adults was available through five cohort [13–17] and four case-controlled studies [18–21]. As shown in Figure 2, the pooled mean prevalence of headache in adults with CD was 26% (95% CI 19.5–33.9%). The meta-analysis of the four case-controlled studies is summarized in Figure 3; the odds of having a headache were significantly higher in the CD groups when compared to controls (OR 2.7, 95% CI 1.7–4.3, $p < 0.0001$).

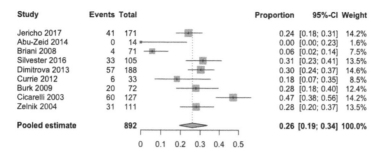

Figure 2. Pooled mean prevalence of headache in adults with coeliac disease.

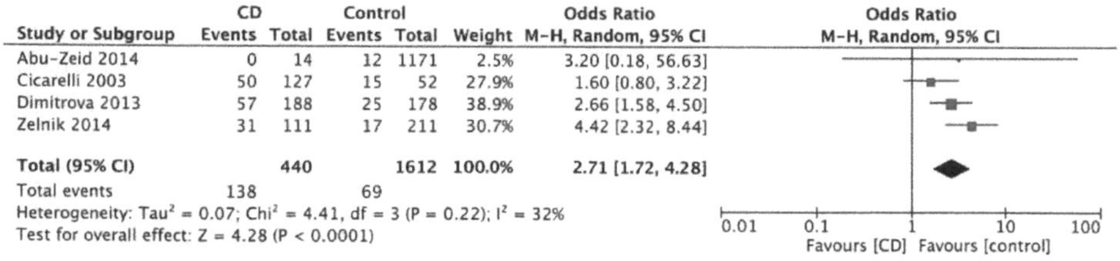

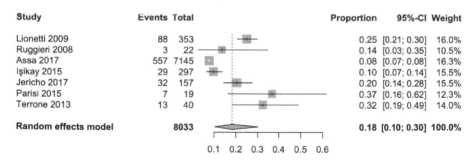

Figure 3. Meta-analysis results as illustrated in the forest plot regarding the odds of having headache in adults with coeliac disease compared to controls.

Information about prevalence of headache in children and adolescents, was available through five cohort [17,22–25], one case-controlled [26], and one population-based study [27]. As shown in Figure 4, the pooled mean prevalence of headache in children and adolescents with CD was 18.3% (95% CI 10.4–30.2%). A cross-sectional, population-based study that was conducted by Assa et al. [27] investigated the association between CD and various comorbidities, demonstrating that the odds of suffering from headache were significantly higher in children and adolescents with CD when compared to controls (OR 2.3, 95% CI 2.1–2.5, $p < 0.0001$).

Study	Events	Total	Proportion	95%-CI	Weight
Lionetti 2009	88	353	0.25	[0.21; 0.30]	16.0%
Ruggieri 2008	3	22	0.14	[0.03; 0.35]	10.5%
Assa 2017	557	7145	0.08	[0.07; 0.08]	16.3%
Işikay 2015	29	297	0.10	[0.07; 0.14]	15.5%
Jericho 2017	32	157	0.20	[0.14; 0.28]	15.5%
Parisi 2015	7	19	0.37	[0.16; 0.62]	12.3%
Terrone 2013	13	40	0.32	[0.19; 0.49]	14.0%
Random effects model		**8033**	**0.18**	**[0.10; 0.30]**	**100.0%**

Figure 4. Pooled mean prevalence of headache in children with coeliac disease.

3.3. Prevalence of CD in Patients with Idiopathic Headache

Headache, usually migraine, has been reported as the first manifestation of CD in several case reports [28–36].

In a case-controlled study, Gabrielli et al. [37] investigated the prevalence of CD amongst 90 adults with idiopathic migraine when compared to blood donor controls. Of them, 4.4% were found to have CD against 0.4% of controls ($p < 0.05$).

Information about prevalence of CD in children with headache was available through two case-control [38,39] and two cohort studies [26,40]. As demonstrated in Figure 5, the pooled mean prevalence of CD in children with idiopathic headache is 2.4% (95% CI 1.5–3.7%), which is significantly higher as compared to the prevalence of CD in the general population in the same age group. Although in one of these studies the authors conclude that that the prevalence of CD was not higher in patients with migraine relative to the control group [38], the other three studies concluded that the odds of a child with headache having CD is significantly higher than in children without headaches, with OR ranging from 1.7 to 8.3 [26,39,40].

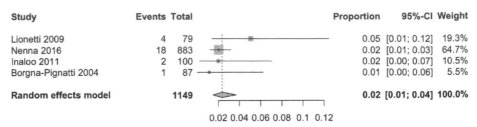

Figure 5. Pooled mean prevalence of coeliac disease in children with idiopathic headache.

3.4. Imaging Findings

Sixteen papers provided information regarding imaging findings [7,14,22,26,28–31,33–37,41–43].

3.4.1. Computed Tomography (CT)

Although brain CT scans in patients with CD and headache are usually normal, there have been cases described of migraine-like headaches with occipital [29,30] or parieto-occipital [33,35] calcifications in both adult and children patients. The two patients with headache and parieto-occipital calcifications being described in the literature were adults, with no evidence of epilepsy or epileptiform activity on EEG. By contrast, all three patients with headache and occipital calcifications were children, of which two also had epilepsy. Cerebral calcifications in the context of CD have been associated with epilepsy [3], which is most commonly known as "epilepsy and cerebral calcification (CEC) syndrome". However, although the available evidence is limited, there are cases with calcifications and migraine-like headaches in the absence of epilepsy. Therefore, patients who present with idiopathic headache in the presence of calcifications in the occipital or parieto-occipital areas of the brain should be screened for CD.

3.4.2. Magnetic Resonance Imaging (MRI)

MRI findings have been reported in isolated case reports and small case series. In a consecutive cohort of 33 adult patients with CD who were referred for a neurological opinion, Currie et al. reported that 12 patients (36%) had white matter abnormalities (WMA) on MRI [14]. When looking specifically into patients with headache, four out of six (67%) had WMA on MRI. In children, one out of six patients with headaches and CD that have been reported to date [22,42,43] was found to have WMA on MRI.

Hadjivassiliou et al. has presented the largest series of patients with CD or GS and WMA on MRI to date [7]. Among 40 adult patients with symptoms and signs of central nervous system dysfunction, most of which had cerebellar ataxia, ten patients (four with CD and six with GS) were found to have WMA. All patients had episodic migraine-like headache. In children with GS the available evidence is limited, however Alehan et al. reported that WMA were present in one out of four TG positive patients [41]. Therefore, patients of all ages who present with idiopathic headache and have non-specific WMA on MRI should be screened for CD and GS.

3.4.3. Single Photon Emission Computed Tomography (SPECT)

Gabrielli et al. conducted a case-controlled study of four adult patients with migraine and newly diagnosed CD and five control patients with migraine, but no CD who underwent a brain SPECT study, which was performed by the administration of 740 MBq of ^{99m}Tc hexemethyl-propylene-amineoxime using a brain-dedicated tomograph [37]. All SPECT studies were performed in the headache free period. All four patients that were affected by both migraine and CD showed evident abnormalities in regional cerebral blood flow. In all cases, a circumscribed area of cortical hypoperfusion was present, whereas there were no interhemispheric asymmetries of cortical regional blood flow in the five migraine patients without evidence of CD.

3.4.4. Positron Emission Tomography (PET)

Lionetti et al. studied the cerebral perfusion in four children headaches and CD with an eight-ring whole-body PET scanner using 2-[18F]-fluoro-2-deoxy-D-glucose, without identifying any abnormalities [26]. This could be because of a selection bias, as the patients that underwent PET had normal standard cerebral imaging, or it might suggest that cerebral hypoperfusion is not present in children with headaches and CD.

3.5. Effect of Gluten-Free Diet

The effect of a gluten-free diet (GFD) has been reported in numerous cohort studies [7,15,17,20,24–26,28,37,40]. In adults, a positive response, defined as a significant reduction in headache frequency, varies from 51.6% [20] to 100% [7,37] of the patients who embarked on a GFD. In up to 75% of adult patients [15] with CD, GFD led to the total resolution of headache. In children, the response rates range between 69.2% [24] and 100% [25,28,40]. In up to 71.3% of paediatric patients [25] with CD, GFD resulted in headache resolution.

As well as direct clinical improvement, it has been demonstrated that a GFD can normalize the cortical hypoperfusion abnormalities that are seen in SPECT [37]. Although, WMA and brain calcifications are not reversible when present, patients on a strict GFD have a lower incidence of WMA [14].

In a survey of pediatric patients with CD that was conducted by Rashid et al., it was reported that up to 13% of patients experience headache after accidental gluten ingestion [44]. In a similar survey of predominantly adults (patients > 16 years old) with CD, Zarkadas et al. found that 23% of patients experienced a headache when they knowingly consumed gluten [45]. In their study, Faulkner-Hogg et al. reported that dietary analysis of patients with persistent symptoms, including headaches, showed that up to 56% of patient still consume traces of gluten. When such patients switched to a strict GFD their symptoms improved [46]. Therefore, specialist dietician advice should always be offered to patients with CD and headaches, and their compliance with the diet should be routinely checked (i.e., AGA titre monitoring).

3.6. Gluten-Related Intracranial Hypertension

Some case reports describe patients who presented with headache secondary to increased intracranial pressure and CD. Dotan et al. reported two cases of boys (three and four years old) who presented with idiopathic intracranial hypertension (IIH). Diagnostic work-up revealed low serum vitamin A titres and further diagnostic work-up led to a diagnosis of CD [43]. A therapeutic regimen of vitamin A supplements, GFD, and acetazolamide proved very effective. Rani et al. reported a single case of a 14-year-old girl with IIH, whose diagnostic work-up revealed CD [42]. Despite the fact that the patient was overweight (BMI 30) a GFD proved to be beneficial, even before the patient started to lose weight and without requiring administration of acetazolamide. Although these data are limited and the evidence is currently weak, the potential link between CD and intracranial hypertension should be investigated further.

3.7. Gluten–Encephalopathy

Gluten encephalopathy is a term that is used to describe a combination of frequent, often intractable, headaches, and cognitive complaints (which patients sometimes describe as a "foggy brain"). Crosato et al. were the first to describe a case of a nine-year-old boy with a history of seizures, headaches, episodes of drowsiness and cerebral calcification on CT who, because of his very low folate levels, was eventually diagnosed with CD [29]. Kakoraç et al. reported a case of a 48-year old man who presented with two episodes of headache, confusion, and seizures and normal MRI, and because of carnitine deficiency, was eventually diagnosed with CD [34].

3.8. NCGS/GS and Headache

A link between headache and NCGS or GS has been also demonstrated in a smaller number of studies.

Information about prevalence of GS in children with headache (all reporting migraine), was available through three case-controlled studies [41,47,48]. As shown in Figure 6, the pooled mean prevalence of GS in children with idiopathic migraine is 6.2% (95% CI 2.6–14.1%). Figure 7 demonstrates that the odds of having migraine are higher (trend for statistical significance) in children with CD as compared to controls (OR 2.8, 95% CI 0.9–8.6, $p = 0.06$).

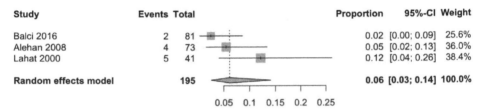

Figure 6. Pooled mean prevalence of serologically confirmed gluten sensitivity in children with idiopathic migraine.

Information about the prevalence of headache in patients with NCGS was available through two studies [49,50]. In a cohort of 486 patients (children and adults), 54% presented with headaches [50]. In a cohort of 78 children with NCGS, 32% presented with headaches, when not on a GFD [49]. It is of interest that 56% of patients with NCGS, when not on a GFD, have positive AGA. This highlights the need to test patients for AGA, the only currently available biomarker of GS.

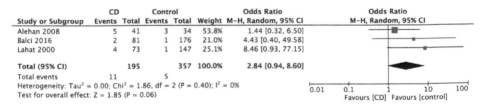

Figure 7. Meta-analysis results as illustrated in the forest plot regarding the odds of having migraine in children with coeliac disease compared to controls.

4. Conclusions and Future Directions

This systematic review, highlights the following key points:

1. There is an increased prevalence of headache amongst patients with CD and an increased prevalence of CD amongst those with idiopathic headache. Such an increased prevalence is evident in both child and adult populations; however, the figures are higher in the latter.

2. Headaches that are associated with CD are predominantly migraines. However, many studies that were used in this report tended to report headaches without specifying the exact type (i.e., tension, cluster, migraine, etc.) making the interpretation of the findings more difficult.

3. CT calcifications and WMA are frequent in patients with headaches that are related to CD, and therefore patients with such imaging findings in in the context of idiopathic headache require further testing for CD.

4. GFD is a very effective treatment for headaches associated with CD and should therefore be offered as soon as possible. This is highly consistent with other neurological GRD, such as the observation that GFD is associated with a significant reduction of pain in patients with gluten neuropathy and an improvement of their quality of life [51,52]. Specialist dietary advise should always be offered, as often patients consume gluten, whilst believe that they are on a strict GFD. Serological testing (i.e., AGA titre) can help in monitoring compliance with diet.

5. Further studies of the prevalence of GS in patients with idiopathic headache are needed. Currently, to our knowledge, no such studies in adults exist.

6. Although there is some evidence that brain hypoperfusion and perivascular inflammation might play a role in the pathogenesis of GS-related headaches more studies on the likely pathogenetic mechanisms are needed.

7. Serum positivity for TG6 antibodies has been identified as a sensitive measure of neurological involvement in GS [53,54] Therefore, a study of the prevalence of TG6 antibodies in patients with headaches that are related to CD and GS should be conducted.

Author Contributions: This work was carried out in collaboration between the authors. P.Z and M.H conceived and designed the study. P.Z and T.J performed the search and collected the data. P.Zdrafted the main part of the manuscript and it was edited by P.Z, T.J and M.H. All authors read and have approved the final manuscript and take full responsibility for its content.

Funding: This research received no external funding.

Acknowledgments: This is a summary of independent research carried out at the NIHR Sheffield Biomedical Research Centre (Translational Neuroscience). The views expressed are those of the authors and not necessarily those of the NHS, the NIHR or the Department of Health. Zis is sincerely thankful to the Ryder Briggs Fund. We are sincerely thankful to the Statistical Services Unit, University of Sheffield, for their valuable help with the statistical analysis.

Conflicts of Interest: The authors declare no conflict of interest.

References

1. Fasano, A.; Catassi, C. Current approaches to diagnosis and treatment of celiac disease: An evolving spectrum. *Gastroenterology* **2001**, *120*, 636–651. [CrossRef] [PubMed]
2. Sapone, A.; Bai, J.C.; Ciacci, C.; Dolinsek, J.; Green, P.H.R.; Hadjivassiliou, M.; Kaukinen, K.; Rostami, K.; Sanders, D.S.; Schumann, M.; et al. Spectrum of gluten-related disorders: Consensus on new nomenclature and classification. *BMC Med.* **2012**, *10*, 13. [CrossRef] [PubMed]
3. Julian, T.; Hadjivassiliou, M.; Zis, P. Gluten sensitivity and epilepsy: A systematic review. *J. Neurol.* **2018**. Epub ahead of print. [CrossRef] [PubMed]
4. Hadjivassiliou, M.; Grünewald, R.A.; Chattopadhyay, A.K.; Davies-Jones, G.A.; Gibson, A.; Jarratt, J.A.; Kandler, R.H.; Lobo, A.; Powell, T.; Smith, C.M.L. Clinical, radiological, neurophysiological, and neuropathological characteristics of gluten ataxia. *Lancet* **1998**, *352*, 1582–1585. [CrossRef]
5. Hadjivassiliou, M.; Grünewald, R.A.; Kandler, R.H.; Chattopadhyay, A.K.; Jarratt, J.A.; Sanders, D.S.; Sharrack, B.; Wharton, S.B.; Davies-Jones, G.A.B. Neuropathy associated with gluten sensitivity. *J. Neurol. Neurosurg. Psychiatry* **2006**, *77*, 1262–1266. [CrossRef] [PubMed]
6. Vinagre-Aragón, A.; Zis, P.; Grunewald, R.A.; Hadjivassiliou, M. Movement Disorders Related to Gluten Sensitivity: A Systematic Review. *Nutrients* **2018**, *10*, 1034. [CrossRef] [PubMed]

7. Hadjivassiliou, M.; Grünewald, R.A.; Lawden, M.; Davies-Jones, G.A.; Powell, T.; Smith, C.M. Headache and CNS white matter abnormalities associated with gluten sensitivity. *Neurology* **2001**, *56*, 385–388. [CrossRef] [PubMed]
8. Moher, D.; Liberati, A.; Tetzlaff, J.; Altman, D.G.; PRISMA Group. Preferred reporting items for systematic reviews and meta-analyses: The PRISMA statement. *PLoS Med.* **2009**, *6*, e1000097. [CrossRef] [PubMed]
9. Jadad, A.R.; Moore, R.A.; Carroll, D.; Jenkinson, C.; Reynolds, D.J.; Gavaghan, D.J.; McQuay, H.J. Assessing the quality of reports of randomized clinical trials: Is blinding necessary? *Control Clin. Trials* **1996**, *17*, 1–12. [CrossRef]
10. Team, RC. *R: A Language and Environment for Statistical Computing*; R Foundation for Statistical Computing: Vienna, Austria, 2013.
11. The Cochrane Collaboration. *Review Manager*; Version 5.3; The Nordic Cochrane Centre: Copenhagen, Denmark, 2014.
12. Lebwohl, B.; Roy, A.; Alaedini, A.; Green, P.H.R.; Ludvigsson, J.F. Risk of Headache-Related Healthcare Visits in Patients With Celiac Disease: A Population-Based Observational Study. *Headache* **2016**, *56*, 849–858. [CrossRef] [PubMed]
13. Silvester, J.A.; Graff, L.A.; Rigaux, L.; Walker, J.R.; Duerksen, D.R. Symptomatic suspected gluten exposure is common among patients with coeliac disease on a gluten-free diet. *Aliment. Pharmacol. Ther.* **2016**, *44*, 612–619. [CrossRef] [PubMed]
14. Currie, S.; Hadjivassiliou, M.; Clark, M.J.R.; Sanders, D.S.; Wilkinson, I.D.; Griffiths, P.D.; Hoggard, N. Should we be "nervous" about coeliac disease? Brain abnormalities in patients with coeliac disease referred for neurological opinion. *J. Neurol. Neurosurg. Psychiatry* **2012**, *83*, 1216–1221. [CrossRef] [PubMed]
15. Bürk, K.; Farecki, M.-L.; Lamprecht, G.; Roth, G.; Decker, P.; Weller, M.; Rammensee, H.-G.; Oertel, W. Neurological symptoms in patients with biopsy proven celiac disease. *Mov. Disord.* **2009**, *24*, 2358–2362. [CrossRef] [PubMed]
16. Briani, C.; Zara, G.; Alaedini, A.; Grassivaro, F.; Ruggero, S.; Toffanin, E.; Albergoni, M.P.; Luca, M.; Giometto, B.; Ermani, M.; et al. Neurological complications of celiac disease and autoimmune mechanisms: A prospective study. *J. Neuroimmunol.* **2008**, *195*, 171–175. [CrossRef] [PubMed]
17. Jericho, H.; Sansotta, N.; Guandalini, S. Extraintestinal Manifestations of Celiac Disease: Effectiveness of the Gluten-Free Diet. *J. Pediatr. Gastroenterol. Nutr.* **2017**, *65*, 75–79. [CrossRef] [PubMed]
18. Dimitrova, A.K.; Ungaro, R.C.; Lebwohl, B.; Lewis, S.K.; Tennyson, C.A.; Green, M.W.; Babyatsky, M.W.; Green, P.H. Prevalence of migraine in patients with celiac disease and inflammatory bowel disease. *Headache* **2013**, *53*, 344–355. [CrossRef] [PubMed]
19. Cicarelli, G.; Della Rocca, G.; Amboni, M.; Ciacci, C.; Mazzacca, G.; Filla, A.; Barone, P. Clinical and neurological abnormalities in adult celiac disease. *Neurol. Sci.* **2003**, *24*, 311–317. [CrossRef] [PubMed]
20. Zelnik, N.; Pacht, A.; Obeid, R.; Lerner, A. Range of neurologic disorders in patients with celiac disease. *Pediatrics* **2004**, *113*, 1672–1676. [CrossRef] [PubMed]
21. Abu-Zeid, Y.A.; Jasem, W.S.; Lebwohl, B.; Green, P.H.; ElGhazali, G. Seroprevalence of celiac disease among United Arab Emirates healthy adult nationals: A gender disparity. *World J. Gastroenterol.* **2014**, *20*, 15830–15836. [CrossRef] [PubMed]
22. Ruggieri, M.; Incorpora, G.; Polizzi, A.; Parano, E.; Spina, M.; Pavone, P. Low prevalence of neurologic and psychiatric manifestations in children with gluten sensitivity. *J. Pediatr.* **2008**, *152*, 244–249. [CrossRef] [PubMed]
23. Işikay, S.; Kocamaz, H. The neurological face of celiac disease. *Arq. Gastroenterol.* **2015**, *52*, 167–170. [CrossRef] [PubMed]
24. Terrone, G.; Parente, I.; Romano, A.; Auricchio, R.; Greco, L.; Del Giudice, E. The Pediatric Symptom Checklist as screening tool for neurological and psychosocial problems in a paediatric cohort of patients with coeliac disease. *Acta Paediatr.* **2013**, *102*, e325–e328. [CrossRef] [PubMed]
25. Parisi, P.; Pietropaoli, N.; Ferretti, A.; Nenna, R.; Mastrogiorgio, G.; Del Pozzo, M.; Principessa, L.; Bonamico, M.; Villa, M.P. Role of the gluten-free diet on neurological-EEG findings and sleep disordered breathing in children with celiac disease. *Seizure* **2015**, *25*, 181–183. [CrossRef] [PubMed]
26. Lionetti, E.; Francavilla, R.; Maiuri, L.; Ruggieri, M.; Spina, M.; Pavone, P.; Francavilla, T.; Magistà, A.M.; Pavone, L. Headache in Pediatric Patients With Celiac Disease and Its Prevalence as a Diagnostic Clue. *J. Pediatr. Gastroenterol. Nutr.* **2009**, *49*, 202–207. [CrossRef] [PubMed]

27. Assa, A.; Frenkel-Nir, Y.; Tzur, D.; Katz, L.H.; Shamir, R. Large population study shows that adolescents with celiac disease have an increased risk of multiple autoimmune and nonautoimmune comorbidities. *Acta Paediatr.* **2017**, *106*, 967–972. [CrossRef] [PubMed]
28. Diaconu, G.; Burlea, M.; Grigore, I.; Anton, D.T.; Trandafir, L.M. Celiac disease with neurologic manifestations in children. *Rev. Med. Chir. Soc. Med. Nat. Iasi.* **2013**, *117*, 88–94. [PubMed]
29. Crosato, F.; Senter, S. Cerebral occipital calcifications in celiac disease. *Neuropediatrics* **1992**, *23*, 214–217. [CrossRef] [PubMed]
30. Battistella, P.A.; Mattesi, P.; Casara, G.L.; Carollo, C.; Condini, A.; Allegri, F.; Rigon, F. Bilateral cerebral occipital calcifications and migraine-like headache. *Cephalalgia* **1987**, *7*, 125–129. [CrossRef] [PubMed]
31. Serratrice, J.; Disdier, P.; de Roux, C.; Christides, C.; Weiller, P.J. Migraine and coeliac disease. *Headache* **1998**, *38*, 627–628. [CrossRef] [PubMed]
32. Mingomataj, E.Ç.; Gjata, E.; Bakiri, A.; Xhixha, F.; Hyso, E.; Ibranji, A. Gliadin allergy manifested with chronic urticaria, headache and amenorrhea. *BMJ Case Rep.* **2011**, *2011*, bcr1020114907. [CrossRef] [PubMed]
33. La Mantia, L.; Pollo, B.; Savoiardo, M.; Costa, A.; Eoli, M.; Allegranza, A.; Boiardi, A.; Cestari, C. Meningo-cortical calcifying angiomatosis and celiac disease. *Clin. Neurol. Neurosurg.* **1998**, *100*, 209–215. [CrossRef]
34. Karakoç, E.; Erdem, S.; Sökmensüer, C.; Kansu, T. Encephalopathy due to carnitine deficiency in an adult patient with gluten enteropathy. *Clin. Neurol. Neurosurg.* **2006**, *108*, 794–797. [CrossRef] [PubMed]
35. D'Amico, D.; Rigamonti, A.; Spina, L.; Bianchi-Marzoli, S.; Vecchi, M.; Bussone, G. Migraine, celiac disease, and cerebral calcifications: A new case. *Headache* **2005**, *45*, 1263–1267. [CrossRef] [PubMed]
36. Benjilali, L.; Zahlane, M.; Essaadouni, L. A migraine as initial presentation of celiac disease. *Rev. Neurol.* **2012**, *168*, 454–456. [CrossRef] [PubMed]
37. Gabrielli, M.; Cremonini, F.; Fiore, G.; Addolorato, G.; Padalino, C.; Candelli, M.; Gasbarrini, A.; Pola, P.; Gasbarrini, A. Association between migraine and Celiac disease: Results from a preliminary case-control and therapeutic study. *Am. J. Gastroenterol.* **2003**, *98*, 625–629. [CrossRef] [PubMed]
38. Inaloo, S.; Dehghani, S.M.; Farzadi, F.; Haghighat, M.; Imanieh, M.H. A comparative study of celiac disease in children with migraine headache and a normal control group. *Turk. J. Gastroenterol.* **2011**, *22*, 32–35. [CrossRef] [PubMed]
39. Borgna-Pignatti, C.; Fiumana, E.; Milani, M.; Calacoci, M.; Soriani, S. Celiac disease in children with migraine. *Pediatrics* **2004**, *114*, 1371. [CrossRef] [PubMed]
40. Nenna, R.; Petrarca, L.; Verdecchia, P.; Florio, M.; Pietropaoli, N.; Mastrogiorgio, G.; Bavastrelli, M.; Bonamico, M.; Cucchiara, S. Celiac disease in a large cohort of children and adolescents with recurrent headache: A retrospective study. *Dig. Liver Dis.* **2016**, *48*, 495–498. [CrossRef] [PubMed]
41. Alehan, F.; Ozçay, F.; Erol, I.; Canan, O.; Cemil, T. Increased risk for coeliac disease in paediatric patients with migraine. *Cephalalgia* **2008**, *28*, 945–949. [CrossRef] [PubMed]
42. Rani, U.; Imdad, A.; Beg, M. Rare Neurological Manifestation of Celiac Disease. *Case Rep. Gastroenterol.* **2015**, *9*, 200–205. [CrossRef] [PubMed]
43. Dotan, G.; Goldstein, M.; Stolovitch, C.; Kesler, A. Pediatric Pseudotumor Cerebri Associated With Low Serum Levels of Vitamin A. *J. Child. Neurol.* **2013**, *28*, 1370–1377. [CrossRef] [PubMed]
44. Rashid, M.; Cranney, A.; Zarkadas, M.; Graham, I.D.; Switzer, C.; Case, S.; Molloy, M.; Warren, R.E.; Burrows, V.; Butzner, J.D. Celiac disease: Evaluation of the diagnosis and dietary compliance in Canadian children. *Pediatrics* **2005**, *116*, e754–e759. [CrossRef] [PubMed]
45. Zarkadas, M.; Cranney, A.; Case, S.; Molloy, M.; Switzer, C.; Graham, I.D.; Butzner, J.D.; Rashid, M.; Warren, R.E.; Burrows, V. The impact of a gluten-free diet on adults with coeliac disease: Results of a national survey. *J. Hum. Nutr. Diet.* **2006**, *19*, 41–49. [CrossRef] [PubMed]
46. Faulkner-Hogg, K.B.; Selby, W.S.; Loblay, R.H. Dietary analysis in symptomatic patients with coeliac disease on a gluten-free diet: The role of trace amounts of gluten and non-gluten food intolerances. *Scand. J. Gastroenterol.* **1999**, *34*, 784–789. [CrossRef] [PubMed]
47. Lahat, E.; Broide, E.; Leshem, M.; Evans, S.; Scapa, E. Prevalence of celiac antibodies in children with neurologic disorders. *Pediatr. Neurol.* **2000**, *22*, 393–396. [CrossRef]
48. Balcı, O.; Yılmaz, D.; Sezer, T.; Hızlı, Ş. Is Celiac Disease an Etiological Factor in Children With Migraine? *J. Child. Neurol.* **2016**, *31*, 929–931. [CrossRef] [PubMed]

49. Volta, U.; Tovoli, F.; Cicola, R.; Parisi, C.; Fabbri, A.; Piscaglia, M.; Fiorini, E.; Caio, G. Serological tests in gluten sensitivity (nonceliac gluten intolerance). *J. Clin. Gastroenterol.* **2012**, *46*, 680–685. [CrossRef] [PubMed]

50. Volta, U.; Bardella, M.T.; Calabrò, A.; Troncone, R.; Corazza, G.R.; Study Group for Non-Celiac Gluten Sensitivity. An Italian prospective multicenter survey on patients suspected of having non-celiac gluten sensitivity. *BMC Med.* **2014**, *12*, 85. [CrossRef] [PubMed]

51. Zis, P.; Sarrigiannis, P.G.; Rao, D.G.; Hadjivassiliou, M. Gluten neuropathy: Prevalence of neuropathic pain and the role of gluten-free diet. *J. Neurol.* **2018**, *265*, 2231–2236. [CrossRef] [PubMed]

52. Zis, P.; Sarrigiannis, P.G.; Rao, D.G.; Hadjivassiliou, M. Quality of Life in Patients with Gluten Neuropathy: A Case-Controlled Study. *Nutrients* **2018**, *10*, 662. [CrossRef] [PubMed]

53. Zis, P.; Rao, D.G.; Sarrigiannis, P.G.; Aeschlimann, P.; Aeschlimann, D.P.; Sanders, D.; Grünewald, R.A.; Hadjivassiliou, M. Transglutaminase 6 antibodies in gluten neuropathy. *Dig. Liver Dis.* **2017**, *49*, 1196–1200. [CrossRef] [PubMed]

54. Hadjivassiliou, M.; Aeschlimann, P.; Sanders, D.S.; Mäki, M.; Kaukinen, K.; Grünewald, R.A.; Bandmann, O.; Woodroofe, N.; Haddock, G.; Aeschlimann, D.P. Transglutaminase 6 antibodies in the diagnosis of gluten ataxia. *Neurology* **2013**, *80*, 1740–1745. [CrossRef] [PubMed]

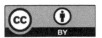

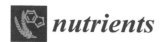

Review

Fatigue as an Extra-Intestinal Manifestation of Celiac Disease: A Systematic Review

Lars-Petter Jelsness-Jørgensen [1,2], Tomm Bernklev [3,4] and Knut E. A. Lundin [5,6,*]

1   Department of Health Science, Østfold University College, N-1757 Halden, Norway;
    lars.p.jelsness-jorgensen@hiof.no
2   Department of Gastroenterology, Østfold Hospital Trust Kalnes, N-1714 Grålum, Norway
3   Department of Research and Innovation, Vestfold Hospital Trust, N-3103 Tønsberg, Norway;
    tomm.bernklev@medisin.uio.no
4   Faculty of Medicine, Institute of Clinical Medicine, University of Oslo, N-0318 Oslo, Norway
5   K.G. Jebsen Coeliac Disease Research Centre, University of Oslo, N-0318 Oslo, Norway
6   Department of gastroenterology, Oslo University Hospital Rikshospitalet, N-0372 Oslo, Norway
*   Correspondence: knut.lundin@medisin.uio.no; Tel.: +4723072400; Fax: +4723072410

Received: 28 September 2018; Accepted: 26 October 2018; Published: 3 November 2018

Abstract: Celiac disease may present with a range of different symptoms, including abdominal problems in a broader sense, iron deficiency and "constant tiredness". All of these symptoms should consequently lead the clinicians to consider celiac disease as a potential etiopathogenetic cause. Although the pathophysiology of celiac disease is well documented, the actual mechanisms for disease presentation(s) are less well understood. We here address the topic of fatigue in celiac disease. A systematic literature search identified 298 papers of which five met the criteria for full evaluation. None of the reviewed papers were of high quality and had several methodological weaknesses. We conclude that there is an unmet need to study the contributing factors and management of fatigue in celiac disease.

Keywords: fatigue; energy; celiac disease; extra-intestinal manifestations

---

1. Introduction

Celiac disease is by definition an inflammatory disorder in the small intestine that is driven by dietary gluten from wheat, rye and barley [1]. The disease is often also termed an autoimmune disease due to a hallmark of the disease; autoantibodies to the endogenous enzyme tissue transglutaminase TG2. The crucial importance of intestinal inflammation and the most frequent presentation of the disease as a severe malabsorption syndrome led most clinicians to think of the disease as mainly an intestinal disorder. However, we now know that a very large proportion of the patients do not primarily display intestinal complaints, but that their disease presentation is more coloured by extra-intestinal manifestations [2,3]. In a recent review by Leffler et al. [3] this is well described, including anaemia, musculoskeletal, skin, neurological and organ-specific manifestations. Some of these manifestations are caused by the intestinal disorder, others may be caused by systemic inflammation and/or genetic overlap to other immune disorders [4]. Today we consider that symptoms like abdominal problems in the wider sense, unexplained iron deficiency and "constant tiredness" should all prompt the clinicians to consider celiac disease [5,6].

From our own clinical practice, we experience many patients with untreated celiac disease that suffer from fatigue. In most cases fatigue improves with diet, but far from always. In addition, these patients also present with a significant reduction in their health-related quality of life [2]. Fatigue is described as a "persistent, overwhelming sense of tiredness, weakness or exhaustion resulting in a decreased capacity for physical and/or mental work". While fatigue may be a natural and transient part of life, a typical feature in chronic disease is that these symptoms are unrelieved by adequate sleep or rest [7]. The aetiopathogenesis of fatigue in chronic disease appears to result from a complex inter-relationship of biological, psychosocial and behavioural processes [8].

The aim of this review was consequently to address the aspect of fatigue in celiac disease and to systematically summarise the existing literature on this topic.

2. Materials and Methods

Multiple searches were undertaken using MEDLINE, CINAHL, EMBASE, Psychinfo, Academic Search Premiere, and Cochrane. Both medical subject heading (MeSH) searching and free-text searching were used to maximize citation retrieval (Table 1). The searches were performed independently by a university librarian, and one of the co-authors (L.-P.J.-J.).

Table 1. Search terms used for literature search.

Fatigue	Coeliac Disease
Fatigue (MeSH)	Coeliac disease
Mental fatigue	
Chronic fatigue	
Tiredness	
Exhaustion	
Weariness	
Vitality	
Asthenia	
Low energy	

Due to the limited number of publications on fatigue in coeliac disease, no time limit was set for the papers. The searches were performed between April and June 2018, and the most recent search was performed on August 5th, 2018. The searches were limited to "humans", "adult" and English language since there was no scope for translation.

Studies with all types of designs were included if they had measured and reported data on fatigue in patients with celiac disease. Reviews, commentaries, abstracts/posters, case reports, protocols and letters to editors were excluded. The review was conducted in line with the PRISMA guidelines [9].

3. Results

The search yielded 298 references in total, of which 248 were excluded on title (Figure 1). After removing duplicates and screening the remaining 42 papers, a total of 16 papers were examined in full. Of these 16 papers, 11 did not report any specific methodology for fatigue measurement and were consequently excluded. Hence, a total of five papers were included in full review. Figure 1 describes the citation retrieval and the handling process in detail.

3.1. Quality Assessment

The quality of the included papers was assessed using the Joanna Briggs Institute Critical Appraisal Checklist, specific to the methodological design of each paper. The studies were classified as being of high, medium or low quality. A quality score was reduced if the paper did not define fatigue, report the sample size, if the sample size was judged inadequate according to study design, if the response rate was low or not reported, if the questionnaires used were not validated, if the methods and statistical analysis was insufficiently described or if there were indications of selective reporting. Two researchers (T.B./L.-P.J.-J.) performed quality assessment independently to ensure optimal assessment of the included papers. Based on these criteria, all of the reviewed papers had several methodological weaknesses, and none were judged to be of high quality. However, due to the low number of publications on fatigue and celiac disease, none of the papers were excluded from full-review based on quality.

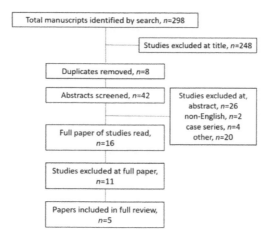

Figure 1. Citation retrieval and handling process.

3.2. Outline of the Included Papers

In total, three papers assessed fatigue as the primary endpoint, one study investigated extra-intestinal symptoms and health-related quality of life (HRQoL), while one study assessed quality of sleep. An overview of the included papers is presented in Table 2.

Table 2. Summary of the included articles.

Study (Ref. No.)	Study Population and Setting	Study Design and Participants	Questionnaires Measuring Fatigue	Strengths and Limitations
Häuser et al., 2006 [10]	A subgroup of members (1000/18,355) from the German Coeliac Society (GZG) ≥18 years was invited to participate Every 18th person on the membership list was invited in order to ensure a geographically representative sample Normative data were collected from the handbooks of the SF-36, GBB-24 and HADS-D Exclusion criteria: <18 years of age	Cross-sectional design Available for analyses: n = 446	SF-36 (Vitality subscale) GBB-24 (Fatigue subscale)	L: Fatigue not specified as aim, merely reported as parts of the questionnaire results L: No definition of fatigue L: Sample consisting of members of a patient society only L: Low response rate S: Normative data for comparison L: Self-reported information on comorbidity L: Single centre study S: Validated instruments used L: Coeliac disease diagnosis self-reported only
Siniscalchi et al., 2005 [11]	Caucasion adults ≥18 years of age from Campania, Italy, were consecutively recruited from an outpatient clinic Participants divided into two groups (Group 1: Patients on gluten containing diet, Group 2: Patients on gluten-free diet) Control group consisted of volunteers recruited from medical an non-medical hospital staff Exclusion criteria: <18 years of age, lack of informed consent, major psychiatric disease, active thyroid gland disease	Cross-sectional design Coeliac disease: n = 130 Control group: n = 80	CFS FSS VAS	S: Definition of fatigue. L: Inadequate language L: Groups not comparable due to differences in BMI, Ferritin, Haemoglobin L: No evidence of appropriate matching of groups L: Inadequate statistical control for differences between groups L: Methods used to collect socio-demographic and clinical data is lacking L: Unclear presentation of results L: Procedure for questionnaire handling insufficiently described L: Lack of information about validity and reliability on the study questionnaires, both in Italian and in the target group L: No clear identification and control of potential confounding factors L: Data not presented in line with study aims

Table 2. *Cont.*

Study (Ref. No.)	Study Population and Setting	Study Design and Participants	Questionnaires Measuring Fatigue	Strengths and Limitations
Jordá et al., 2010 [12]	Patients with celiac disease seen between March 2008 and April 2009 were prospectively invited to participate in the study Included patients stratified in two groups (Group 1: Following gluten-free diet, Group 2: Untreated)	Cross-sectional study n = 51 Group 1: n = 38 Group 2: n = 13	D-FIS	L: No definition of fatigue. S: Validated fatigue questionnaire used L: Small sample and small subgroups L: Lack of information on recruitment procedure L: Lack of information concerning the collection of socio-demographic and clinical data L: No information on ethical approval L: No information about response rate or number of patients approached for inclusion L: Characteristics differ between groups
Ciacci et al., 2007 [13]	Patients with CD screened for inclusion at the Department of Clinical and Experimental Medicine, Federico II University—Naples, Italy6 0 patients randomized following a 30-day gluten-free diet	Randomized, double blind, parallel study n = 60 (L-Carnitine group n = 30, placebo n = 30)	Scott-Huskisson VAS VSA SF-36 (Vitality subscale)	S: Definition of fatigue S: Randomized groups S: Allocation concealment S: Clear definition of coeliac disease L: Large number of participants did not complete study (n = 13 (22%)) L: Single centre L: Lack of calculation of effect size L: No information on validity/reliability of fatigue questionnaires
Zingone et al., 2010 [14]	Adult coeliac disease patients consecutively recruited from September 2009 to March 2010 from Frederico II University (Naples, Italy) Participants divided into two groups (Group 1: Coeliac patients at diagnosis on gluten containing diet. Group 2: Coeliac patients at follow up on gluten-free diet) Gender- and age-matched control group Inclusion criteria: Informed consent, 19–60 years Exclusion criteria: Major psychiatric disease, cancer, pregnancy or children blow 3 years of age	Case Control study Group 1: n = 30 Group 2: n = 30 Control group: n = 30	Fatigue-VAS	L: Fatigue not specified as aim, merely reported as parts of the questionnaire results. L: No definition of fatigue L: No information about response rate or number of patients approached for inclusion L: Large numeric differences in characteristics between coeliac groups L: No control for confounding variables S: Gender- and age-matched controls

Table legends and abbreviations: L; Limitation., S; Strength., SF-36; Short Form-36 Health Survey., D-FIS; Daily Fatigue Impact Scale., FSS; Fatigue Severity Scale., CFS; Chronic Fatigue Syndrome Questionnaire., GBB-24., Geißener Symptom Check List., VSA; Verbal Scale for Asthenia, VSA. CD; Coeliac disease, HADS-D; Hospital anxiety and depression scale – depression.

3.3. Definition and Measurement of Fatigue

In two out of five papers, a definition or a more detailed description of fatigue was provided. Both Siniscalchi et al. [11] and Ciacci et al. [13] defined fatigue as "difficulty in initiating or sustaining regular activities". However, in none of these studies a reference to the definition were provided.

In total, six different ways of measuring fatigue have been used in the five studies reviewed. Five of these instruments have only been used once. In addition, one study has used the sub-scale vitality from the health-related quality of life questionnaire SF-36.

In a majority of the papers, there is lack of information about the validity and reliability of the instruments used to measure fatigue. While Häuser et al. [10] and Jordá et al. [12] provide references to adequate psychometrical testing of the SF-36, Giessener Symptom Checklist (GBB-24) and Daily Fatigue Impact Scale (D-FIS), none of the Italian studies provide clear reference to adequate testing. In fact, in two of the latter studies one of the instruments seem to have been labeled differently while referring to the same reference by Wessely et al. [15]. While Siniscalchi et al. [11] use the label Chronic Fatigue Syndrome (CFS) questionnaire, Ciacci et al. [13] use the label Verbal Scale for Asthenia. Moreover, when investigating the original study by Wessely et al. [15] in depth, it seems like this instrument was developed for this particular study and that the necessary tests for validity and reliability were not performed, and at least not published.

3.4. Prevalence of Fatigue and Its Associations

None of the reviewed studies present prevalence data, even though one of the aims in the study by Siniscalchi et al. [11] were to evaluate the prevalence of fatigue in celiac disease. When looking at fatigue in patients on normal versus gluten-free diet, results also differ. While Zingone et al. [14] and Siniscalchi et al. [11] found no significant differences, Jordá et al. [12] found that untreated patients reported significantly worse fatigue. In addition, when comparing celiac disease patients and healthy controls, both Häuser et al. [10] and Zingone et al. [14] found impaired scores in celiac disease.

While Zingone et al. [14] found impaired sleep to be associated with increased fatigue, Jordá et al. [12] found that increased fatigue was associated with impaired HRQoL. Merely two studies [11,12] investigated potential socio-demographic and clinical factors associated with fatigue, finding that there is no association between fatigue and factors such as gender, age, or GI symptoms in celiac disease. While Jordá et al. [12] reported that lower haemoglobin levels were correlated with worse scores of the D-FIS fatigue scale, Siniscalchi et al. [11] were not able to identify any association.

3.5. Interventions to Alleviate Fatigue

Only one of the studies were designed as an intervention. The study by Ciacci et al. [13] aimed to investigate the effect on fatigue of a long L-Carnitine treatment in adult celiac disease patients. While there were no reports of serious adverse events, abdominal and skin problems were registered in a total of six patients (10%). Moreover, a large number of patients did not complete the study (n = 13), of which three were dropouts. The main finding is that fatigue scores were significantly more improved in the intervention versus placebo group. However, even though fatigue scores in the intervention group displayed a larger decrease than in the placebo group, patients in the intervention group had a higher fatigue scores than the placebo group at baseline (T0). Moreover, the mean fatigue VAS at the end of study (T2) was 2.40 (SD 1.80) versus 2.93 (SD 1.85) in the intervention versus placebo group, respectively. While Ciacci et al. does not report any measures of effect size, calculation of Cohens d [16] on the differences between the intervention and placebo group at T2 reveal a small effect size (0.29).

4. Discussion

In this review we were only able to identify 16 papers that, to some extent, had investigated fatigue in celiac disease. Of these, 11 papers [6,17–26] did not report any specific methodology concerning fatigue assessment. Of the remaining five papers [10–14], in which fatigue assessment had been described methodologically, merely three investigated fatigue as the primary endpoint [11–13]. In addition, critical assessment revealed that none of the included studies held high scientific quality.

A basic problem in fatigue research is the lack of a common accepted definition [27]. Indeed, lack of definition and conceptual clarification was also observed in this review, where only two studies provided a definition of fatigue [11,13]. On the other hand, the fatigue definitions presented in those two papers both lacked a clear reference to existing literature.

Fatigue is frequently reported by patients as well as observed by clinicians in celiac disease [23,25,26]. However, a vast majority of the published literature base their reports merely on clinical consultation rather than rigorous methodological research (i.e., using validated measurement tools). Thus, the actual prevalence of fatigue in celiac disease remains unclear. However, there are indications that the level of fatigue is higher in these patients than in control groups and the background population [10,14]

We were only able to identify one single study that reported on potential socio-demographic and clinical factors associated with fatigue symptoms in celiac disease [11]. Of the factors studied, none were significantly associated with fatigue. However, since data is not shown, it is unclear whether this finding was true for all of the different fatigue measures used in the study. Furthermore, two of the included studies found that fatigue was associated with reduced HRQoL and increased sleep problems, respectively [12,14]. Although there is currently very limited documentation on these associations, this appears to coincide with findings in other patient populations [28–32]. In addition, our review only found one study that was designed as an intervention with fatigue as the primary endpoint. Even though Ciacci et al. [13] conclude that L-Carnitine therapy is safe and effective in ameliorating fatigue in celiac disease, these results should be interpreted with extreme caution. Firstly, the study is hampered by the fact that it does not reach its own power estimates due to a large number of patients not completing the study (21.6%). Secondly, the study does not use fatigue measurement tools that has been adequately tested for validity and reliability. In addition, the absolute difference in mean fatigue VAS between the groups at end of study revealed a small effect size according to Cohen's d [16,33].

Several studies in other populations have shown that anaemia is associated with increased fatigue symptoms [7,34]. The pathogenesis of anaemia-related fatigue remains unclear, but some suggest that abnormalities in energy metabolism play a role in inducing fatigue [35]. Moreover, while some studies have shown that haemoglobin response is associated with meaningful improvements in fatigue, others have not been able to reveal any significant association between the use of erythropoiesis-stimulating agents and fatigue symptom [36,37]. In the current review we were unable to identify studies that specifically looked at anaemia as predictor of fatigue in celiac disease. However, Siniscalchi et al. [11] noted that the included celiac patients in their study had significantly lower haemoglobin levels. A similar observation was reported in Jordá et al. [12]. In the latter study, a significant correlation between worse fatigue scores and lower haemoglobin levels was reported. However, even though Jordá et al. [12] report that their regression analysis show that haemoglobin levels may be involved in the perception of fatigue, the data presented in the paper does not justify such a conclusion. In fact, the dependent variable used in their study was not fatigue, but HRQoL (EQ-5D-VAS). Consequently, the current observation on the potential association between fatigue and anaemia was based on a univariate analysis only.

This review is not without limitations. The fact that we chose to limit our focus to adults and English publications only may have influenced our identification of relevant publications. On the other hand, a strength is the rigorous literature search in several databases, as well as the blinded quality assessment of each of the papers by two of the authors.

5. Conclusions

Although frequently reported in clinical practice, fatigue has been scarcely studied in celiac disease. In addition, existing literature is characterized by significant methodological weaknesses. Consequently, there is an unmet need to understand contributing factors for fatigue as well as the impact of fatigue in celiac disease.

Author Contributions: K.E.A.L. identified the topic of this review and prepared a first draft. L.-P. J.-J. and T.B. performed the literature review and prepared the manuscript. All authors finalized the manuscript.

Funding: The authors did not receive any specific funding for this study.

Acknowledgments: Trine Tingelholm Karlsen (Østfold University College) is acknowledged for her contribution to the literature search.

Conflicts of Interest: The authors declare no conflict of interest.

References

1. Ludvigsson, J.F.; Leffler, D.A.; Bai, J.C.; Biagi, F.; Fasano, A.; Green, P.H.; Hadjivassiliou, M.; Kaukinen, K.; Kelly, C.P.; Leonard, J.N.; et al. The Oslo definitions for coeliac disease and related terms. *Gut* **2013**, *62*, 43–52. [CrossRef] [PubMed]
2. Ludvigsson, J.F.; Bai, J.C.; Biagi, F.; Card, T.R.; Ciacci, C.; Ciclitira, P.J.; Green, P.H.R.; Hadjivassiliou, M.; Holdoway, A.; van Heel, D.A.; et al. Diagnosis and management of adult coeliac disease: Guidelines from the British Society of Gastroenterology. *Gut* **2014**, *63*, 1210–1228. [CrossRef] [PubMed]

3. Leffler, D.A.; Green, P.H.; Fasano, A. Extraintestinal manifestations of coeliac disease. *Nat. Rev. Gastroenterol. Hepatol.* **2015**, *12*, 561–571. [CrossRef] [PubMed]

4. Lundin, K.E.; Wijmenga, C. Coeliac disease and autoimmune disease-genetic overlap and screening. *Nat. Rev. Gastroenterol. Hepatol.* **2015**, *12*, 507–515. [CrossRef] [PubMed]

5. Hin, H.; Bird, G.; Fisher, P.; Mahy, N.; Jewell, D. Coeliac disease in primary care: Case finding study. *BMJ* **1999**, *318*, 164–167. [CrossRef] [PubMed]

6. Sanders, D.S.; Patel, D.; Stephenson, T.J.; Ward, A.M.; McCloskey, E.V.; Hadjivassiliou, M.; Lobo, A.J. A primary care cross-sectional study of undiagnosed adult coeliac disease. *Eur. J. Gastroenterol. Hepatol.* **2003**, *15*, 407–413. [CrossRef] [PubMed]

7. Jelsness-Jorgensen, L.P.; Bernklev, T.; Henriksen, M.; Torp, R.; Moum, B.A. Chronic fatigue is more prevalent in patients with inflammatory bowel disease than in healthy controls. *Inflamm. Bowel Dis.* **2011**, *17*, 1564–1572. [CrossRef] [PubMed]

8. Van Langenberg, D.R.; Gibson, P.R. Systematic review: Fatigue in inflammatory bowel disease. *Aliment. Pharmacol. Ther.* **2010**, *32*, 131–143. [CrossRef] [PubMed]

9. Moher, D.; Liberati, A.; Tetzlaff, J.; Altman, D.G. Preferred reporting items for systematic reviews and meta-analyses: The PRISMA statement. *Ann. Intern. Med.* **2009**, *151*, 264–269. [CrossRef] [PubMed]

10. Hauser, W.; Gold, J.; Stein, J.; Caspary, W.F.; Stallmach, A. Health-related quality of life in adult coeliac disease in Germany: Results of a national survey. *Eur. J. Gastroenterol. Hepatol.* **2006**, *18*, 747–754. [CrossRef] [PubMed]

11. Siniscalchi, M.; Iovino, P.; Tortora, R.; Forestiero, S.; Somma, A.; Capuano, L.; Franzese, M.D.; Sabbatini, F.; Ciacci, C. Fatigue in adult coeliac disease. *Aliment. Pharmacol. Ther.* **2005**, *22*, 489–494. [CrossRef] [PubMed]

12. Jorda, F.C.; Lopez Vivancos, J. Fatigue as a determinant of health in patients with celiac disease. *J. Clin. Gastroenterol.* **2010**, *44*, 423–427. [CrossRef] [PubMed]

13. Ciacci, C.; Peluso, G.; Iannoni, E.; Siniscalchi, M.; Iovino, P.; Rispo, A.; Tortora, R.; Bucci, C.; Zingone, F.; Margarucci, S.; et al. L-Carnitine in the treatment of fatigue in adult celiac disease patients: A pilot study. *Dig. Liver. Dis.* **2007**, *39*, 922–928. [CrossRef] [PubMed]

14. Zingone, F.; Siniscalchi, M.; Capone, P.; Tortora, R.; Andreozzi, P.; Capone, E.; Ciacci, C. The quality of sleep in patients with coeliac disease. *Aliment. Pharmacol. Ther.* **2010**, *32*, 1031–1036. [CrossRef] [PubMed]

15. Wessely, S.; Powell, R. Fatigue syndromes: A comparison of chronic "postviral" fatigue with neuromuscular and affective disorders. *J. Neurol. Neurosurg. Psychiatr.* **1989**, *52*, 940–948. [CrossRef]

16. Cohen, J. *Statistical Power Analysis for The Behavioral Sciences*, 2nd ed.; Lawrence Erlbaum Associates: Mahwah, NJ, USA, 1988.

17. Zarkadas, M.; Cranney, A.; Case, S.; Molloy, M.; Switzer, C.; Graham, I.D.; Butzner, J.D.; Rashid, M.; Warren, R.E.; Burrows, V. The impact of a gluten-free diet on adults with coeliac disease: Results of a national survey. *J. Hum. Nutr. Diet.* **2006**, *19*, 41–49. [CrossRef] [PubMed]

18. Spijkerman, M.; Tan, I.L.; Kolkman, J.J.; Withoff, S.; Wijmenga, C.; Visschedijk, M.C.; Weersma, R.K. A large variety of clinical features and concomitant disorders in celiac disease—A cohort study in the Netherlands. *Dig. Liver Dis.* **2016**, *48*, 499–505. [CrossRef] [PubMed]

19. Silvester, J.A.; Graff, L.A.; Rigaux, L.; Walker, J.R.; Duerksen, D.R. Symptomatic suspected gluten exposure is common among patients with coeliac disease on a gluten-free diet. *Aliment. Pharmacol. Ther.* **2016**, *44*, 612–619. [CrossRef] [PubMed]

20. Jericho, H.; Sansotta, N.; Guandalini, S. Extraintestinal manifestations of celiac disease: Effectiveness of the gluten-free diet. *J. Pediatr. Gastroenterol. Nutr.* **2017**, *65*, 75–79. [CrossRef] [PubMed]

21. Sansotta, N.; Amirikian, K.; Guandalini, S.; Jericho, H. Celiac disease symptom resolution: Effectiveness of the gluten-free diet. *J. Pediatr. Gastroenterol. Nutr.* **2018**, *66*, 48–52. [CrossRef] [PubMed]

22. Catassi, C.; Kryszak, D.; Louis-Jacques, O.; Duerksen, D.R.; Hill, I.; Crowe, S.E.; Brown, A.R.; Procaccini, N.J.; Wonderly, B.A.; Hartley, P.; et al. Detection of Celiac disease in primary care: A multicenter case-finding study in North America. *Am. J. Gastroenterol.* **2007**, *102*, 1454–1460. [CrossRef] [PubMed]

23. Nurminen, S.; Kivela, L.; Huhtala, H.; Kaukinen, K.; Kurppa, K. Extraintestinal manifestations were common in children with coeliac disease and were more prevalent in patients with more severe clinical and histological presentation. *Acta Paediatr.* **2018**. [CrossRef] [PubMed]

24. Barratt, S.M.; Leeds, J.S.; Sanders, D.S. Factors influencing the type, timing and severity of symptomatic responses to dietary gluten in patients with biopsy-proven coeliac disease. *JGLD* **2013**, *22*, 391–396. [PubMed]

25. Ford, S.; Howard, R.; Oyebode, J. Psychosocial aspects of coeliac disease: A cross-sectional survey of a UK population. *Br. J. Health Psychol.* **2012**, *17*, 743–757. [CrossRef] [PubMed]

26. Francavilla, R.; Cristofori, F.; Castellaneta, S.; Polloni, C.; Albano, V.; Dellatte, S.; Indrio, F.; Cavallo, L.; Catassi, C. Clinical, serologic, and histologic features of gluten sensitivity in children. *J. Pediatr.* **2014**, *164*, 463–467. [CrossRef] [PubMed]

27. DeLuca, J. *Fatigue: As a Window to the Brain*, 1st ed.; MIT Press: Cambridge, MA, USA, 2005.

28. Jelsness-Jorgensen, L.P.; Bernklev, T.; Henriksen, M.; Torp, R.; Moum, B.A. Chronic fatigue is associated with impaired health-related quality of life in inflammatory bowel disease. *Aliment. Pharmacol. Ther.* **2011**, *33*, 106–114. [CrossRef] [PubMed]

29. Frigstad, S.O.; Hoivik, M.L.; Jahnsen, J.; Cvancarova, M.; Grimstad, T.; Berset, I.P.; Huppertz-Hauss, G.; Hovde, Ø.; Bernklev, T.; Moum, B.; et al. Fatigue is not associated with vitamin D deficiency in inflammatory bowel disease patients. *WJG* **2018**, *24*, 3293–3301. [CrossRef] [PubMed]

30. Kotterba, S.; Neusser, T.; Norenberg, C.; Bussfeld, P.; Glaser, T.; Dorner, M.; Schürks, M. Sleep quality, daytime sleepiness, fatigue, and quality of life in patients with multiple sclerosis treated with interferon beta-1b: Results from a prospective observational cohort study. *BMC Nephrol.* **2018**, *18*. [CrossRef] [PubMed]

31. Rupp, I.; Boshuizen, H.C.; Jacobi, C.E.; Dinant, H.J.; van den Bos, G.A.M. Impact of fatigue on health-related quality of life in rheumatoid arthritis. *Arthritis Rheum.* **2004**, *51*, 578–585. [CrossRef] [PubMed]

32. Opheim, R.; Fagermoen, M.S.; Bernklev, T.; Jelsness-Jorgensen, L.P.; Moum, B. Fatigue interference with daily living among patients with inflammatory bowel disease. *Qual. Life Res.* **2014**, *23*, 707–717. [CrossRef] [PubMed]

33. Cohen, J. A power primer. *Psychol. Bull.* **1992**, *112*, 155–159. [CrossRef] [PubMed]

34. Romberg-Camps, M.J.; Bol, Y.; Dagnelie, P.C.; Hesselink-van de Kruijs, M.A.; Kester, A.D.; Engels, L.G.; van Deursen, C.; Hameeteman, W.H.A.; Pierik, M.; Pierik, F.; et al. Fatigue and health-related quality of life in inflammatory bowel disease: Results from a population-based study in the Netherlands: The IBD-South Limburg cohort. *Inflamm. Bowel Dis.* **2010**, *16*, 2137–2147. [CrossRef] [PubMed]

35. Sobrero, A.; Puglisi, F.; Guglielmi, A.; Belvedere, O.; Aprile, G.; Ramello, M.; Grossi, F.A.O.U. San Martino—IST, Istituto Nazionale Ricerca sul Cancro (GENOVA) Fatigue: A main component of anemia symptomatology. *Semin. Oncol.* **2001**, *28*, 15–18. [CrossRef]

36. Bohlius, J.; Tonia, T.; Nuesch, E.; Juni, P.; Fey, M.F.; Egger, M.; Bernhard, J. Effects of erythropoiesis-stimulating agents on fatigue- and anaemia-related symptoms in cancer patients: Systematic review and meta-analyses of published and unpublished data. *Br. J. Cancer* **2014**, *111*, 33–45. [CrossRef] [PubMed]

37. Cella, D.; Kallich, J.; McDermott, A.; Xu, X. The longitudinal relationship of hemoglobin, fatigue and quality of life in anemic cancer patients: Results from five randomized clinical trials. *Ann. Oncol.* **2004**, *15*, 979–986. [CrossRef] [PubMed]

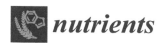

Review

Gluten-Induced Extra-Intestinal Manifestations in Potential Celiac Disease—Celiac Trait

Alina Popp [1,2] and Markku Mäki [2,*]

[1] University of Medicine and Pharmacy "Carol Davila" and National Institute for Mother and Child Health "Alessandrescu-Rusescu", Bucharest 020395, Romania; alina.popp@uta.fi

[2] Faculty of Medicine and Health Technology, Tampere University and Tampere University Hospital, 33520 Tampere, Finland

* Correspondence: markku.maki@uta.fi; Tel.: +358-50-3656668

Received: 21 December 2018; Accepted: 29 January 2019; Published: 1 February 2019

Abstract: Celiac disease patients may suffer from a number of extra-intestinal diseases related to long-term gluten ingestion. The diagnosis of celiac disease is based on the presence of a manifest small intestinal mucosal lesion. Individuals with a normal biopsy but an increased risk of developing celiac disease are referred to as potential celiac disease patients. However, these patients are not treated. This review highlights that patients with normal biopsies may suffer from the same extra-intestinal gluten-induced complications before the disease manifests at the intestinal level. We discuss diagnostic markers revealing true potential celiac disease. The evidence-based medical literature shows that these potential patients, who are "excluded" for celiac disease would in fact benefit from gluten-free diets. The question is why wait for an end-stage disease to occur when it can be prevented? We utilize research on dermatitis herpetiformis, which is a model disease in which a gluten-induced entity erupts in the skin irrespective of the state of the small intestinal mucosal morphology. Furthermore, gluten ataxia can be categorized as its own entity. The other extra-intestinal manifestations occurring in celiac disease are also found at the latent disease stage. Consequently, patients with celiac traits should be identified and treated.

Keywords: gluten; latent celiac disease; potential celiac disease; extra-intestinal manifestations; mild enteropathy; early developing celiac disease; genetic gluten intolerance; natural history; celiac trait

1. Introduction

Celiac disease is an autoimmune systemic disorder in genetically susceptible persons perpetuated by the daily ingestion of gluten cereals (wheat, rye, and barley) with manifestations in the small intestine and organs outside the gut. Patients diagnosed with celiac disease show gluten-induced and gluten-dependent duodenal mucosal lesions (i.e., the typical crypt hyperplastic lesion with villous atrophy). Clinically these newly diagnosed patients may or may not be suffering from gastrointestinal symptoms. A gluten-driven extra-intestinal manifestation is often the only clue for the disease. In the primary care and within different medical disciplines, physicians should suspect celiac disease and perform case finding by serum autoantibody screening. Positive serology is often the only way to identify potential patients for a diagnostic upper intestinal endoscopy [1–3]. In fact, less than half of all adult patients diagnosed with celiac disease complain of gastrointestinal symptoms at an initial diagnosis [4]. This knowledge comes from Finland, where adult celiac disease diagnoses have increased 20 times in recent decades and 0.8% of the total population has a biopsy-confirmed diagnosis [5–7].

Patients diagnosed with celiac disease including a duodenal mucosal lesion may suffer from a number of extra-intestinal diseases [2,3]. Dermatitis herpetiformis manifests outside the gut, is gluten driven and dependent [8,9], has the same genetic background, and occurs within the same families as celiac disease [9,10]. In fact, one identical twin may have celiac disease while the other suffers from dermatitis herpetiformis [11]. Other gluten-driven extra-intestinal manifestations in celiac disease include osteopenia, osteoporosis, fractures [12–14], permanent tooth enamel defects [6,15], arthritis, and arthralgia [16–18] as well as further central and peripheral nervous system [19–22], liver [23–25], and reproductive system involvements [26,27]. Even autoimmune diseases may be gluten driven [28,29], and there is a risk for malignant complications, especially non-Hodgkin lymphoma, in untreated celiac disease [30,31].

By definition, celiac disease is excluded in patients who have normal small intestinal mucosal morphology at their first diagnostic endoscopy if they have been following a normal gluten-containing diet. However, it seems evident that this is not accurate. In a review in 2001, we wrote that gluten-induced extra-intestinal manifestations may develop at the latent disease stage when the mucosa is still morphologically normal [32], citing several observations [19,33–36]. Today such patients are often referred to as having "potential celiac disease" because they are found to be "normal" on biopsy [37]. Meanwhile, dermatitis herpetiformis is our model disease, in which an extra-intestinal manifestation is treated with a gluten-free diet irrespective of the mucosal finding (diseased or not). We reviewed the literature for evidence for extra-intestinal gluten-dependent manifestations in patients "excluded" for celiac disease. In this paper, we also discuss tools for identifying these "potential" treatable patients.

2. Latent or Potential Celiac Disease

The "pre-celiac" state has been described in patients with dermatitis herpetiformis, in whom small intestinal mucosal deterioration was shown to occur after adding extra gluten to the diet [38–40]. An extra gluten load also induced mucosal lesions in healthy individuals [39,41]. The concept of latent celiac disease, without having an extra load of gluten, was shown to be part of the gluten sensitivity spectrum and natural history of celiac disease [42–45]. Specifically, this was shown in Finland in celiac patients who, by chance, had previously undergone a small intestinal biopsy that was reported as normal or who were followed up because of positive serum autoantibody results.

We chose to use the term "latent celiac disease", which is similar to Weinstein [38], when referring to patients with a normal biopsy who later exhibited mucosal deterioration and were diagnosed as celiac disease patients. For us, "latent" means existing but not manifest (i.e., the disease exists but is not manifest at the mucosal level). Based on our early descriptions, Ferguson et al. (1993) defined latent celiac disease as follows: "This term should only be applied to patients who fulfill the following conditions: (i) have a normal jejunal biopsy while taking a normal diet, (ii) at some other time, before or since, have had a flat jejunal biopsy which recovers on a gluten free diet" [46]. Following the first reports on existing celiac disease latency, a numbers of other results have been published, with early papers by Troncone [47] and Corazza et al. [48]. It is now clear that oral tolerance towards gluten can be kept for longer periods, even for decades and into older age [49].

The term "potential celiac disease" has been used interchangeably with latent celiac disease, and this has led to confusion in the celiac disease literature. Thus, the Oslo task force discouraged the use of the term "latent celiac disease", and individuals with a normal outcome from a small intestinal biopsy but who are at increased risk of developing celiac disease based on positive celiac disease serology should be referred to as having potential celiac disease [37]. These "potential patients" are not treated as celiac. The question is, what should a gluten-triggered and gluten-dependent treatable disease outside the gut be called, when the extra-intestinal manifestation occurs at the latent stage of the disease and when conventional diagnostic biopsy criteria have excluded celiac disease? We infer that such patients should not be categorized as having potential celiac disease. Rather, they require proper treatment [50,51].

In Figure 1, we summarize the lifespan natural history of celiac gluten sensitivity, where each line represents a single individual. The term celiac gluten sensitivity encompasses celiac traits, latent celiac disease, genetic gluten intolerance, mild enteropathy celiac disease, early developing celiac disease, and celiac disease itself [1,32,50–53]. The gluten-induced mucosal damage develops rapidly or gradually from normal mucosal morphology to a manifest mucosal lesion. The tolerance towards gluten is individual, and it may be broken after only months or years (childhood celiac disease) but also at adolescence, adulthood, and even after decades of gluten ingestion in old age. The latent celiac disease patients, the "true potential" patients in Figure 1 (i.e., normal on biopsy showing villus height crypt depth ratio >2), are classified as having celiac disease only when the disease has deteriorated to the degree of a manifest mucosal lesion (i.e., villus height crypt depth ratio <2).

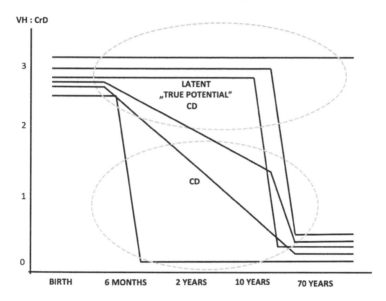

Figure 1. Natural history of developing celiac disease (CD) at the small intestinal mucosal level. Each line represents one individual. We are born with a normal mucosal morphology, a villus height (VH), and a crypt depth (CrD) ratio of approximately three and villi three times taller than crypts are deep. Upon gluten ingestion, mucosal injury proceeds rapidly or gradually at different ages, in childhood or only at an older age. Before developing a manifest mucosal lesion (diseased mucosa on biopsy, VH:CrD <2) every CD patient belongs to the category latent "true potential" CD (normal on biopsy, VH:CrD >2).

3. Markers of Existing Early Disease

An existing gluten-dependent disease without evidence of enteropathy until a later age - latent celiac disease - includes in its definition the susceptibility genes for celiac disease and the genes encoding the *human leukocyte antigen* (HLA) DQ2 or DQ8 molecules [1,32,54]. This is a check that clinicians may perform when there are symptoms and signs suggestive of celiac disease, but the biopsy is normal or does not show clear crypt hyperplasia. It shows only inflammation and descriptive mild villus atrophy. Positivity for DQ2 or DQ8 does not mean very much, since 30% to 40% of the citizens in the country are positive, but double negative means that no celiac disease will develop.

Patients positive for *celiac disease serology* with normal biopsies should be considered to have potential celiac disease [37]. However, gliadin antibody positivity, which is a frequent finding in celiac disease control patients and even in healthy individuals, does not correlate with celiac disease susceptibility genes [55]. Currently, tissue transglutaminase autoantibody (TG2-ab) testing is used to screen for celiac disease. It should be noted, however, that not all serum TG2-abs predict celiac disease [56]. TG2-abs have been described in other autoimmune diseases as well as in infections, tumors, myocardial damage, liver disorders, and psoriasis [54]. These antibodies are not associated with endomysial autoantibodies and may occur in persons negative both for HLA DQ2 and DQ8. The serum endomysial antibody test is the gold standard, and the presence of these autoantibodies predicts impending celiac disease [1,45,50,53,55]. In celiac disease in patients with extra-intestinal manifestations, other autoantibodies play a role in diagnosis and potentially in disease mechanisms [57].

At the mucosal level, inflammation, as measured as the density of intraepithelial T cells (*IELs*), is a very unspecific finding, but is also gluten-dependent in cases of celiac disease [58]. Marsh 1 lesions with increased IELs were shown to have a sensitivity of 59% and specificity of 57% in predicting forthcoming celiac disease [59]. However, when searched for, an autoimmune insult to the morphologically normal intestinal mucosa is, in fact, present. A high density of $\gamma\delta$ *T-cell-receptor-bearing IELs* in patients with morphologically normal mucosa who also carry the susceptibility genes for celiac disease seems to be a prerequisite for developing celiac disease [43,60,61]. Yet, even if an increased density of $\gamma\delta$ T cells is found in latent celiac disease, such a finding is not pathognomonic for the disease [59,61]. In the small intestine, the gluten-dependent autoantibodies target extracellular TG2 and may be detected as *IgA deposits* in biopsy tissues at the latent disease stage [62–64] (Figure 2). In fact, the IgA deposits in the duodenal biopsies accurately predicted forthcoming celiac disease better than IELs, $\gamma\delta^+$ IELs, or serum autoantibodies [59]. The detection of intestinal TG2-abs by phage-antibody libraries is another possibility for diagnosis [52]. However, intestinal TG2-ab production is not only found in celiac disease [65]. Again, when finding an increased density of $\gamma\delta^+$ IELs or IgA deposits in a patient with normal small intestinal mucosal morphology, it is recommended to check whether the patient belongs to the "celiac family" (i.e., are carrying either the HLA DQ2 or DQ8 molecules).

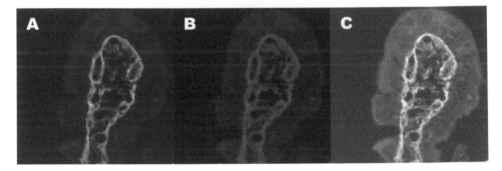

Figure 2. Small intestinal mucosal immunoglobulin (Ig) A deposits are shown in a villus tip from a dermatitis herpetiformis patient with normal mucosal morphology. IgA is stained with green (**A**), transglutaminase 2 (TG2) with red (**B**), and subepithelial colocalisation of IgA and TG2 can be seen in yellow (**C**).

4. Extraintestinal Manifestations

4.1. Dermatitis Herpetiformis

In dermatitis herpetiformis, a gluten-induced and gluten-dependent manifestation occurs outside the gut even in the absence of intestinal mucosal villous atrophy [8,66]. Today, up to 30% of patients with dermatitis herpetiformis have a normal small intestinal mucosal lining [67]. Typically, the disease manifests with itchy papules and vesicles on the elbows, knees and buttocks, and overt gastrointestinal symptoms are rare [67,68]. When patients without enteropathy are challenged with extra gluten, their small intestinal mucosae deteriorate in a way typical of celiac disease [38–40]. When no enteropathy is present, patients only test positively for serum TG2-abs and endomysial antibodies in 40% of cases [67]. However, the patients could be serum endomysial autoantibody positive already while having normal small intestinal mucosa prior to any evidence of skin eruptions [44]. If searched for, the autoimmune effect to the morphologically normal intestinal mucosa caused by an environmental trigger—the daily ingestion of gluten—is, in fact, present. Mucosal inflammatory markers (i.e., the high density of $\gamma\delta^+$ IELs) shows this [35]. Furthermore, in patients who are negative for serum autoantibodies, the antibodies are found at the mucosal level targeting extracellular TG2 [62,69,70], which is a finding typical for an existing disease that is not manifest at the mucosal architectural level (Figure 2).

We infer that patients with gluten-triggered extra-intestinal manifestations, who are now classified as having dermatitis herpetiformis but show a normal small intestinal mucosa, do not belong to the category of potential celiac disease. These patients may even be suffering from osteoporosis and experience bone fractures. Clearly, it is a treatable disease [67,68,71]. In the following, we use parallel reasoning for patients having other gluten-dependent extra-intestinal manifestations occurring at the latent stage of celiac disease.

4.2. Central and Peripheral Nervous System

Gluten-induced neurological manifestations including gluten ataxia are common in adult celiac disease [19–22] and occur in children [2]. Hadjivassiliou et al. noticed that gluten sensitivity was found in patients with neurological disease, and they screened the patients with gliadin antibodies [72]. They also showed that neurological complications occurred during the latent stage of celiac disease. Their use of gliadin antibodies created some skepticism toward the findings, but today gluten ataxia has become a gluten-induced entity in itself, similar to dermatitis herpetiformis [20,73]. In fact, it was shown that gluten ataxia might respond to a strict gluten-free diet even in the absence of an enteropathy [74,75]. Serum transglutaminase 6 antibodies are used for detecting gluten ataxia in patients with and without small intestinal mucosal lesions. Negative seroconversion results from a gluten-free diet [75]. Further evidence that gluten ataxia without enteropathy belongs to the celiac spectrum comes from the finding that TG2-specific autoantibody deposits were detected in the intestinal mucosa [74]. The patients were HLA DQ2-positive or DQ8-positive. All of the control ataxia patients were negative for celiac-type HLA, and they had no IgA deposits in the mucosa [74]. In one gluten ataxia patient, similar TG2-targeted IgA deposits were found in the small vessels of the brain [74]. In a different cohort of idiopathic ataxia patients, the TG2-targeted IgA deposits were again detected, even in the absence of circulating TG2-abs [76].

Gluten-induced peripheral nervous system involvement often expresses as a symmetrical sensorimotor axonal peripheral neuropathy [77]. In patients with or without enteropathy, neuropathies cannot be differentiated based on clinical, genetic, or immunological grounds [78,79].

4.3. Bone Disease

Bone diseases, osteopenia, osteoporosis, and even fractures are highly prevalent in untreated celiac disease [14,80,81]. Strict gluten-free diets improve bone health in celiac disease and are an effective therapy for long-term bone mineral recovery [13,82].

Latent celiac disease patients, before manifesting an overt disease, might suffer from gluten-dependent symptoms as well as osteopenia and osteoporosis [62,83–86]. Kaukinen et al. showed that eight of 10 patients without villous atrophy had a bone disease, and they all were DQ2 positive [83]. On biopsy, it was shown that they belonged to the celiac spectrum since they had increased densities of $\gamma\delta^+$ IELs. Furthermore, their initial TG2 and endomysial antibodies normalized with a gluten-free diet. Dickey et al. again measured bone mineral density in 31 endomysial antibody-positive patients who were excluded for celiac disease (i.e., classified as having Marsh 0 or Marsh 1 lesions). They found osteopenia to be present in 30% and osteoporosis in 10% of these patients, and the degree of bone disease did not differ from that found in patients diagnosed with overt celiac disease. Negative seroconversion followed upon implementation of a gluten-free diet in the 26 of the 27 patients with normal biopsies. On the contrary, eight patients continued their gluten-containing diet, and seven of them evolved toward villous atrophy compatible with celiac disease within one to two years [84]. Kurppa et al. proved that the gluten-free diet had a positive effect on the bone mineral density in endomysial antibody-positive patients with normal villous morphology, which is similar to those with celiac-type enteropathy [85]. Zanini et al. concluded that celiac disease patients with mild enteropathy have various markers of existing malabsorption including bone disease, and, thus, require treatment with a gluten-free diet [86].

Patients with true potential celiac disease are also a risk of fractures. Pasternack et al. showed that dermatitis herpetiformis patients reported earlier fractures in 45 out of 222 cases at diagnosis. Altogether, 16% of the fractures had occurred in patients with normal small intestinal histology, 35% occurred in patients with partial villous atrophy, and 49% occurred in patients with subtotal villous atrophy in Reference [71].

4.4. Liver Diseases

Celiac disease may initially present as a monosymptomatic liver disease, such as cryptogenic hypertransaminasaemia or autoimmunue-type of liver damage [23–25,87]. There are few reports of liver injury in potential or latent celiac disease. Zanini et al. observed that celiac disease with mild enteropathy and positive celiac disease-related serology is not a mild disease. Moreover, they showed alanine aminotransferase serum values to be elevated in 9/121 (8%), γ-glutamyltransferase in 5/102 (5%), and alkaline phosphatase in 6/101 (6%) of patients. The authors concluded that these patients should also be treated [86].

4.5. Other Extraintestinal Manifestations

4.5.1. Permanent Tooth Dental Enamel Defects

Adult patients with celiac disease and dermatitis herpetiformis, as well as children with dermatitis herpetiformis, show celiac-type dental enamel defects in their permanent dentition [15,88–90]. Typical enamel defects were found in all healthy family members of celiac disease patients found to have manifest mucosal lesions. Furthermore, these celiac-type enamel defects occurred without small intestinal changes and were strongly associated with the HLA DR3 [34]. Importantly, these permanent tooth enamel defects are induced by gluten ingestion in early childhood, when the enamel is developing (i.e., at the latent stage of celiac disease and dermatitis herpetiformis).

4.5.2. Malignancies

In 1986, Freeman and Chiu reported that intestinal lymphoma might appear at the latent stage of celiac disease when the mucosa is morphologically normal [33]. However, it is not known whether untreated patients without a manifest mucosal lesion carry an increased risk of malignancy. However, there are many complications, including malignancies, that may occur in adulthood when the patient is undiagnosed by ingesting gluten. Celiac disease patients diagnosed at an adult and elderly age have not had manifest mucosal lesions from early childhood (Figure 1) [42–45,48,49].

Figure 3 indicates that all the extra-intestinal manifestations induced by gluten in untreated celiac disease can be detected in the latent stage of the disease.

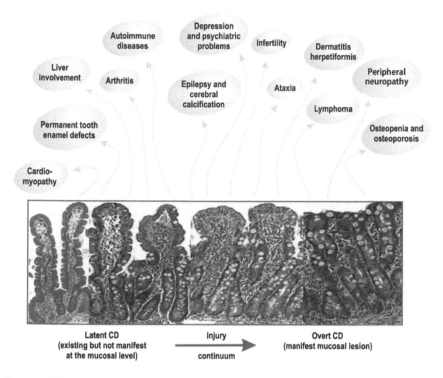

Figure 3. Celiac trait. Gluten-induced extra-intestinal manifestations exist in both patients with normal (latent celiac disease, CD) and diseased small intestinal mucosa (overt CD). Drawing adapted from the "cooking pot" of splashing extra-intestinal manifestations, which is first presented at the International Celiac Disease Symposium in Dublin 1992, and from drawings in references No. 34, 53, and 54.

5. Celiac Trait

Celiac disease diagnosis requires a gluten-induced small intestinal mucosal lesion. As indicated in Figure 3, the so-called "flat" lesion is the end stage of the mucosal injury. Figure 3 also summarizes our review and shows that, when there is a gluten-induced and gluten-dependent extra-intestinal manifestation in celiac disease, the manifestation can be found in patients before the mucosa is diseased or when it shows only minor non-specific changes. For susceptible persons, upon gluten ingestion, celiac disease develops gradually from normal mucosal morphology through mucosal inflammation, crypt hyperplasia, and villous atrophy to the "flat" mucosal lesions [91]. When the mucosa is morphologically normal and, for example, bones are already fracturing due to gluten ingestion, we should not call this condition potential celiac disease [38]. Moreover, we should not wait for the manifest mucosal lesion to develop (i.e., celiac disease). The patient deserves accurate treatment early. The benefit of treating these patients may be due to correction of micronutrient deficiencies having an impact on extra-intestinal manifestations [58]. We suggest that the term celiac trait be used in these cases [1,32,51].

Author Contributions: Both authors searched the literature and contributed equally in writing the review.

Funding: A.P. and M.M. were financially supported by the Competitive State Research Financing of the Expert Responsibility Area of Tampere University Hospital, Grant No. 9V041.

Conflicts of Interest: The authors declare no conflict of interest.

References

1. Mäki, M.; Collin, P. Celiac disease. *Lancet* **1997**, *349*, 1755–1759. [CrossRef]
2. Laurikka, P.; Nurminen, S.; Kivelä, L.; Kurppa, K. Extraintestinal manifestations of celiac disease: Early detection for better long-term outcomes. *Nutrients* **2018**, *10*, 1015. [CrossRef] [PubMed]
3. Pinto-Sanchez, M.I.; Bercik, P.; Verdu, E.F.; Bai, J.C. Extraintestinal manifestations of celiac disease. *Dig. Dis.* **2015**, *33*, 147–154. [CrossRef] [PubMed]
4. Kaukinen, K.; Collin, P.; Mäki, M. Celiac disease-a diagnostic and therapeutic challenge. *Duodecim* **2010**, *126*, 245–254. [PubMed]
5. Collin, P.; Reunala, T.; Rasmussen, M.; Kyrönpalo, S.; Pehkonen, E.; Laippala, P.; Mäki, M. High incidence and prevalence of adult celiac disease: Augmented diagnostic approach. *Scand. J. Gastroenterol.* **1997**, *32*, 1129–1133. [CrossRef] [PubMed]
6. Lohi, S.; Mustalahti, K.; Kaukinen, K.; Laurila, K.; Collin, P.; Rissanen, H.; Lohi, O.; Bravi, E.; Gasparin, M.; Reunanen, A.; et al. Increasing prevalence of celiac disease over time. *Aliment. Pharmacol. Ther.* **2007**, *26*, 1217–1225. [CrossRef] [PubMed]
7. Virta, L.J.; Kaukinen, K.; Collin, P. Incidence and prevalence of diagnosed celiac disease in Finland: Results of effective case finding in adults. *Scand. J. Gastroenterol.* **2009**, *44*, 933–938. [CrossRef] [PubMed]
8. Fry, L.; Riches, D.J.; Seah, P.P.; Hoffbrand, A.V. Clearance of skin lesions in dermatitis herpetiformis after gluten withdrawal. *Lancet* **1973**, *301*, 288–291. [CrossRef]
9. Reunala, T.; Kosnai, I.; Karpati, S.; Kuitunen, P.; Török, E.; Savilahti, E. Dermatitis herpetiformis: Jejunal findings and skin response to gluten-free diet. *Arch. Dis. Child.* **1984**, *59*, 517–522. [CrossRef]
10. Reunala, T.; Mäki, M. Dermatitis herpetiformis: A genetic disease. *Eur. J. Dermatol.* **1993**, *3*, 519–526.
11. Hervonen, K.; Karell, K.; Holopainen, P.; Collin, P.; Partanen, J.; Reunala, T. Concordance of dermatitis herpetiformis and celiac disease in monozygous twins. *J. Investig. Dermatol.* **2000**, *115*, 990–993. [CrossRef] [PubMed]
12. Molteni, N.; Caraceni, M.P.; Bardella, M.T.; Ortolani, S.; Gandolini, G.G.; Bianchi, P. Bone mineral density in adult celiac patients and the effect of gluten-free diet from childhood. *Am. J. Gastroenterol.* **1990**, *85*, 51–53. [PubMed]
13. Mustalahti, K.; Collin, P.; Sievänen, H.; Salmi, J.; Mäki, M. Osteopenia in patients with clinically silent celiac disease warrants screening. *Lancet* **1999**, *354*, 744–745. [CrossRef]
14. Heikkilä, K.; Pearce, J.; Mäki, M.; Kaukinen, K. Celiac disease and bone fractures: A systematic review and meta-analysis. *J. Clin. Endocrinol. Metab.* **2015**, *100*, 25–34. [CrossRef] [PubMed]
15. Trotta, L.; Biagi, F.; Bianchi, P.I.; Marchese, A.; Vattiato, C.; Balduzzi, D.; Collesano, V.; Corazza, G.R. Dental enamel defects in adult celiac disease: Prevalence and correlation with symptoms and age at diagnosis. *Eur. J. Intern. Med.* **2013**, *24*, 832–834. [CrossRef] [PubMed]
16. Mäki, M.; Hällström, O.; Verronen, P.; Reunala, T.; Lahdeaho, M.L.; Holm, K.; Visakorpi, J.K. Reticulin antibody, arthritis, and celiac disease in children. *Lancet* **1988**, *1*, 479–480. [CrossRef]
17. Collin, P.; Korpela, M.; Hällström, O.; Viander, M.; Keyriläinen, O.; Mäki, M. Rheumatic complaints as a presenting symptom in patients with celiac disease. *Scand. J. Rheumatol.* **1992**, *21*, 20–23. [CrossRef] [PubMed]
18. Daron, C.; Soubrier, M.; Mathieu, S. Occurrence of rheumatic symptoms in celiac disease: A meta-analysis: Comment on the article "Osteoarticular manifestations of celiac disease and non-celiac gluten hypersensitivity" by Dos Santos and Lioté. *Jt. Bone Spine* **2017**, *84*, 645–646. [CrossRef]
19. Gobbi, G.; Bouquet, F.; Greco, L.; Lambertini, A.; Tassinari, C.A.; Ventura, A.; Zaniboni, M.G. Celiac disease, epilepsy and cerebral calcifications. The Italian Working Group on Celiac Disease and Epilepsy. *Lancet* **1992**, *340*, 439–443.
20. Hadjivassiliou, M.; Grunewald, R.A.; Chattopadhyay, A.K.; Davies-Jones, G.A.; Gibson, A.; Jarrat, J.A.; Kandler, R.H.; Lobo, A.; Powell, T.; Smith, C.M. Clinical, radiological, neurophysiological, and neuropathological characteristics of gluten ataxia. *Lancet* **1998**, *352*, 1582–1585. [CrossRef]
21. Luostarinen, L.; Pirttilä, T.; Collin, P. Celiac disease presenting with neurological disorders. *Eur. Neurol.* **1999**, *42*, 132–135. [CrossRef] [PubMed]
22. Zis, P.; Sarrigiannis, P.G.; Rao, D.G.; Hadjivassiliou, M. Gluten neuropathy: Prevalence of neuropathic pain and the role of gluten-free diet. *J. Neurol.* **2018**, *265*, 2231–2236. [CrossRef] [PubMed]

23. Volta, U.; De Franceschi, L.; Lari, F.; Molinaro, N.; Zoli, M.; Bianchi, F.B. Celiac disease hidden by cryptogenic hypertransaminasaemia. *Lancet* **1998**, *352*, 26–29. [CrossRef]
24. Kaukinen, K.; Halme, L.; Collin, P.; Färkkilä, M.; Mäki, M.; Vehmanen, P.; Partanen, J.; Höckerstedt, K. Celiac disease in patients with severe liver disease: Gluten-free diet may reverse hepatic failure. *Gastroenterology* **2002**, *122*, 881–888. [CrossRef] [PubMed]
25. Korpimäki, S.; Kaukinen, K.; Collin, P.; Haapala, A.-M.; Holm, P.; Laurila, K.; Kurppa, K.; Saavalainen, P.; Haimila, K.; Partanen, J.; et al. Gluten-sensitive hypertransaminasemia in celiac disease: An infrequent and often subclinical finding. *Am. J. Gastroenterol.* **2011**, *106*, 1689–1696. [CrossRef] [PubMed]
26. Sher, K.S.; Jayanthi, V.; Probert, C.S.; Stewart, C.R.; Mayberry, J.F. Infertility, obstetric and gynaecological problems in celiac sprue. *Dig. Dis.* **1994**, *12*, 186–190. [CrossRef]
27. Tersigni, C.; Castellani, R.; de Waure, C.; Fattorossi, A.; De Spirito, M.; Gasbarrini, A.; Scambia, G.; Di Simone, N. Celiac disease and reproductive gdisorders: Meta-analysis of epidemiologic associations and potential pathogenic mechanisms. *Hum. Reprod. Update* **2014**, *20*, 582–593. [CrossRef]
28. Ventura, A.; Magazzu, G.; Greco, L. Duration of exposure to gluten and risk for autoimmune disorders in patients with celiac disease. *Gastroenterology* **1999**, *117*, 297–303. [CrossRef]
29. Cosnes, J.; Cellier, C.; Viola, S.; Colombel, J.F.; Michaud, L.; Sarles, J.; Hugot, J.P.; Ginies, J.L.; Dabadie, A.; Mouterde, O. Groupe D'Etude et de Recherche Sur la Maladie Coeliaque. Incidence of autoimmune diseases in celiac disease: Protective effect of the gluten-free diet. *Clin. Gastroenterol. Hepatol.* **2008**, *6*, 753–758. [CrossRef]
30. Holmes, G.K.T.; Prior, P.; Lane, M.R.; Pope, D.; Allan, R.N. Malignancy in celiac disease—Effect of a gluten free diet. *Gut* **1989**, *30*, 333–338. [CrossRef]
31. Tio, M.; Cox, M.R.; Eslick, G.D. Meta-analysis: Celiac disease and the risk of all-cause mortality, any malignancy and lymphoid malignancy. *Aliment. Pharmacol. Ther.* **2012**, *35*, 540–551. [CrossRef] [PubMed]
32. Mäki, M. Celiac disease. In *Gastrointestinal Functions*; Delvin, E.E., Lentze, M.J., Eds.; Nestlé Nutrition Workshop Series, Pediatric Program; Lippincott Williams & Wilkins: Vevey, Switzerland, 2001; Volume 46, pp. 257–274. ISBN 0-7817-3208-5.
33. Freeman, H.J.; Chiu, B.K. Multifocal small bowel lymphoma and latent celiac sprue. *Gastroenterology* **1986**, *90*, 1992–1997. [CrossRef]
34. Mäki, M.; Aine, L.; Lipsanen, V.; Koskimies, S. Dental enamel defects in first-degree relatives of celiac disease patients. *Lancet* **1991**, *337*, 763–764. [CrossRef]
35. Savilahti, E.; Reunala, T.; Mäki, M. Increase of lymphocytes bearing the gamma/delta T-cell receptor in the jejunum of patients with dermatitis herpetiformis. *Gut* **1992**, *33*, 206–211. [CrossRef] [PubMed]
36. Maki, M.; Huupponen, T.; Holm, K.; Hallstrom, O. Seroconversion of reticulin autoantibodies predicts celiac disease in insulin-dependent diabetes mellitus. *Gut* **1995**, *36*, 239–242. [CrossRef] [PubMed]
37. Ludvigsson, J.F.; Leffler, D.A.; Bai, J.C.; Biagi, F.; Fasano, A.; Green, P.H.; Hadjivassiliou, M.; Kaukinen, K.; Kelly, C.P.; Leonard, J.N.; et al. The Oslo definitions for celiac disease and related terms. *Gut* **2013**, *62*, 43–52. [CrossRef] [PubMed]
38. Weinstein, W.M. Latent celiac sprue. *Gastroenterology* **1974**, *66*, 489–493.
39. Ferguson, A.; Blackwell, J.N.; Barnetson, R.S. Effects of additional dietary gluten on the small-intestinal mucosa of volunteers and of patients with dermatitis herpetiformis. *Scand. J. Gastroenterol.* **1987**, *22*, 543–549. [CrossRef]
40. Chorzelski, T.P.; Rosinska, D.; Beutner, E.H.; Sulej, J.; Kumar, V. Aggressive gluten challenge of dermatitis herpetiformis cases converts them from seronegative to seropositive for IgA-class endomysial antibodies. *J. Am. Acad. Dermatol.* **1988**, *18*, 672–678. [CrossRef]
41. Doherty, M.; Barry, R.E. Gluten-induced mucosal changes in subjects without overt small-bowel disease. *Lancet* **1981**, *1*, 517–520. [CrossRef]
42. Mäki, M.; Holm, K.; Koskimies, S.; Hallstrom, O.; Visakorpi, J.K. Normal small bowel biopsy followed by celiac disease. *Arch. Dis. Child.* **1990**, *65*, 1137–1141. [CrossRef] [PubMed]
43. Mäki, M.; Holm, K.; Collin, P.; Savilahti, E. Increase in γ/δ T cell receptor bearing lymphocytes in normal small bowel mucosa in latent celiac disease. *Gut* **1991**, *32*, 1412–1414. [CrossRef] [PubMed]
44. Mäki, M.; Holm, K.; Lipsanen, V.; Hällström, O.; Viander, M.; Collin, P.; Savilahti, E.; Koskimies, S. Serological markers and HLA genes among healthy first-degree relatives of patients with celiac disease. *Lancet* **1991**, *338*, 1350–1353. [CrossRef]

45. Collin, P.; Helin, H.; Mäki, M.; Hällström, O.; Karvonen, A.L. Follow-up of patients positive in reticulin and gliadin antibody tests with normal small-bowel biopsy findings. *Scand. J. Gastroenterol.* **1993**, *28*, 595–598. [CrossRef] [PubMed]
46. Ferguson, A.; Arranz, E.; O'Mahony, S. Clinical and pathological spectrum of celiac disease—Active, silent, latent, potential. *Gut* **1993**, *34*, 150–151. [CrossRef] [PubMed]
47. Troncone, R. Latent celiac disease in Italy. *Acta Paediatr.* **1995**, *84*, 1252–1257. [CrossRef] [PubMed]
48. Corazza, G.R.; Andreani, M.L.; Biagi, F.; Bonvicini, F.; Bernardi, M.; Gasbarrini, G. Clinical, pathological, and antibody pattern of latent celiac disease: Report of three adult cases. *Am. J. Gastroenterol.* **1996**, *91*, 2203–2207.
49. Vilppula, A.; Kaukinen, K.; Luostarinen, L.; Kerkelä, I.; Patrikainen, H.; Valve, T.; Mäki, M.; Collin, P. Increasing prevalence and high incidence of celiac disease in elderly people: A population-based study. *BMC Gastroenterol.* **2009**, *9*, 49. [CrossRef]
50. Kaukinen, K.; Collin, P.; Mäki, M. Latent celiac disease or celiac disease beyond villous atrophy? *Gut* **2007**, *56*, 1339–1340. [CrossRef]
51. Mäki, M. Lack of consensus regarding definitions of celiac disease. *Nat. Rev. Gastroenterol. Hepatol.* **2012**, *9*, 305–306. [CrossRef]
52. Not, T.; Ziberna, F.; Vatta, S.; Quaglia, S.; Martelossi, S.; Villanacci, V.; Marzari, R.; Florian, F.; Vecchiet, M.; Sulic, A.M.; et al. Cryptic genetic gluten intolerance revealed by intestinal antitransglutaminase antibodies and response to gluten-free diet. *Gut* **2011**, *60*, 1487–1493. [CrossRef] [PubMed]
53. Kurppa, K.; Collin, P.; Viljamaa, M.; Haimila, K.; Saavalainen, P.; Partanen, J.; Laurila, K.; Huhtala, H.; Paasikivi, K.; et al. Diagnosing mild enteropathy celiac disease: A randomized, controlled clinical study. *Gastroenterology* **2009**, *136*, 816–823. [CrossRef] [PubMed]
54. Husby, S.; Koletzko, S.; Korponay-Szabó, I.R.; Mearin, M.L.; Phillips, A.; Shamir, R.; Troncone, R.; Giersiepen, K.; Branski, D.; Catassi, C.; et al. European Society for Pediatric Gastroenterology, Hepatology, and Nutrition Guidelines for the Diagnosis of Celiac Disease. *J. Pediatr. Gastroenterol. Nutr.* **2012**, *54*, 136–160. [CrossRef] [PubMed]
55. Mäki, M. The humoral immune system in celiac disease. *Baillière's Clin. Gastroenterol.* **1995**, *9*, 231–249. [CrossRef]
56. Simon-Vecsei, Z.; Király, R.; Bagossi, P.; Tóth, B.; Dahlbom, I.; Caja, S.; Csősz, E.; Lindfors, K.; Sblattero, D.; Nemes, E.; et al. A single conformational transglutaminase 2 epitope contributed by three domains is critical for celiac antibody binding and effects. *Proc. Natl. Acad. Sci. USA* **2012**, *109*, 431–436. [CrossRef] [PubMed]
57. Yu, X.B.; Uhde, M.; Green, P.H.; Alaedini, A. Autoantibodies in the extraintestinal manifestations of celiac disease. *Nutrients* **2018**, *10*, 1123. [CrossRef] [PubMed]
58. Rostami, K.; Aldulaimi, D.; Holmes, G.; Johnson, M.W.; Robert, M.; Srivastava, A.; Fléjou, J.-F.; Sanders, D.S.; Volta, U.; Derakhshan, M.H.; et al. Microscopic enteritis: Bucharest consensus. *World J. Gastroenterol.* **2015**, *21*, 2593–2604. [CrossRef] [PubMed]
59. Salmi, T.T.; Collin, P.; Järvinen, O.; Haimila, K.; Partanen, J.; Laurila, K.; Korponay-Szabo, I.R.; Huhtala, H.; Reunala, T.; Mäki, M.; et al. Immunoglobulin A autoantibodies against transglutaminase 2 in the small intestinal mucosa predict forthcoming celiac disease. *Aliment. Pharmacol. Ther.* **2006**, *24*, 541–552. [CrossRef] [PubMed]
60. Holm, K.; Mäki, M.; Savilahti, E.; Lipsanen, V.; Laippala, P.; Koskimies, S. Intraepithelial gamma/delta T-cell-receptor lymphocytes and genetic susceptibility to celiac disease. *Lancet* **1992**, *339*, 1500–1503. [CrossRef]
61. Iltanen, S.; Holm, K.; Partanen, J.; Laippala, P.; Mäki, M. Increased density of jejunal $\gamma\delta+$ T cells in patients having normal mucosa—Marker of operative autoimmune mechanisms? *Autoimmunity* **1999**, *29*, 1787–1791. [CrossRef]
62. Korponay-Szabo, I.R.; Halttunen, T.; Szalai, Z.; Laurila, K.; Király, R.; Kovács, J.B.; Fésüs, L.; Mäki, M. In vivo targeting of intestinal and extraintestinal transglutaminase 2 by celiac autoantibodies. *Gut* **2004**, *53*, 641–648. [CrossRef] [PubMed]
63. Kaukinen, K.; Peräaho, M.; Collin, P.; Partanen, J.; Woolley, N.; Kaartinen, T.; Nuutinen, T.; Halttunen, T.; Mäki, M.; Korponay-Szabo, I. Small-bowel mucosal transglutaminase 2-specific IgA deposits in celiac disease without villous atrophy: A prospective and randomized clinical study. *Scand. J. Gastroenterol.* **2005**, *40*, 564–572. [CrossRef] [PubMed]

64. Koskinen, O.; Collin, P.; Korponay-Szabo, I.; Salmi, T.; Iltanen, S.; Haimila, K.; Partanen, J.; Mäki, M.; Kaukinen, K. Gluten-dependent small bowel mucosal transglutaminase 2-specific IgA deposits in overt and mild enteropathy celiac disease. *J. Pediatr. Gastroenterol. Nutr.* **2008**, *47*, 436–442. [CrossRef] [PubMed]

65. Maglio, M.; Ziberna, F.; Aitoro, R.; Discepolo, V.; Lania, G.; Bassi, V.; Miele, E.; Not, T.; Troncone, R.; Auricchio, R. Intestinal production of anti-tissue transglutaminase 2 antibodies in patients with diagnosis other than celiac disease. *Nutrients* **2017**, *9*, 1050. [CrossRef] [PubMed]

66. Reunala, T.; Blomqvist, K.; Tarpila, S.; Halme, H.; Kangas, K. Gluten-free diet in dermatitis herpetiformis. I. Clinical response of skin lesions in 81 patients. *Br. J. Dermatol.* **1977**, *97*, 473–480. [CrossRef] [PubMed]

67. Mansikka, E.; Hervonen, K.; Kaukinen, K.; Collin, P.; Huhtala, H.; Reunala, T.; Salmi, T. Prognosis of dermatitis herpetiformis patients with and without villous atrophy at diagnosis. *Nutrients* **2018**, *10*, 641. [CrossRef] [PubMed]

68. Reunala, T.; Salmi, T.T.; Hervonen, K.; Kaukinen, K.; Collin, P. Dermatitis herpetiformis: A common extraintestinal manifestation of celiac disease. *Nutrients* **2018**, *10*, 602. [CrossRef]

69. Salmi, T.T.; Hervonen, K.; Laurila, K.; Collin, P.; Mäki, M.; Koskinen, O.; Huhtala, H.; Kaukinen, K.; Reunala, T. Small bowel transglutaminase 2-specific IgA deposits in dermatitis herpetiformis. *Acta Derm. Venereol.* **2014**, *94*, 393–397. [CrossRef]

70. Salmi, T.; Collin, P.; Korponay-Szabo, I.R.; Laurila, K.; Partanen, J.; Huhtala, H.; Kiraly, R.; Lorand, L.; Reunala, T.; Mäki, M.; et al. Endomysial antibody-negative celiac disease: Clinical characteristics and intestinal autoantibody deposits. *Gut* **2006**, *55*, 1746–1753. [CrossRef]

71. Pasternack, C.; Mansikka, E.; Kaukinen, K.; Hervonen, K.; Reunala, T.; Collin, P.; Huhtala, H.; Mattila, V.M.; Salmi, T. Self-reported fractures in dermatitis herpetiformis compared to celiac disease. *Nutrients* **2018**, *10*, 351. [CrossRef]

72. Hadjivassiliou, M.; Gibson, A.; Davies-Jones, G.A.; Lobo, A.J.; Stephenson, T.J.; Milford-Ward, A. Does cryptic gluten sensitivity play a part in neurological illness? *Lancet* **1996**, *347*, 369–371. [CrossRef]

73. Hadjivassiliou, M.; Grünewald, R.A.; Sanders, D.S.; Zis, P.; Croall, I.; Shanmugarajah, P.D.; Sarrigiannis, P.G.; Trott, N.; Wild, G.; Hoggard, N. The significance of low titre antigliadin antibodies in the diagnosis of gluten ataxia. *Nutrients* **2018**, *10*, 1444. [CrossRef] [PubMed]

74. Hadjivassiliou, M.; Davies-Jones, G.A.B.; Sanders, D.S.; Grunewald, R.A. Dietary treatment of gluten ataxia. *J. Neurol. Neurosurg. Psychiatry* **2003**, *74*, 1221–1224. [CrossRef] [PubMed]

75. Hadjivassiliou, M.; Mäki, M.; Sanders, D.S.; Williamson, C.A.; Grunewald, R.A.; Woodroofe, N.M.; Korponay-Szabo, I.R. Antibody targeting of brain and intestinal trasnglutaminase in gluten ataxia. *Neurology* **2006**, *66*, 373–377. [CrossRef] [PubMed]

76. Hadjivassiliou, M.; Aeschlimann, P.; Sanders, D.S.; Maki, M.; Kaukinen, K.; Grünewald, R.A.; Bandmann, O.; Woodroofe, N.; Haddock, G.; Aeschlimann, D.P. Transglutaminase 6 antibodies in the diagnosis of gluten ataxia. *Neurology* **2013**, *80*, 1740–1745. [CrossRef] [PubMed]

77. Zis, P.; Sarrigiannis, P.G.; Rao, D.G.; Hadjivassiliou, M. Quality of life in patients with gluten neuropathy: A case-controlled study. *Nutrients* **2018**, *10*, 662. [CrossRef] [PubMed]

78. Hadjivassiliou, M.; Grünewald, R.A.; Kandler, R.H.; Chattopadhyay, A.K.; Jarratt, J.A.; Sanders, D.S.; Sharrack, B.; Wharton, S.B.; Davies-Jones, G.A. Neuropathy associated with gluten sensitivity. *J. Neurol. Neurosurg. Psychiatry* **2006**, *77*, 1262–1266. [CrossRef]

79. Hadjivassiliou, M.; Kandler, R.H.; Chattopadhyay, A.K.; Davies-Jones, A.G.; Jarratt, J.A.; Sanders, D.S.; Sharrack, B.; Grünewald, R.A. Dietary treatment of gluten neuropathy. *Muscle Nerve* **2006**, *34*, 762–766. [CrossRef]

80. Larussa, T.; Suraci, E.; Nazionale, I.; Abenavoli, L.; Imeneo, M.; Luzza, F. Bone mineralization in celiac disease. *Gastroenterol. Res. Pract.* **2012**, 198025. [CrossRef]

81. Zanchetta, M.B.; Longobardi, V.; Bai, J.C. Bone and celiac disease. *Curr. Osteoporos. Rep.* **2016**, *14*, 43–48. [CrossRef]

82. Grace-Farfaglia, P. Bones of contention: Bone mineral density recovery in celiac disease—A systematic review. *Nutrients* **2015**, *7*, 3347–3369. [CrossRef] [PubMed]

83. Kaukinen, K.; Mäki, M.; Partanen, J.; Sievänen, H.; Collin, P. Celiac disease without villous atrophy: Revision of criteria called for. *Dig. Dis. Sci.* **2001**, *46*, 879–887. [CrossRef] [PubMed]

84. Dickey, W.; Hughes, D.F.; McMillan, S.A. Patients with serum IgA endomysial antibodies and intact duodenal villi: Clinical characteristics and management options. *Scand. J. Gastroenterol.* **2005**, *40*, 1240–1243. [CrossRef] [PubMed]

85. Kurppa, K.; Collin, P.; Sievänen, H.; Huhtala, H.; Mäki, M.; Kaukinen, K. Gastrointestinal symptoms, quality of life and bone mineral density in mild enteropathic celiac disease: A prospective clinical trial. *Scand. J. Gastroenterol.* **2010**, *45*, 305–314. [CrossRef] [PubMed]

86. Zanini, B.; Caselani, F.; Magni, A.; Turini, D.; Ferraresi, A.; Lanzarotto, F.; Villanacci, V.; Carabellese, N.; Ricci, C.; Lanzini, A. Celiac disease with mild enteropathy is not mild disease. *Clin. Gastroenterol. Hepatol.* **2013**, *11*, 253–258. [CrossRef] [PubMed]

87. Volta, U. Pathogenesis and clinical significance of liver injury in celiac disease. *Clin. Rev. Allergy Immunol.* **2009**, *36*, 62–70. [CrossRef] [PubMed]

88. Aine, L.; Mäki, M.; Collin, P.; Keyriläinen, O. Dental enamel defects in celiac disease. *J. Oral Pathol. Med.* **1990**, *19*, 241–245. [CrossRef]

89. Aine, L.; Reunala, T.; Mäki, M. Dental enamel defects in children with dermatitis herpetiformis. *J. Pediatr.* **1991**, *118*, 572–574. [CrossRef]

90. Aine, L.; Mäki, M.; Reunala, T. Celiac-type dental enamel defects in patients with dermatitis herpetiformis. *Acta Derm. Venereol.* **1992**, *72*, 25–27.

91. Marsh, M.N. Gluten, major histocompatibility complex, and the small intestine. A molecular and immunologic approach to the spectrum of gluten sensitivity ('celiac sprue'). *Gastroenterology* **1992**, *102*, 330–354. [CrossRef]

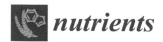

Review

Neurological Manifestations of Neuropathy and Ataxia in Celiac Disease: A Systematic Review

Elizabeth S. Mearns [1,†], **Aliki Taylor** [2,†], **Kelly J. Thomas Craig** [1,*,†], **Stefanie Puglielli** [1], **Allie B. Cichewicz** [1], **Daniel A. Leffler** [3], **David S. Sanders** [4], **Benjamin Lebwohl** [5] and **Marios Hadjivassiliou** [4]

1   IBM Watson Health, Cambridge, MA 02142, USA; elizabethmearns@gmail.com (E.S.M.);
     stefanie.puglielli@gmail.com (S.P.); allie.cichewicz@gmail.com (A.B.C.)
2   Takeda Development Centre Europe Ltd., London WC2B 4AE, UK; aliki28@me.com
3   Takeda Pharmaceuticals International Co, Cambridge, MA 02139, USA; daniel.leffler@takeda.com
4   Royal Hallamshire Hospital and University of Sheffield, Sheffield S10 2RX, UK;
     david.sanders@sth.nhs.uk (D.S.S.); m.hadjivassiliou@sheffield.ac.uk (M.H.)
5   Department of Medicine, Celiac Disease Center, Columbia University Medical Center,
     New York, NY 10032, USA; bl114@cumc.columbia.edu
*   Correspondence: kelly.jean.craig@ibm.com; Tel.: +1-(970)-261-3366
†   These authors contributed equally to this work.

Received: 23 January 2019; Accepted: 7 February 2019; Published: 12 February 2019

Abstract: Celiac disease (CD) is an immune-mediated gastrointestinal disorder driven by innate and adaptive immune responses to gluten. Patients with CD are at an increased risk of several neurological manifestations, frequently peripheral neuropathy and gluten ataxia. A systematic literature review of the most commonly reported neurological manifestations (neuropathy and ataxia) associated with CD was performed. MEDLINE, Embase, the Cochrane Library, and conference proceedings were systematically searched from January 2007 through September 2018. Included studies evaluated patients with CD with at least one neurological manifestation of interest and reported prevalence, and/or incidence, and/or clinical outcomes. Sixteen studies were included describing the risk of gluten neuropathy and/or gluten ataxia in patients with CD. Gluten neuropathy was a neurological manifestation in CD (up to 39%) in 13 studies. Nine studies reported a lower risk and/or prevalence of gluten ataxia with a range of 0%–6%. Adherence to a gluten free diet appeared to improve symptoms of both neuropathy and ataxia. The prevalence of gluten neuropathy and gluten ataxia in patients with CD varied in reported studies, but the increased risk supports the need for physicians to consider CD in patients with ataxia and neurological manifestations of unknown etiology.

Keywords: celiac disease; gluten neuropathy; gluten ataxia; prevalence; incidence; gluten-free diet

1. Introduction

Celiac disease (CD) is a chronic, immune-mediated enteropathy in which dietary gluten triggers an inflammatory reaction of the small intestine in genetically predisposed individuals [1–3]. The clinical presentation of the disease varies broadly and may include an array of intestinal symptoms and extra-intestinal manifestations, such as iron-deficiency anemia, osteoporosis, dermatitis herpetiformis, and neurologic disorders [4].

Over the last several decades, the clinical presentation of CD has changed [5] with the proportion of patients presenting with classical CD symptoms decreasing and a corresponding increase in the frequency of extra-intestinal symptoms in children and adults [5–7]. This increasing proportion of extra-intestinal symptoms at presentation can result in lengthened diagnostic delay [8]. Active case-finding to facilitate prompt detection of CD and life-long adherence to a strict gluten-free diet (GFD) among patients with confirmed CD is recommended to reduce symptoms and the likelihood of disease of potentially serious manifestations [1].

Manifestations of CD can include a broad spectrum of musculoskeletal, neurological, cardiovascular, and autoimmune disorders. Most notably, peripheral neuropathies and gluten ataxia are frequent neurological manifestations of CD [9,10]. Many patients who present with neurological manifestations of CD have no gastrointestinal symptoms [11]. Peripheral neuropathy in patients with CD presents with tingling, pain, and numbness from nerve damage, initially in the hands and feet. Otherwise known as gluten neuropathy, it is defined as apparently sporadic idiopathic neuropathy in the absence of an alternative etiology and in the presence of serological evidence of gluten sensitivity. It is a slowly progressive disease with a mean age at onset of 55 years. Only one-third of patients have evidence of enteropathy on biopsy, but the presence or absence of enteropathy does not predetermine the effect of a GFD [12].

CD patients with ataxia often present with difficulty with arm and leg control, gait instability, poor coordination, loss of fine motor skills such as writing, problems with talking, and visual issues. Gluten ataxia usually has an insidious onset with a mean age at onset of 53 years [11]. Patients with gluten ataxia can show signs of cerebellar atrophy which can be irreversible and difficult to treat. Other neurological symptoms include encephalopathy, myopathy, myelopathy, ataxia with myoclonus, and chorea [9,10]. Gluten ataxia was first defined in 1996 as apparently idiopathic sporadic ataxia in patients with positive anti-gliadin antibodies (AGA). CD patients with gluten ataxia also often have oligoclonal bands in their cerebrospinal fluid, evidence of perivascular inflammation in the cerebellum, and anti-Purkinje cell antibodies [13].

Although these neurological manifestations of CD have been described over the last 30 years in the literature, there are still diagnostic delays often resulting in permanent neurological disability. Such delays are attributed to "controversies" arising from some variation in reported prevalence and poor understanding of the use of appropriate serological testing [14–16]. To examine the recent evidence, a systematic literature review was conducted to evaluate the prevalence and outcomes of the two most commonly reported neurological manifestations of CD: gluten neuropathy and gluten ataxia.

2. Materials and Methods

A systematic review of literature indexed in MEDLINE (via PubMed), Embase, and the Cochrane Library from January 2007 to August 2018 was performed in accordance with Preferred Reporting Items for Systematic Reviews and Meta-Analyses (PRISMA) guidelines [17]. The search strategy conducted in MEDLINE (via PubMed) is provided in Table 1. Manual backwards citation tracking of references from included studies and systematic review articles was performed to identify additional relevant studies. Searches were also performed in proceedings of the past three meetings (2015–2018) of the following conferences: Digestive Disease Week, American College of Gastroenterology, and United European Gastroenterology Week.

Table 1. MEDLINE (via PubMed.com) Search Strategy.

Search No.	Search Terms	Search Results (28 August 2018)
1	celiac*[tiab] OR coeliac*[tiab] OR celiac disease[MeSH]	31,137
2	((coeliac OR celiac) AND (trunk* OR axis OR node*)) OR "coeliac artery" OR "celiac artery"	7348
3	#1 NOT #2	25,521
4	(cerebellar ataxia[MeSH] OR "cerebellar ataxia"[tiab] OR ((cerebellum* OR cerebellar) AND ataxi*) OR "gluten ataxia" OR "gluten-sensitive ataxia")	17,238
5	neuropathy[tiab] OR neuropathies[tiab] OR neuropathic[tiab]	88,749
6	#3 AND #4	141
7	#3 AND #5	213
8	#6 OR #7	309
9	case reports[pt]	1,893,340
10	#8 NOT #9	238
11	mice OR mouse OR murine OR rodent*	1,754,334
12	#10 NOT #11	227
13	review[pt] NOT (systematic OR Cochrane OR meta-analy*)	2,162,485
14	#12 NOT #13	160
15	#14; Filter: published 2007 or later	99
16	#15; Filter: abstract	96

Footnotes: *, wildcard search term; #, search number. Abbreviations: tiab, title/abstract; pt, publication type.

To be included, studies (primary studies or systematic reviews with or without meta-analyses) had to be conducted in patients with CD, published from 2007 or later (or last three meetings for conference abstracts) in English, and report the incidence, prevalence, and/or clinical outcomes of ataxia and/or neuropathy. Neuropathy, which is often used synonymously with peripheral neuropathy, is classified according to the type of damage to the nerve. In this systematic review, the terms "neuropathy" and "peripheral neuropathy" are stated as the authors have used them in their studies, recognizing that "neuropathy" may include a wider range of symptoms than peripheral neuropathy, which would represent a large proportion of neuropathy cases overall.

A single investigator screened titles and abstracts to determine if the citation met inclusion criteria, with validation by a second reviewer required for exclusion. Two investigators independently reviewed all potentially relevant full-text citations, with discrepancies resolved by a third reviewer. Screening, data extraction, and validation were performed using DistillerSR (Evidence Partners Inc., Kanata, Ottawa, Canada). One investigator abstracted all data using a standardized tool, and a second reviewer verified entries.

Two independent investigators assessed the quality of included studies using the Oxford Levels of Evidence Instrument [18]. Reviewers used the "Differential diagnosis/symptom prevalence study" section to assess the overall grade of the evidence. Details regarding the categorization of the study designs are available in Table 2.

Table 2. Oxford Levels of Evidence & Grades of Recommendation.

Level	Differential Diagnosis/Symptom Prevalence Study
1a	Systematic review (with homogeneity) of prospective cohort studies
1b	Prospective cohort study with good follow-up
1c	All or none case-series
2a	Systematic review (with homogeneity) of 2b and better studies
2b	Retrospective cohort study, or poor follow-up
2c	Ecological studies
3a	Systematic review (with homogeneity) of 3b and better studies
3b	Non-consecutive cohort study, or very limited population
4	Case-series or superseded reference standards
5	Expert opinion without explicit critical appraisal, or based on physiology, bench research or "first principles"
Grade	**Levels of Individual Studies**
A	Consistent level 1 studies
B	Consistent level 2 or 3 studies or extrapolations from level 1 studies
C	Level 4 studies or extrapolations from level 2 or 3 studies
D	Level 5 evidence or troublingly inconsistent or inconclusive studies of any level

Table adapted from the Oxford Centre for Evidence-Based Medicine [18].

3. Results

The searches identified 441 citations, 299 conference abstracts, and 1 additional citation identified through backwards citation tracking. After removal of duplicates and screening of titles and abstracts screening, 45 were eligible for full-text review. A total of 16 studies met all eligibility criteria and were included in the systematic review (Figure 1, Table 3) [10,19–33]. Nine studies on gluten ataxia [10,20–23,26,28,31,32] and 13 articles on gluten neuropathy were included [10,19,20,22,24–30,32,33].

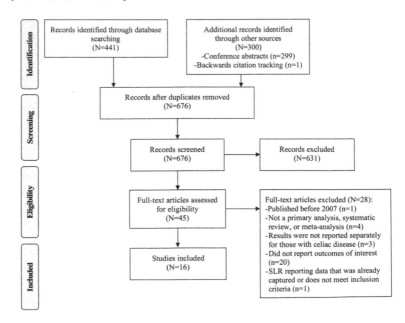

Figure 1. Flow Diagram Showing the Results of the Literature Search.

Table 3. Characteristics of Included Studies.

Author (year)	Study Design	Country	Population	Neurological Complication
Briani and Doria et al. (2008) [19]	Prospective, single-center, cross-sectional	Italy	Patients with CD	Neuropathy
Briani and Zara et al. (2008) [20]	Prospective, single-center, cross-sectional	Italy	Unselected, consecutive patients with CD treated at the University of Padova	Ataxia, neuropathy
Burk et al. (2013) [21]	Prospective, single-center, cross-sectional	Germany	Patients with CD on a GFD recruited from advertisements in the official journal of the German Celiac Society or personal contact	Ataxia
Cakir et al. (2007)[22]	Prospective, multi-center, cross-sectional	Turkey	Children with CD treated at the outpatient follow-up program of celiac patients in the pediatric gastroenterology and nutrition division of Ege University Hospital from 1998–2002	Ataxia, neuropathy
Diaconu et al. (2013) [23]	Prospective, single-center, cross-sectional	Romania	Children (2–18 years) diagnosed with CD from 2000–2010	Ataxia
Hadjivassiliou et al. (2016) [10]	Retrospective, single-center, cohort	UK	Patients with CD and neurological manifestations presenting to the Neuroscience Department at Royal Hallamshire Hospital from 1994–2014	Ataxia, neuropathy
Hadjivassiliou et al. (2017) [31]	Prospective, single-center, observational case series	UK	Patients diagnosed with gluten ataxia at the Sheffield Ataxia Centre	Ataxia
Isikay (2015) [24]	Prospective, single-center, cross-sectional, case-control	Turkey	Asymptomatic children with CD diagnosed at a pediatric gastroenterology outpatient clinic from September 2012–August 2014	Ataxia, neuropathy
Jericho et al. (2017) [25]	Retrospective, single-center, chart review	US	Patients with CD registered at the University of Chicago Celiac Center clinic from January 2002–October 2014	Ataxia, neuropathy
Ludvigsson et al. (2007) [26]	Retrospective, multi-center, database	Sweden	Patients in the Swedish national inpatient register with a hospital-based discharge diagnosis of CD from 1964–2003	Ataxia, neuropathy
Mukherjee et al. (2010) [27]	Retrospective, single-center, database	US	Patients with CD from a prospectively generated database at a university-based referral center	Neuropathy
Ruggieri et al. (2008) [28]	Prospective, single-center, cross-sectional	Italy	Children with CD and neurological dysfunction evaluated at the gluten sensitivity clinic at the Department of Pediatrics at the University of Catania from January 1991–December 2004	Ataxia, neuropathy
Sangat et al. (2017) [32]	Retrospective, single-center, medical record review	Not reported	Children with and without gluten-related disorders between July 2013 and May 2016	Ataxia, neuropathy
Shen et al. (2012) [29]	Questionnaire-based, multi-center, cross-sectional, case-control	US	Patients with CD recruited from the Celiac Disease Center at Columbia University and support groups in New York and California	Neuropathy
Thawani et al. (2015) [30]	Retrospective, multi-center	Sweden	Patients with CD from one of Sweden's pathology departments from June 1969–February 2008	Neuropathy
Thawani et al. (2017) [33]	Retrospective, nationwide registry	Sweden	Patients diagnosed with T1DM between 1964 and 2009, with and without CD (based on biopsies between 1969 and 2008) in the Swedish National Patient Register	Neuropathy

Abbreviations: CD, celiac disease; GFD, gluten-free diet; T1DM, type 1 diabetes mellitus; US, United States; UK, United Kingdom.

The PRISMA flow diagram depicts the flow of information through the different phases of this systematic review. It maps out the number of records identified, included and excluded, and the reasons for exclusions.

Of the studies included, 50% (eight out of 16) were full-text, prospective analyses that reported global prevalence or incidence rates of gluten neuropathy and gluten ataxia [19–24,28,29]. See Box 1 for the definitions of CD, gluten ataxia, and gluten neuropathy. Most studies were performed in Europe (9; Germany, Italy, Romania, Sweden, and United Kingdom (UK)), while four were from the United States (US), two from Turkey, and one multinational study. Findings reported on adults (5), children (5), and both children and adults (6). Clinical outcomes of CD manifestations were reported in 50% (8 out of 16) of the included studies, while the remainder only addressed epidemiology.

Box 1. Definitions of gluten-sensitivity spectrum disorders used in this study.

celiac disease – autoimmune disorder whereby gluten ingestion damages the portion of the small intestine responsible for nutrient absorption; also referred to as gluten-sensitive enteropathy.
gluten ataxia – autoimmune disorder whereby gluten ingestion damages the cerebellum, which controls gait and muscle coordination, and fine control of voluntary movements is compromised.
gluten neuropathy – autoimmune disorder whereby gluten ingestion damages the nerves of the peripheral nervous system, which disrupts communication from the brain and spinal cord to the rest of the body.

3.1. Gluten Neuropathy

Thirteen articles reported gluten neuropathy as a manifestation of CD [10,19,20,22,24–30,32,33]. Estimates of the prevalence of neuropathy in these patients ranged from 0% to 39%, with an increased prevalence/risk in older and female patients. In retrospective and prospective studies of patients with CD in the US and Europe, prevalence of neuropathy ranged from 4% to 23% of adults [20,25,27], 0% to 7% of children [22,24,25,28,32], and 0.7% to 39% of combined/unspecified populations [20,29,30,32]. While these ranges appear to overlap, a few studies directly compared the prevalence and risk of neuropathy by age and indicated that neuropathy occurs more frequently in older populations [27]. In a retrospective US study of adults (n = 171) and children (n = 157) with CD, gluten neuropathy was reported in 23% of adults with a follow-up period of >24 months between 2002 and 2014; however, no cases were reported in children [25]. Another retrospective US study found that significantly more elderly patients aged $\geq$65 years (11%) had gluten neuropathy compared with younger patients aged 18–30 years (4%; p = 0.023) [27]. Similar to young adults, gluten neuropathy was identified in 3 to 4.5% of children with CD in two studies [28,32]. Another questionnaire-based US study found that the risk of gluten neuropathy rose significantly with every ten-year increase in age (OR, 1.13; 95% CI, 1.04–1.23; p = 0.006). This study also reported a higher risk of gluten neuropathy in females (OR, 1.71; 95% CI, 1.25–2.33; p = 0.001) [29].

Gluten neuropathy may account for approximately one-quarter of neurological manifestations in those with CD. In two studies (one retrospective (n = 228) and one prospective (n = 72)) examining patients with CD and neurological conditions, gluten neuropathy accounted for 19% to 30% of neurological manifestations [10,20]. Patients with CD have a higher risk of gluten neuropathy and experience more severe neuropathic symptoms compared with non-CD controls (p < 0.01) [29]. In three studies (two retrospective and one questionnaire-based) from the US and Sweden, patients with CD had a significantly higher (2.3–5.6 times) risk of peripheral neuropathy compared with control populations [26,29,30]. The risk of polyneuropathy appears highest (4.4–5.6 times) during the first year of follow-up after CD diagnosis [26,30], compared with overall risk, or risk excluding the first year of follow-up (2.3–3.4 times) [26,30]. The risk estimate for neuropathy was only marginally affected after adjustment for education, socioeconomic status, type 1 diabetes mellitus (T1DM), type 2 diabetes mellitus (T2DM), thyroid disease, rheumatologic diseases, pernicious anemia, vitamin deficiencies, and alcoholic disorders (Hazard Ratio (HR), 2.3; 95% Confidence Interval (CI), 1.9–2.7) [30]. Notably, two of these studies adjusted their design to control for the rate of T1DM, as peripheral neuropathy is a long-term manifestation of T1DM [26,30]. However, Thawani et al. (2017) observed there was no significant increased risk of neuropathy for biopsy-confirmed CD patients with T1DM after examining neuropathy incidence in the first five years of CD diagnosis when compared to patients with T1DM only [33].

Symptoms from gluten neuropathy improve when patients with CD follow a GFD, although the diet may not prevent its development, and longer adherence to a GFD may not completely reverse neuropathy. One retrospective US study found that among patients who developed gluten neuropathy (*n* = 39), there was a significant improvement on a GFD (*p* < 0.05) [25]. Two prospective Italian studies also reported that in patients with gluten neuropathy, dietary adherence led to improvement in neuropathy and non-adherence led to worsening [20,28]. However, it should be noted that only one to two patients developed neuropathy in each of these Italian studies. While a GFD may improve symptoms of gluten neuropathy, one questionnaire-based US study found that duration of the diet (<5 vs. 5–9 vs. ≥10 years) did not significantly change the proportion of patients who developed the manifestation [29]. Similar proportions of patients developed neuropathy regardless of whether patients were reported to be following a GFD [10,22,25]. In the studies that did document GFD status, the extent of GFD adherence was not reported, limiting assessment of the relationship between neuropathy and degree of gluten exposure.

The severity of gluten neuropathy is variable. With a follow-up period of >20 years, one retrospective British study found that patients with CD on a GFD who developed gluten neuropathy, severity was mild (confined to the legs) in 27%, moderate (involvement of arms but sparing radial nerve) in 40%, and severe (involvement of radial nerve) in 33% [10]. A questionnaire-based US study suggested that the severity of neuropathy is not associated with duration on the GFD [29].

3.2. Gluten Ataxia

Upon physical examination for neurological deficits in patients with CD, estimates of the prevalence of gluten ataxia varied from 0% to 6% [20–23,28,32]. However, in studies among CD patients with neurological manifestations, gluten ataxia was reported in 19% to 41% of patients [10,23]. While studies tended to use similar definitions of ataxia, prevalence estimates varied. Six of the ten included studies used standard neurological exams with combinations of either magnetic resonance imaging (MRI) or magnetic resonance spectroscopy (MRS), or computed tomography (CT) to confirm the diagnosis of ataxia by examination of the vermis, eliminating other potential common causes of ataxia such as thyroid dysfunction, vitamin E deficiency, toxicity, and genetic forms of ataxia (spinocerebellar and Friedrich's) [20–23,28,31].

Of the prospective European studies that used diagnostic CT or MRI/MRS, gluten ataxia was diagnosed in two studies [21,23]. One study of adults (*n* = 72) [21] and one of children (*n* = 48) [23] each reported a prevalence of 6% in patients with CD. The study of 48 children attributed the prevalence of gluten ataxia and the presence of the comorbidities of mental retardation and developmental delays to nutritional deficiencies and toxic effects of severe malnutrition [23]. The other three studies utilizing CT or MRI to define ataxia, one in adults (*n* = 71) [20] and two in children (*n* = 27 and *n* = 835) [22,28], reported that no patients (0%) developed ataxia.

Two included retrospective studies did not report a prevalence of gluten ataxia [10,26]. One study used International Classification of Diseases (ICD, 7–10) codes to identify the symptom of ataxia (excluding trauma or toxicity as main diagnoses) or hereditary ataxia to determine the risk of ataxia in patients with CD [26]. The remaining study had less transparency in the diagnosis of ataxia as the diagnostic criteria were not described, where authors reported that a standard neurological assessment was performed and only reported on the severity of ataxia [10].

One British study suggested that most cases (69%) of gluten ataxia in patients with CD are mild, and patients could walk without assistance [10]. Of the remaining ataxia cases, 17% were moderate (requiring walking aids/support), and 14% were severe (needing a wheelchair). All patients were reported to be following a GFD [10].

In the nine included studies [10,20–23,26,28,31,32], gluten ataxia accounted for up to half of all neurological manifestations observed in people with CD. Definitive conclusions cannot be made regarding age-related differences in CD-associated ataxia from included studies, but available data suggest that gluten ataxia accounts for a smaller proportion of neurological manifestations in children with CD compared with adults.

The risk of gluten ataxia appears to vary over time after CD diagnosis. A retrospective population-based registry study from Sweden evaluated the risk of gluten ataxia in patients with a hospital-based diagnosis of CD (n = 14,371), and found a greater risk of ataxia compared with controls without CD when patients were followed during the first year after discharge (HR, 2.6; 95% CI, 1.0–6.5; p = 0.042) [26]. However, if the first year of follow-up was excluded, the higher risk of ataxia was no longer statistically significant (HR, 1.9; 95% CI, 0.6–6.2; p > 0.05) based upon 14,371 patients with CD and 70,155 reference individuals [26].

The observed effect of GFD on ataxia may be dependent upon the methodological tests to monitor adherence to a GFD and the metrics utilized to assess neurological improvement. A quantitative assessment of the effect of GFD on gluten ataxia was provided by cerebellar MRS in Hadjivassiliou et al. (2017) [31]. In this study, CD patients with gluten ataxia (n = 117) were reviewed for response to GFD: 63 were on strict GFD with the elimination of AGAs, 35 were on GFD but still positive for AGAs, and 19 patients were not on a GFD. GFD adherence was monitored by serological assessments. On MRS, there was a significant improvement in the cerebellum in 62 out of 63 (98%) patients on a strict GFD, in nine of 35 (26%) patients on GFD with positive AGAs, but in only one of 19 (5%) patients not on GFD. Notably, the presence of enteropathy (CD), usually required for the diagnosis of CD, in addition to positive serology, was not found to be a prerequisite for improvement in the cerebellum. The authors concluded that patients with positive serology results and negative duodenal biopsy should still be treated with strict GFD and noted that improved cerebellar function with GFD adherence was associated with clinical improvement [31]. In contrast, a prospective Romanian study in 48 children reported that none of the patients with gluten ataxia had improved symptoms while on a GFD [23]. However, Diaconu et al. (2014) did not state how GFD adherence was monitored and ataxia assessments were self-reported by the parents of the children affected [23].

3.3. Quality Assessment

Based on Oxford Levels of Evidence, the evidence in this review has an overall grade of B. Only one study provided Level 1b evidence [19]. Seven studies [10,25–27,30,32,33] were retrospective cohort studies, which represented Level 2b evidence. One study was a prospective case series, representing level 4 evidence [31]. The remaining seven studies [20–24,28,29] were cross-sectional studies, which we have categorized as Level 2c. The levels of evidence for individual studies are shown in Table 4.

Table 4. Quality Assessment of Included Studies.

Study Identifier	Oxford Level of Evidence
Briani and Doria et al. (2008) [19]	2c. Ecological study *
Briani and Zara et al. (2008) [20]	1b. Prospective cohort study
Burk et al. (2013) [21]	2c. Ecological study *
Cakir et al. (2007) [22]	2c. Ecological study *
Diaconu et al. (2013) [23]	2c. Ecological study *
Hadjivassiliou et al. (2016) [10]	2b. Retrospective cohort study
Hadjivassiliou et al. (2017) [31]	4. Case-series or superseded reference standards
Isikay et al. (2015) [24]	2c. Ecological study *
Jericho et al. (2017) [25]	2b. Retrospective cohort study
Ludvigsson et al. (2007) [26]	2b. Retrospective cohort study
Mukherjee et al. (2010) [27]	2b. Retrospective cohort study
Ruggieri et al. (2008) [28]	2c. Ecological study *
Sangal et al. (2017) [32]	2b. Retrospective cohort study
Shen et al. (2012) [29]	2c. Ecological study *
Thawani et al. (2015) [30]	2b. Retrospective cohort study
Thawani et al. (2017) [33]	2b. Retrospective cohort study

*, Note that this was a cross-sectional study, not an ecological study; there is no Oxford Level of Evidence for cross-sectional studies [18].

4. Discussion

This systematic review demonstrates that gluten neuropathy was reported more often than gluten ataxia (81.25% of included studies reported neuropathy), although the prevalence of gluten neuropathy varied widely (0%–39%). Both ataxia and neuropathy were more prevalent in patients with CD compared with controls. Symptoms of neuropathy were most commonly categorized as moderate, affecting extremities. Prevalence of gluten ataxia in patients with diagnosed CD varied from 0–6%; symptoms were often described as mild, in which patients were still able to walk, although in some cases could be very severe and persistent. The variations in prevalence rates across studies of both gluten ataxia and gluten neuropathy may be related to study design and inclusion criteria, retrospective nature of data collection, quality of assessment of adherence to a GFD, clinical assessment of neurological symptoms, and the age of the populations included.

The prevalence of idiopathic neuropathy in the general population is low but the risk is increased in CD. A literature review of 28 studies reported the prevalence of neuropathy in the general middle-aged and elderly population between 0.1% and 3.3% [34]. Increased neuropathy prevalence was reported in a US study published in 2003 using retrospective data from 400 patients with neuropathy, whereby neuropathy rates for CD were between 2.5% and 8% (compared to 1% in the healthy population) [35]. In a large Swedish population-based study that examined the risk of neurological disease, polyneuropathy was found to be significantly associated with CD (odds ratio 5.4; 95% CI 3.6–8.2) [36]. In further support of this, an age- and sex-matched control study, identified in this review, comparing patients with CD to controls found that CD was associated with a 2.5-fold increased risk of later neuropathy [30]. The highest risk for gluten neuropathy was just after diagnosis of CD, but there was also a consistent excess risk of neuropathy beyond five years after a diagnosis of CD. Two other included studies compared patients with CD of different ages and found that younger patients were less likely to experience neuropathy [25,27]. However, these studies examined established patients with CD and their findings may be an underestimation of risk of neuropathy in young patients. The presentation of atypical symptoms, such as neurological complications, at time of CD diagnosis in children, reported neuropathy prevalence of 10.5% in this small study population [32].

Similar to trends for neuropathy, the prevalence of ataxia in the general population is very low, but this risk is increased in patients with CD. A UK based population-based study estimated the prevalence of late-onset cerebellar ataxia as 0.01% in the general population [37]. Three studies identified in this review reported no cases (0%) of ataxia in both adults and children [20,22,28]; however, estimates of ataxia prevalence ranged from 0-6% across all ages [21,23,32]. In studies that determined ataxia prevalence in children, neurological manifestations were the initial symptoms of CD in 25%–33.33% of patients, and ataxia accounted for 5.26%–18.8% of those cases. [23,32]. The risk of ataxia in those with CD was estimated to be 1.9- to 2.6-fold compared with controls during the first year after diagnosis [26].

Although the prevalence of ataxia in CD is thought to be low, it may be underestimated. A recent UK study of 500 patients diagnosed with progressive ataxia and evaluated over a period of 13 years, found that 101 of 215 (47%) patients with idiopathic sporadic ataxia had serological evidence of gluten reactivity [38]. A study of 1500 patients with cerebellar ataxia referred to the Sheffield Ataxia Centre, UK assessed over 20 years found that 20% had a family history of ataxia, and the remaining 80% had sporadic ataxia. Of sporadic ataxias, gluten ataxia was the most common cause (25%); followed by genetic causes (13%), alcohol excess (12%), and a cerebellar variant of multiple system atrophy (11%) [39]. In a review of gluten sensitivity by Hadjivassiliou et al. (2010) [11], many studies reported that a high proportion of patients with sporadic ataxias (12%–47%) tested positive for AGA compared with 2%–12% of healthy controls [11,38–48]. These studies suggest that even though ataxia is rare, gluten ataxia is a common subtype of sporadic ataxia.

Adherence to a strict GFD can result in clinical improvement in both gluten neuropathy and gluten ataxia. Publications which met criteria for inclusion in this review unanimously support a beneficial effect of the GFD on neuropathy, however, a benefit in ataxia is less clear. Some studies report that ataxia persists in patients on a GFD, while others demonstrated improvement on GFD [10,21,23,31].

This heterogeneity is most likely due to differences in study design, including the assessment of GFD adherence and ataxia symptoms. Severity of ataxia can be assessed with a variety of instruments including self-report and clinician determination using scales for the assessment and rating of ataxia (e.g., Brief Ataxia Rating Scale (BARS), Scale for the Assessment and Rating of Ataxia (SARA), International Cooperative Ataxia Rating Scale (ICARS), modified ICARS (MICARS)), and imaging studies (e.g., MRS, MRI, EEG). Objective quantitation of motor deficits in ataxia is fundamental for measurement of clinical severity but was not commonly reported in studies examining the association between improvements of ataxia and GFD adherence. One study by Hadjivassiliou et al. (2017) utilized a quantitative methodology via MRS to monitor ataxia severity by cerebellar atrophy and assessed GFD adherence with AGA testing [31]. This study demonstrated a beneficial effect of strict GFD adherence on ataxia and benefits were seen in all AGA positive individuals, regardless of baseline enteropathy [31].

It is important to clarify the differences between CD and gluten sensitivity in the context of gluten ataxia and gluten neuropathy. This systematic review primarily concentrated on patients with CD and these two common neurological manifestations. These manifestations, however, may exist in the presence of AGA alone (gluten sensitivity) without evidence of enteropathy (CD), and such patients benefit equally from GFD. Indeed Hadjivassiliou et al. (2016) demonstrated there are no distinguishing features (e.g., type of neurological manifestation, severity, and response to GFD) between those patients with neurological manifestations and CD and those with just positive AGA (no enteropathy) [10]. Despite this, the majority of immunological laboratories have abandoned the use of native AGA assays due to poor specificity in diagnosing CD. Estimation of specificity, however, is based on the presence of a gold standard, in this case, the presence of enteropathy. Given that sensitivity to gluten exists in the absence of enteropathy, then AGA remains probably the only serological marker in diagnosing the whole spectrum of extraintestinal manifestations. Another important consideration when using AGA is the serological cut-off for positive AGA. Such assays are calibrated using serology from patients with CD as the gold standard, and consequently, the serological cut-off tends to be high. It has recently been shown that by recalibrating the serological cut-off of a commercially available AGA assay based on the ability to diagnose GA, the sensitivity of AGA in diagnosing CD became 100% [49].

There were a small number of studies identified that did not meet our inclusion criteria but described the association between gluten neuropathy and enteropathy, and the effects of strict GFD on gluten neuropathy. Of note, a study published by Hadjivassiliou et al. (2006) reported that of 100 patients with clinical immunological characteristics of gluten neuropathy, 29% of patients had evidence of enteropathy [50]. A prospective study published in 2006, followed 35 patients with gluten neuropathy, 25 of which were assigned to strict adherence to a GFD with the remaining ten patients as controls. Strict GFD adherence was defined by the elimination of AGA after one year. When asked, 16/25 patients on the GFD said their neuropathy was better compared to 0/10 in the control group. Eight out of ten patients in the control group stated that their neuropathy was worse [12]. Gluten neuropathy can be associated with significant chronic pain and negatively impact mental health. A recent study assessed neuropathic pain in 60 patients with gluten neuropathy. Neuropathic pain was present in 33 patients and painless neuropathy was more common in patients on a strict GFD (55.6% versus 21.2%, $p = 0.006$). Patients with painful gluten neuropathy presented with significantly worse mental health status [12]. Multivariate analysis showed that, after adjusting for age, gender and mental health index-5, strict GFD was associated with an 89% reduction in risk of peripheral neuropathic pain ($p = 0.006$) [51].

Gluten ataxia and neuropathy were selected for this review because they are the most common neurological manifestations in CD. However, there are other neurological manifestations not assessed (a systematic review of movement disorders related to gluten sensitivity by Vinagre-Aragon et al. (2017) is available [52] for reference). A prospective study reported that up to 22% of patients with CD ($n = 71$) developed some form of neurologic or psychiatric dysfunction (headache, depression, entrapment syndromes, peripheral neuropathy, and epilepsy) [20]. In a British study published in 1998,

57% of patients with neurological dysfunction of unknown cause had serological evidence of gluten sensitivity, compared with 12% of healthy blood donors [53]. Neurological manifestations can have a significant impact on patients' quality of life, and a greater understanding of these complications is needed.

There are several limitations to this systematic review. Both clinical and methodological heterogeneity among reviewed studies limited comparisons of the data. Across all studies included, it is not possible to determine whether factors such as the timing of diagnosis, presentation of CD, or differences diagnostic techniques, affect rates of ataxia and peripheral neuropathy. Lastly, there is potential for publication bias and missed eligible articles in any literature review. However, this risk is assumed to be minimal due to strict adherence to standards for systematic search methodology.

5. Conclusions

In conclusion, this systematic review provides important evidence on the substantially increased risk of gluten ataxia and gluten neuropathy in patients with CD, although estimates across studies vary. These results indicate that adherence to a GFD appears to improve symptoms of both neuropathy and ataxia. The scarcity of data from this global search highlights the need for additional well-designed studies to improve the understanding of neurological manifestations in patients with CD. Given that these results suggest an increased risk of ataxia and neuropathy among patients with CD, clinicians should evaluate for gluten sensitivity in patients with ataxia and neuropathy of unknown origin.

Author Contributions: Conceptualization: E.S.M., A.T., D.A.L., M.H.; Formal analysis: S.P., K.J.T.C., A.B.C.; Funding Acquisition: K.J.T.C.; Methodology: E.S.M., A.B.C., S.P., K.J.T.C.; Project Administration: E.S.M., K.J.T.C.; Supervision: E.S.M., A.T., K.J.T.C.; Validation: K.J.T.C., S.P., A.B.C.; Writing—original draft: E.S.M., A.T., K.J.T.C., S.P.; Writing—review & editing: all authors.

Funding: IBM Watson Health received a research contract from Takeda Pharmaceuticals International Co. to conduct the study and prepare this manuscript.

Acknowledgments: The authors would like to thank Lynne Stoecklein for assisting with screening of titles/abstracts and full texts, data collection, and language editing; Talia Boulanger for the conceptualization and design of the systematic review; Jennifer Drahos for critical reading and feedback; and Nicole Fusco for assisting in data collection and proofreading.

Conflicts of Interest: E.S.M., A.B.C., S.P. and K.J.T.C. were employees of IBM Watson Health during the completion of this study. A.T., M.G. and D.A.L. were employees of Takeda Pharmaceuticals International Co during the completion of this study. D.S.S., B.L. and M.H. serve as consultants for Takeda Pharmaceuticals International Co. The authors declare no conflict of interest.

References

1. Rubio-Tapia, A.; Hill, I.D.; Kelly, C.P.; Calderwood, A.H.; Murray, J.A. ACG clinical guidelines: Diagnosis and management of celiac disease. *Am. J. Gastroenterol.* **2013**, *108*, 656–676. [CrossRef] [PubMed]
2. Tonutti, E.; Bizzaro, N. Diagnosis and classification of celiac disease and gluten sensitivity. *Autoimmun. Rev.* **2014**, *13*, 472–476. [CrossRef]
3. Ludvigsson, J.F.; Leffler, D.A.; Bai, J.C.; Biagi, F.; Fasano, A.; Green, P.H.; Hadjivassiliou, M.; Kaukinen, K.; Kelly, C.P.; Leonard, J.N.; et al. The Oslo definitions for coeliac disease and related terms. *Gut* **2013**, *62*, 43–52. [CrossRef] [PubMed]
4. Green, P.H.; Lebwohl, B.; Greywoode, R. Celiac disease. *J. Allergy Clin. Immunol.* **2015**, *135*, 1099–1106. [CrossRef] [PubMed]
5. Reilly, N.R.; Green, P.H. Epidemiology and clinical presentations of celiac disease. *Semin. Immunopathol.* **2012**, *34*, 473–478. [CrossRef]
6. Roma, E.; Panayiotou, J.; Karantana, H.; Constantinidou, C.; Siakavellas, S.I.; Krini, M.; Syriopoulou, V.P.; Bamias, G. Changing pattern in the clinical presentation of pediatric celiac disease: A 30-year study. *Digestion* **2009**, *80*, 185–191. [CrossRef]
7. Ludvigsson, J.F.; Rubio-Tapia, A.; van Dyke, C.T.; Melton, L.J., 3rd; Zinsmeister, A.R.; Lahr, B.D.; Murray, J.A. Increasing incidence of celiac disease in a North American population. *Am. J. Gastroenterol.* **2013**, *108*, 818–824. [CrossRef] [PubMed]

8. Fuchs, V.; Kurppa, K.; Huhtala, H.; Collin, P.; Maki, M.; Kaukinen, K. Factors associated with long diagnostic delay in celiac disease. *Scand. J. Gastroenterol.* **2014**, *49*, 1304–1310. [CrossRef]
9. Leffler, D.A.; Green, P.H.; Fasano, A. Extraintestinal manifestations of coeliac disease. *Nat. Rev. Gastroenterol. Hepatol.* **2015**, *12*, 561–571. [CrossRef] [PubMed]
10. Hadjivassiliou, M.; Rao, D.G.; Grinewald, R.A.; Aeschlimann, D.P.; Sarrigiannis, P.G.; Hoggard, N.; Aeschlimann, P.; Mooney, P.D.; Sanders, D.S. Neurological Dysfunction in Coeliac Disease and Non-Coeliac Gluten Sensitivity. *Am. J. Gastroenterol.* **2016**, *111*, 561–567. [CrossRef] [PubMed]
11. Hadjivassiliou, M.; Sanders, D.S.; Grunewald, R.A.; Woodroofe, N.; Boscolo, S.; Aeschlimann, D. Gluten sensitivity: From gut to brain. *Lancet Neurol.* **2010**, *9*, 318–330. [CrossRef]
12. Hadjivassiliou, M.; Kandler, R.H.; Chattopadhyay, A.K.; Davies-Jones, A.G.; Jarratt, J.A.; Sanders, D.S.; Sharrack, B.; Grunewald, R.A. Dietary treatment of gluten neuropathy. *Muscle Nerve* **2006**, *34*, 762–766. [CrossRef] [PubMed]
13. Hadjivassiliou, M.; Williamson, C.A.; Woodroofe, N. The immunology of gluten sensitivity: Beyond the gut. *Trends Immunol.* **2004**, *25*, 578–582. [CrossRef] [PubMed]
14. Rampertab, S.D.; Pooran, N.; Brar, P.; Singh, P.; Green, P.H. Trends in the presentation of celiac disease. *Am. J. Med.* **2006**, *119*, 355.e9–355.e14. [CrossRef] [PubMed]
15. Green, P.H. The many faces of celiac disease: Clinical presentation of celiac disease in the adult population. *Gastroenterology* **2005**, *128*, S74–S78. [CrossRef] [PubMed]
16. Lionetti, E.; Catassi, C. The role of environmental factors in the development of celiac disease: What is new? *Diseases* **2015**, *3*, 282–293. [CrossRef] [PubMed]
17. Moher, D.; Liberati, A.; Tetzlaff, J.; Altman, D.G. Preferred reporting items for systematic reviews and meta-analyses: The PRISMA statement. *Ann. Intern. Med.* **2009**, *151*, 264–269. [CrossRef] [PubMed]
18. Oxford Centre for Evidence-Based Medicine—Levels of Evidence. March 2009. Available online: http://www.cebm.net/blog/2009/06/11/oxford-centre-evidence-based-medicine-levels-evidence-march-2009/ (accessed on 16 January 2018).
19. Briani, C.; Doria, A.; Ruggero, S.; Toffanin, E.; Luca, M.; Albergoni, M.P.; Odorico, A.D.; Grassivaro, F.; Lucchetta, M.; Lazzari, F.D.; et al. Antibodies to muscle and ganglionic acetylcholine receptors (AchR) in celiac disease. *Autoimmunity* **2008**, *41*, 100–104. [CrossRef] [PubMed]
20. Briani, C.; Zara, G.; Alaedini, A.; Grassivaro, F.; Ruggero, S.; Toffanin, E.; Albergoni, M.P.; Luca, M.; Giometto, B.; Ermani, M.; et al. Neurological complications of celiac disease and autoimmune mechanisms: A prospective study. *J. Neuroimmunol.* **2008**, *195*, 171–175. [CrossRef]
21. Burk, K.; Farecki, M.L.; Lamprecht, G.; Roth, G.; Decker, P.; Weller, M.; Rammensee, H.G.; Oertel, W. Neurological symptoms in patients with biopsy proven celiac disease. *Mov. Disord.* **2009**, *24*, 2358–2362. [CrossRef]
22. Cakir, D.; Tosun, A.; Polat, M.; Celebisoy, N.; Gokben, S.; Aydogdu, S.; Yagci, R.V.; Tekgul, H. Subclinical neurological abnormalities in children with celiac disease receiving a gluten-free diet. *J. Pediatr. Gastroenterol. Nutr.* **2007**, *45*, 366–369. [CrossRef]
23. Diaconu, G.; Burlea, M.; Grigore, I.; Anton, D.T.; Trandafir, L.M. Celiac disease with neurologic manifestations in children. *Revista Medico-Chirurgicala A Societatii de Medici si Naturalisti din Iasi* **2014**, *117*, 88–94.
24. Isikay, S.; Isikay, N.; Kocamaz, H.; Hizli, S. Peripheral neuropathy electrophysiological screening in children with celiac disease. *Arq. Gastroenterol.* **2015**, *52*, 134–138. [CrossRef]
25. Jericho, H.; Sansotta, N.; Guandalini, S. Extraintestinal Manifestations of Celiac Disease: Effectiveness of the Gluten-Free Diet. *J. Pediatr. Gastroenterol. Nutr.* **2017**, *65*, 75–79. [CrossRef]
26. Ludvigsson, J.F.; Olsson, T.; Ekbom, A.; Montgomery, S.M. A population-based study of coeliac disease, neurodegenerative and neuroinflammatory diseases. *Aliment. Pharmacol. Ther.* **2007**, *25*, 1317–1327. [CrossRef]
27. Mukherjee, R.; Egbuna, I.; Brar, P.; Hernandez, L.; McMahon, D.J.; Shane, E.J.; Bhagat, G.; Green, P.H. Celiac disease: Similar presentations in the elderly and young adults. *Dig. Dis. Sci.* **2010**, *55*, 3147–3153. [CrossRef]
28. Ruggieri, M.; Incorpora, G.; Polizzi, A.; Parano, E.; Spina, M.; Pavone, P. Low prevalence of neurologic and psychiatric manifestations in children with gluten sensitivity. *J. Pediatr.* **2008**, *152*, 244–249. [CrossRef]
29. Shen, T.C.; Lebwohl, B.; Verma, H.; Kumta, N.; Tennyson, C.; Lewis, S.; Scherl, E.; Swaminath, A.; Capiak, K.M.; DiGiacomo, D.; et al. Peripheral neuropathic symptoms in celiac disease and inflammatory bowel disease. *J. Clin. Neuromuscul. Dis.* **2012**, *13*, 137–145. [CrossRef]

30. Thawani, S.P.; Brannagan, T.H., 3rd; Lebwohl, B.; Green, P.H.; Ludvigsson, J.F. Risk of Neuropathy Among 28,232 Patients with Biopsy-Verified Celiac Disease. *JAMA Neurol.* **2015**, *72*, 806–811. [CrossRef]

31. Hadjivassiliou, M.; Grunewald, R.A.; Sanders, D.S.; Shanmugarajah, P.; Hoggard, N. Effect of gluten-free diet on cerebellar MR spectroscopy in gluten ataxia. *Neurology* **2017**, *89*, 705–709. [CrossRef]

32. Sangal, K.; Camhi, S.; Lima, R.; Kenyon, V.; Fasano, A.; Leonard, M. Prevalence of neurological symptoms in children with gluten related disorders. *J. Pediatr. Gastroenterol. Nutr.* **2017**, *65*, S328–S329. [CrossRef]

33. Thawani, S.; Brannagan, T.H., 3rd; Lebwohl, B.; Mollazadegan, K.; Green, P.H.R.; Ludvigsson, J.F. Type 1 Diabetes, Celiac Disease, and Neuropathy-A Nationwide Cohort Study. *J. Clin. Neuromuscul. Dis.* **2017**, *19*, 12–18. [CrossRef]

34. Hanewinckel, R.; Drenthen, J.; van Oijen, M.; Hofman, A.; van Doorn, P.A.; Ikram, M.A. Prevalence of polyneuropathy in the general middle-aged and elderly population. *Neurology* **2016**, *87*, 1892–1898. [CrossRef]

35. Chin, R.L.; Sander, H.W.; Brannagan, T.H.; Green, P.H.; Hays, A.P.; Alaedini, A.; Latov, N. Celiac neuropathy. *Neurology* **2003**, *60*, 1581–1585. [CrossRef]

36. Luostarinen, L.; Himanen, S.L.; Luostarinen, M.; Collin, P.; Pirttila, T. Neuromuscular and sensory disturbances in patients with well treated coeliac disease. *J. Neurol. Neurosurg. Psychiatry* **2003**, *74*, 490–494. [CrossRef]

37. Muzaimi, M.B.; Thomas, J.; Palmer-Smith, S.; Rosser, L.; Harper, P.S.; Wiles, C.M.; Ravine, D.; Robertson, N.P. Population based study of late onset cerebellar ataxia in south east Wales. *J. Neurol. Neurosurg. Psychiatry* **2004**, *75*, 1129–1134. [CrossRef]

38. Hadjivassiliou, M. Immune-mediated acquired ataxias. *Handb. Clin. Neurol.* **2012**, *103*, 189–199. [CrossRef]

39. Hadjivassiliou, M.; Boscolo, S.; Tongiorgi, E.; Grunewald, R.A.; Sharrack, B.; Sanders, D.S.; Woodroofe, N.; Davies-Jones, G.A. Cerebellar ataxia as a possible organ-specific autoimmune disease. *Mov. Disord.* **2008**, *23*, 1370–1377. [CrossRef]

40. Abele, M.; Burk, K.; Schols, L.; Schwartz, S.; Besenthal, I.; Dichgans, J.; Zuhlke, C.; Riess, O.; Klockgether, T. The aetiology of sporadic adult-onset ataxia. *Brain* **2002**, *125*, 961–968. [CrossRef]

41. Abele, M.; Schols, L.; Schwartz, S.; Klockgether, T. Prevalence of antigliadin antibodies in ataxia patients. *Neurology* **2003**, *60*, 1674–1675. [CrossRef]

42. Burk, K.; Bosch, S.; Muller, C.A.; Melms, A.; Zuhlke, C.; Stern, M.; Besenthal, I.; Skalej, M.; Ruck, P.; Ferber, S.; et al. Sporadic cerebellar ataxia associated with gluten sensitivity. *Brain* **2001**, *124*, 1013–1019. [CrossRef]

43. Bushara, K.O.; Goebel, S.U.; Shill, H.; Goldfarb, L.G.; Hallett, M. Gluten sensitivity in sporadic and hereditary cerebellar ataxia. *Ann. Neurol.* **2001**, *49*, 540–543. [CrossRef]

44. Hadjivassiliou, M.; Grunewald, R.; Sharrack, B.; Sanders, D.; Lobo, A.; Williamson, C.; Woodroofe, N.; Wood, N.; Davies-Jones, A. Gluten ataxia in perspective: Epidemiology, genetic susceptibility and clinical characteristics. *Brain* **2003**, *126*, 685–691. [CrossRef]

45. Ihara, M.; Makino, F.; Sawada, H.; Mezaki, T.; Mizutani, K.; Nakase, H.; Matsui, M.; Tomimoto, H.; Shimohama, S. Gluten sensitivity in Japanese patients with adult-onset cerebellar ataxia. *Intern. Med.* **2006**, *45*, 135–140. [CrossRef]

46. Luostarinen, L.K.; Collin, P.O.; Peraaho, M.J.; Maki, M.J.; Pirttila, T.A. Coeliac disease in patients with cerebellar ataxia of unknown origin. *Ann. Med.* **2001**, *33*, 445–449. [CrossRef]

47. Pellecchia, M.T.; Scala, R.; Filla, A.; De Michele, G.; Ciacci, C.; Barone, P. Idiopathic cerebellar ataxia associated with celiac disease: Lack of distinctive neurological features. *J. Neurol. Neurosurg. Psychiatry* **1999**, *66*, 32–35. [CrossRef]

48. Anheim, M.; Degos, B.; Echaniz-Laguna, A.; Fleury, M.; Grucker, M.; Tranchant, C. Ataxia associated with gluten sensitivity, myth or reality? *Rev. Neurol.* **2006**, *162*, 214–221. [CrossRef]

49. Hadjivassiliou, M.; Grünewald, R.; Sanders, D.; Zis, P.; Croall, I.; Shanmugarajah, P.; Sarrigiannis, P.; Trott, N.; Wild, G.; Hoggard, N. The Significance of Low Titre Antigliadin Antibodies in the Diagnosis of Gluten Ataxia. *Nutrients* **2018**, *10*, 1444. [CrossRef]

50. Hadjivassiliou, M.; Grunewald, R.A.; Kandler, R.H.; Chattopadhyay, A.K.; Jarratt, J.A.; Sanders, D.S.; Sharrack, B.; Wharton, S.B.; Davies-Jones, G.A. Neuropathy associated with gluten sensitivity. *J. Neurol. Neurosurg. Psychiatry* **2006**, *77*, 1262–1266. [CrossRef]

51. Zis, P.; Sarrigiannis, P.G.; Rao, D.G.; Hadjivassiliou, M. Gluten neuropathy: Prevalence of neuropathic pain and the role of gluten-free diet. *J. Neurol.* **2018**, *265*, 2231–2236. [CrossRef]

52. Vinagre-Aragon, A.; Zis, P.; Grunewald, R.A.; Hadjivassiliou, M. Movement Disorders Related to Gluten Sensitivity: A Systematic Review. *Nutrients* **2018**, *10*, 34. [CrossRef]
53. Hadjivassiliou, M.; Gibson, A.; Davies-Jones, G.A.; Lobo, A.J.; Stephenson, T.J.; Milford-Ward, A. Does cryptic gluten sensitivity play a part in neurological illness? *Lancet* **1996**, *347*, 369–371. [CrossRef]

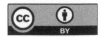